NURSING RESEARCH

SAGE was founded in 1965 by Sara Miller McCune to support the dissemination of usable knowledge by publishing innovative and high-quality research and teaching content. Today, we publish over 900 journals, including those of more than 400 learned societies, more than 800 new books per year, and a growing range of library products including archives, data, case studies, reports, and video. SAGE remains majority-owned by our founder, and after Sara's lifetime will become owned by a charitable trust that secures our continued independence.

Los Angeles | London | New Delhi | Singapore | Washington DC | Melbourne

3RD EDITION

NURSING RESEARCH

AN INTRODUCTION

PAM MOULE, HELEN AVEYARD & MARGARET GOODMAN

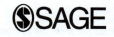

Los Angeles | London | New Delhi
Singapore | Washington DC | Melbourne

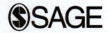

Los Angeles | London | New Delhi
Singapore | Washington DC | Melbourne

SAGE Publications Ltd
1 Oliver's Yard
55 City Road
London EC1Y 1SP

SAGE Publications Inc.
2455 Teller Road
Thousand Oaks, California 91320

SAGE Publications India Pvt Ltd
B 1/I 1 Mohan Cooperative Industrial Area
Mathura Road
New Delhi 110 044

SAGE Publications Asia-Pacific Pte Ltd
3 Church Street
#10-04 Samsung Hub
Singapore 049483

Editor: Becky Taylor
Editorial assistant: Charlène Burin
Production editor: Katie Forsythe
Copyeditor: Christine Bitten
Proofreader: Philippa May
Marketing manager: Tamara Navaratnam
Cover design: Wendy Scott
Typeset by: C&M Digitals (P) Ltd, Chennai, India
Printed and bound by CPI Group (UK) Ltd,
Croydon, CR0 4YY

Library of Congress Control Number: 2016937758

British Library Cataloguing in Publication data

A catalogue record for this book is available from
the British Library

ISBN 978-1-4739-5341-3
ISBN 978-1-4739-5342-0 (pbk)

At SAGE we take sustainability seriously. Most of our products are printed in the UK using FSC papers and boards.
When we print overseas we ensure sustainable papers are used as measured by the PREPS grading system.
We undertake an annual audit to monitor our sustainability.

This book is dedicated to the memory of Gill Hek who inspired many 'nurse researchers'

CONTENTS

ABOUT THE AUTHORS

Professor Pam Moule, Professor in Health Services Research, is based in the Faculty of Health and Life Sciences at the University of the West of England, Bristol. Pam leads the Centre of Health and Clinical Research. She is an active researcher undertaking evaluative projects in a number of areas and using a range of methodological approaches. She has supported the teaching and supervision of nursing research at all levels for a number of years including the supervision of undergraduate, Master's and doctoral students.

Dr Helen Aveyard is a senior lecturer at Oxford Brookes University. Helen leads academic courses in research and evidence-based practice and has written various undergraduate and postgraduate textbooks on research methods, including *Doing a Literature Review in Health and Social Care* which is now in its 3rd edition. Helen has supported the teaching and supervision of nursing research for undergraduate, master's and PhD level students.

Dr Margaret L. Goodman is now retired and her current research lies in organic gardening. Formerly she was an active researcher and Senior Lecturer in Research and NHS Research Facilitator working with healthcare practitioners to help them become research active. Her research projects have been in areas such as clinical practice development, healthcare service evaluation, palliative care and patient safety. Margaret also taught research at postgraduate level and supervised Master's and doctoral students.

PREFACE

Welcome to the third edition of this textbook written as a comprehensive guide to introduce student nurses and practitioners to some of the complexities of nursing research. The book builds on the previous editions and leads the novice nurse researcher through the main techniques and skills required to appreciate and undertake nursing research. We have drawn on our experiences and knowledge of nursing and nursing research to update and enhance the previous edition writing chapters that present key theoretical information in an applied way, drawing on examples from our own research and that of others. We hope that in continuing to take this practical and applied approach the book should help demystify research for readers and encourage appreciation and understanding of research practice and processes.

The book aims to be the only research book you will ever need, including four parts – Appraising Research, Preparing for Research, Doing Research and Sharing Research. It includes 29 chapters covering key aspects of nursing research that introduce the reader to issues of research design, process, dissemination and implementation. The layout is straightforward allowing the readers to negotiate the content to meet their own learning needs. It is possible to read individual chapters without the need to constantly refer to other sections of the book, though in places we have suggested where further materials and explanations may be found.

The chapters are structured to include learning outcomes, content with reference support and up-to-date examples from practice and literature, and a summary. In addition, some chapters offer reflective exercises. A comprehensive glossary is provided towards the end of the text. Each chapter ends with a summary that reminds the reader of the key issues presented. Suggested further reading lists, recommended websites and references are provided.

Part 1 – Appraising Research – includes Chapters 1 and 2 which discuss the position and place of research in nursing knowledge and practice development, emphasising the need for evidence-based practice. Chapter 3 introduces the research process that guides research activity and design, and sets the tone for the content of the subsequent chapters. Chapters 4 to 6 give practical advice on undertaking literature searching, developing the skills of critical appraisal and literature reviewing. The once coveted critical appraisal skills are necessary to support 'research literacy' and an ability to critically appraise and use research in practice.

Part 2 – Preparing for Research – includes Chapters 7 and 8 which cover aspects of research governance and ethics and encourage the reader to think about the processes involved in researching ethically and with potentially vulnerable populations. Ethical issues are complex and need consideration prior to developing a research design.

Chapter 9 provides key information on the development of research questions used to guide the research project.

Many nurses are undertaking undergraduate and postgraduate studies that require them to produce a research proposal. Others are undertaking local or funded projects as part of clinical practice or education roles. To help address these needs Chapter 10 provides guidance and examples of how to develop a research proposal for academic study or to undertake a research project as part of current work or for a funding body.

Part 3 – Doing Research – includes a number of chapters that address 'How to do research', addressing issues of research design, methods, data collection, data analysis and sampling to support the development of a proposal. These aspects of research are covered in Chapters 11 to 27. These chapters provide comprehensive information about a range of research designs, methods and data collection techniques. They explain key research terms and provide examples of use. Chapter 21 describes the use of mixed methods approaches in research that integrates both qualitative and quantitative methods in one design. Mixed methods approaches are commonplace in healthcare research as they enable the team to address different research questions within one design.

We also discuss issues of maintaining quality in the research process – important for integrity, rigour and trustworthiness. Chapter 13 discusses issues of validity and reliability, terms that can cause confusion for research consumers. Chapters 26 and 27 present data analysis techniques, often found difficult by many researchers. Both chapters give information on approaches to data analysis and present the processes of analysis, providing worked examples.

Part 4 – Sharing Research – includes the concluding chapters (28 and 29) addressing the final stages of the research process. Practical guidance regarding dissemination processes are offered in the penultimate chapter, which includes report writing, conference presentation and writing for publication. The final chapter considers how research findings might be used to support nursing practice and brings us to the conclusion of the research journey.

To further aid nurse researchers in the development of research understanding and skills we have developed an accompanying website (https://study.sagepub.com/mouleaveyard3e) that provides additional materials to support learning about research. The site includes a range of materials and learning resources that can be accessed for independent study and/or used to structure formal teaching sessions. These materials are a useful additional resource for personal study or group facilitation.

We hope you find the book and web materials not only provide you with key knowledge and understanding of nursing research, but stimulate you to engage with research as critical appraisers, researchers and implementers of evidence-based practice.

ACKNOWLEDGEMENTS

We are pleased to recognise Gill Hek's input to the conception of the first edition and to the fashioning of three chapters and Dr Margaret Goodman who conceived a number of chapters in the first and second editions. Finally, we are grateful to Mollie Gilchrist and Chris Wright for contributing Chapter 27 in the earlier editions.

PUBLISHER'S ACKNOWLEDGEMENTS

The publishers would like to thank the following individuals for their invaluable feedback on the second edition textbook and companion website, as well as chapters in the third edition:

Nina Dunne, University of Brighton, UK

Jeff Fernandez, Whittington Health NHS, UK

Dr Faridah Hashim, Open University Malaysia, Malaysia

Dr. Julie MacInnes, Canterbury Christ Church University, UK

Dr Yim Wah Mak, The Hong Kong Polytechnic University, Hong Kong

Chris Wheable, University of Wolverhampton, UK

ABOUT THE COMPANION WEBSITE

The third edition of *Nursing Research: An Introduction* is supported by a wealth of online resources for both students and lecturers to aid study and support teaching, which are available at https://study.sagepub.com/mouleaveyard3e.

FOR STUDENTS

- A **flashcard glossary**, which features terms from the book, is an ideal tool to help you get to grips with research, key terms and revise for exams.
- **Read more widely!** A selection of free SAGE journal articles for each chapter to help deepen your knowledge.
- **Web links** provide direct links to the online resources listed at the end of each chapter.

FOR LECTURERS

- **Lesson plans** related to each chapter of the book with discussion questions and ideas for group exercises.
- **PowerPoint slides** for use in teaching, linked to each chapter in the book.

PART 1
APPRAISING RESEARCH

1
RESEARCH IN NURSING

Learning outcomes

This chapter will enable you to:

- Understand the nature and historical context of nursing research
- Define research in nursing
- Understand evidence-based practice
- Reflect on how to involve the public in research
- Appreciate the relationship between research and nurse education

The care provided by nurses must be based on up-to-date knowledge and research that supports the delivery of the highest standards of practice possible. Nurses are developing their own professional knowledge base with strong foundations built on research and evidence. Nurses have a responsibility in some way to contribute to the development of the profession's knowledge through research.

The term 'research literate' or 'research aware' is used by many to describe the way that nurses should be in the twenty-first century. This means:

- having the capacity for critical thought
- possessing analytical skills
- having the skills to gain access to relevant research and evidence
- having a critical understanding of research processes
- being able to read and critically appraise research and other types of evidence
- having an awareness of ethical issues related to research.

By possessing these skills and being 'research literate', nurses should be able to assess the appropriateness of using specific types of evidence in their daily practice. It should be a natural activity for nurses to keep up to date and use research findings and evidence in their work, and being 'research literate' is one of the basic skills.

In this chapter, we consider the historical context of nursing research, the nature of nursing research, including different definitions, and the development of evidence-based practice.

HISTORICAL AND CURRENT CONTEXT

Florence Nightingale is often seen as the very first nurse researcher. Her research in the 1850s focused on soldiers' morbidity and mortality during the Crimean War. Nightingale identified 'research' questions in practice and undertook a systematic collection of data to try to find answers to the problems. Her 'research' eventually led to changes in the environment for sick people, including cleanliness, ventilation, clean water and adequate diet. However, Nightingale's contribution has been described as atypical with Kirby (2004) pointing out that the development of **nursing research** in the United Kingdom really only started with the inception of the National Health Service (NHS) – now the world's largest publicly funded health service – in the late 1940s. Prior to this, the development of nursing research had relied on a few highly determined individuals and was bound up with the professionalisation of nursing, the demands for suitable nurses, and the raising of educational standards for nurses (Kirby, 2004). Furthermore, in the 1950s, sociologists and psychologists were more likely to be undertaking research into nursing and nurses; only a small number of pioneering nurses were researching nursing and nurses themselves, one being Marjorie Simpson, who started the first self-help group for nurse researchers in 1959 called the Research Discussion Group (Hopps, 1994). This went on to become the Royal College of Nursing Research Society, which continues today. The Royal College of Nursing is a body in the UK that represents nurses and nursing, promotes excellence in practice and shapes health policies.

Tierney (1998) presented a picture of the development of nursing research across Europe. She identified the UK, Finland and Denmark as having developed in a similar way over the past 30 years, with Estonia, Lithuania and Slovenia only developing in the last 15 years. Growth was particularly evident in the 1980s and 1990s. It can be seen that, although overall growth has been slow, it has been more rapid in developed European countries. Many factors have affected this growth, such as the lack of resources and funding to support research, slow development of research training, **capacity** and **capability building**, and the low status of nurses relative to other health professions, particularly medicine. Tierney pointed out that there are four elements that support development: 'bottom-up' initiatives by forward looking individuals; 'top-down' initiatives through government support; growth of a research infrastructure as seen through universities; and a strategic approach rather than ad hoc initiatives.

In the 1970s, serious consideration of nursing research in the UK came with the publication of the Briggs report (Committee on Nursing, 1972), which recommended nursing should become a 'research-based' profession. This is often seen as a turning point in the historical context of nursing research, and as something that was badly needed for professional status. However, in the decades following the publication of the Briggs report, many suggested that nursing had not become 'research based', nor had research made an impact on the daily practice of nurses (Hunt, 1981; Thomas, 1985; Webb and Mackenzie, 1993). Specifically, the arguments were that nurses did not read or understand research, nurses did not know how to use research in practice, nurses did not believe research, nurses were not able to use research to change practice, and nurse researchers did not communicate well. It is interesting to think about the current position: Do nurses read research? Do they understand research? Is research impacting on practice?

In 1993 the *Report of the Taskforce on the Strategy for Research in Nursing, Midwifery and Health Visiting* (DH, 1993) was published. It sought to address many of the deficiencies noted earlier about nursing becoming a 'research-based' profession. It was suggested that nurse education, support and research infrastructure needed to be developed to support progress. The report did not suggest that all nurses should be undertaking research; rather it recommended that all nurses should become **research literate**, an essential skill for knowledge-led nursing practice. It became much clearer that all nurses needed to become equipped with the skills of understanding the **research process**, and an ability to retrieve and critically assess research findings, increasing capacity, with only a few nurses needing to be prepared to undertake research, increasing capability.

The impetus to develop evidence-based practice in order to achieve best care delivery has influenced nurse education. It was recognised that nurses needed to be able to critically read and understand research in order to support its use in practice. In addition, it was suggested that some nurses would need to develop greater research capability in order to lead research and contribute to the existing evidence base. This led to a number of changes, such as the funding initiatives by the Higher Education Funding Council for England (2001) and innovations in the delivery of nurse education. Research was fully integrated into the pre-registration curricula in the 1980s (UKCC, 1986) and introduced to post-registration provision shortly after (UKCC, 1994). The move of nurse education into higher education institutions in the 1990s supported ongoing academic development. In 2009, 30 per cent of nurses qualified at degree level or above (Ball and Pike, 2009) and increased numbers studied at Master's and doctoral level. Now all entrants to the profession follow an undergraduate degree level programme (Commission on Nursing and Midwifery, 2010).

The Higher Education Funding Council – a body that promotes and funds high-quality, cost-effective teaching and research in higher education in England (HEFCE, 2001) – provided capability building for both nursing and allied health professionals following the 2001 Research Assessment Exercise (RAE). A further RAE in 2008 also saw some universities secure monies to support capacity building, some of which will have benefitted nurse researchers. The RAE was an audit of research volume and quality used to allocate research funding to higher education institutions based on the quality of research activity. Nursing departments scoring 3a and 3b in the 2001 RAE received funding through the Research Capability Fund. The results of the 2008 RAE showed 36 institutions entered 641 full time equivalent (fte) staff. These results showed a positive impact on patients, families and communities with nursing rising from the bottom to the middle of the table. Of the research, 19 per cent was ranked world leading in terms of originality, significance and rigour (Council of Deans, 2009).

The Research Excellence Framework (REF) exercise submitted in 2013 superseded the RAE. This submission saw nursing and midwifery as part of a larger Unit of Assessment (UoA3), which included other disciplines such as pharmacy and allied health professions. The submissions were judged on research outputs including publications, the research environment, which included doctoral complications, and the impact of the research in a range of areas such as practice, policy and economics. Only the highest levels of quality research received funding, deemed as world leading and internationally excellent in originality, rigour and significance. The results of the 2014 REF submission are encouraging for nursing. Unit of Assessment 3 achieved 81 per cent world leading/internationally excellent research and the quality of the research environment was deemed as world leading in 50.1 per cent of submissions. Outstanding impact was present in a number of areas such as ageing, diabetes, palliative care and rehabilitation. However, it should be noted that there is still some way to go as submitting universities included less than 40 per cent of eligible nursing staff. This suggests nursing research is improving but needs further investment and development.

Attention has also been given to developing research skills amongst the clinical research workforce. The UK Clinical Research Collaboration (UKCRC) reported in 2007 on *Developing the Best Research Professionals. Qualified Graduate Nurses: Recommendations for Preparing and Supporting Clinical Academic Nurses of the Future* (UKCRC, 2007). This report was part of the agenda to modernise nursing careers, developing and preparing nurses to lead in a modernised healthcare system (DH, 2006). The report recommended the establishment of a range of research training opportunities including Master's and doctoral studies and fellowships, career flexibility that allows the combination of research and clinical practice and information provision to promote career opportunities for nursing. Development followed with the launch in 2009 of a funded programme from the National Institute for Health Research and the Chief Nursing Officer to fund Master's degrees in research, doctoral and postdoctoral programmes. This programme still continues and supports the development of clinical academic careers and was promoted by the Commission on Nursing report, *Frontline Care: Report by the Prime Minister's Commission on the Future of Nursing and Midwifery in England* (Commission on Nursing and Midwifery, 2010). It highlighted the need for innovation in nursing and midwifery, promoting capacity building in nursing and midwifery and the future development of research skills through clinical academic career pathways, in addition to changes in undergraduate nurse education which provided only undergraduate degrees in nursing from 2013.

The development of nursing research has also been aided by nursing organisations both nationally and internationally. This is acknowledged by Tierney (1997), who suggests that national nursing associations across Europe have been instrumental in strengthening the support for nursing research. In the UK, the Royal College of Nursing has a well-established research and development (R&D) support resource that can be accessed via the World Wide Web as well as the Research Society and occasional funding for research projects. In the UK, the Foundation of Nursing Studies and the Queen's Nursing Institute are just two of the organisations that support nursing research. The Department of Health has occasional streams of funding specifically for nursing research, as well as multi-disciplinary health research funding opportunities. Nurses now compete on a national basis with other disciplines for research funding.

Rafferty (1997), however, argues that we cannot ignore the 'politics' of nursing research, particularly the economic and organisational factors that influence research priorities. In nursing, these influences are powerful and there is no doubt that they affect the direction and development of nursing research in the UK. Economic, political and organisation factors influence the types of research that nurses undertake and can influence where the research funding is allocated.

Some nurse researchers have benefitted from the Department of Health strategy set out in 2006, which aimed to see the UK as a world-class environment for health research, development and innovation (DH, 2006). The strategy outlined a development plan that aimed to see more patients and healthcare professionals engaged in health research, which increased the evidence base and improved health and healthcare. To support this, the development of research policy and commissioning of research through the NHS R&D programme was recast into key programmes, which are today supported through the National Institute for Health Research (www.nihr.ac.uk), which aims to facilitate research and development that finds new evidence to support health and social care decisions. Many nurses have led and been members of research teams benefitting from these funding initiatives.

Table 1.1   Key strategy documents

Document	Development issues
Making a Difference: Strengthening the Nursing, Midwifery and Health Visiting Contribution to Health and Healthcare (DH, 1999)	● Need for nurses to develop critical research appraisal skills. ● Need for nurses to influence the government's research and development policies.
Towards a Strategy for Nursing Research and Development (DH, 2000)	● Need for monies to support research programmes. ● Need for capability building through collaborative partnerships.
Promoting Research in Nursing and the Allied Health Professions (HEFCE, 2001)	● Need for capability building to support evidence-based practice and the RAE.
Best Research for Best Health: A National Health Service Research Strategy (DH, 2006)	● Need to develop a world-class environment for health research, development and innovation.
Developing the Best Research Professionals (UKCRC, 2007)	● Need to develop clinical research career structures for nurses – suggested models are based on the clinical academic career model.
Frontline Care: Report by the Prime Minister's Commission on the Future of Nursing and Midwifery in England (Commission on Nursing and Midwifery, 2010)	● Need for capacity building in nursing and midwifery and the future development of research skills through clinical academic career pathways, changes in undergraduate nurse education which is to provide only undergraduate degrees in nursing from 2013 onwards and the strengthening of integration between nursing and practice, education and research.

Additionally, there are publications relating to nursing research development within Scotland (*National Guidance for Clinical Academic Research Careers for Nurses, Midwives and Allied Health Professionals*, 2011) and Northern Ireland (*Health and Social Care Research and Development Strategy 2007–2012*, 2007). It should be noted that policy changes rapidly, and readers may find it useful to keep updated by accessing the Department of Health website (www.dh.gov.uk).

HOW DO WE UNDERSTAND THE NATURE OF NURSING RESEARCH?

Though the growth of nursing research has been slow, it continues to develop and is broad-ranging, relating to practice, policy, education and management. It encompasses, for example, research about the effectiveness of nursing practice, the development and evaluation of new types of care delivery, the expansion of nursing theories and concepts, the impact of policy on practice, new roles, and new ways of educating the nursing workforce. Nursing research is interested in what patients and clients feel and experience, how nurses learn and develop throughout their careers, how multi-disciplinary working and learning contributes to the care of patients, and the **outcomes** of nursing practice. The nursing profession is continually striving to develop its own body of research, and to contribute to health services research and the social sciences.

The nature of nursing research is complex. We have already suggested that nursing research is broad and wide ranging, capturing research into practice, care outcomes, education and management issues. Additionally, it should be remembered that nurses work as part of interprofessional teams in different healthcare settings and increasingly for different healthcare providers. A number of research issues and questions might therefore arise that relate to interprofessional working. These factors impact on how nursing research is defined. Definitions of nursing research reflect the perspective of those researching nursing.

Bowling (2014), in describing research on health and health services, views research as a **process** of enquiry that develops explanatory concepts and theories to contribute to a scientific body of knowledge. She then goes on to acknowledge the importance of multi-disciplinary health services research, which includes anthropologists, epidemiologists, health economists, medical sociologists and statisticians, amongst others, who conduct healthcare research. Each discipline can come with their own perspective on what defines research and how it should be conducted. Thus, in defining nursing research there must be recognition of the potential multi-disciplinary nature of research teams and the consequential wide range of 'qualitative' and 'quantitative' research methods that will be employed to address the broad range of research issues.

Before moving on to consider definitions of research, it is important to understand the main research approaches used – qualitative and quantitative – and to appreciate that often to address the complexity of nursing research both approaches can be combined within one study. The research approach is the whole design, which includes the researcher position and assumptions, the process of enquiry and the way data is collected and analysed. Qualitative research is part of an interpretivist or constructivist position that has long been part of social and behavioural sciences (Guba and Lincoln, 1982). The approach is used to describe and understand individual perspectives and experiences. For example, qualitative research may be used to answer questions about the patient experience or staff perceptions of new ways of working or new roles in nursing. Qualitative research can explore questions such as: What are patients' experiences of the cardiac rehabilitation service? How have patients experienced a new nursing role? To gather information about personal views and experiences, research methods such as interviewing and observation are used, collecting textual or visual data for analysis.

Quantitative research has its origins in a scientific paradigm and roots in positivism, which believes human phenomena can be subjected to measurement and objective study. In nursing research quantitative approaches can be used to measure whether one treatment has a better effect than another. For example, quantitative designs might answer research questions such as 'Is treatment A better than treatment B?' The researcher may be guided by a hypothesis, a statement for testing (see Chapter 26) – for example, 'Adults classed as clinically obese receiving an exercise programme of 30 minutes per day will have greater weight loss within two months of starting the programme than those undertaking a 10-minute exercise programme for two months.' Quantitative research takes a formal approach to the collection and analysis of numerical data. Within this approach health economics data may also be collected to show the economic benefit of service delivery for healthcare. For example, the introduction of a new service may require some measure of economic impact or benefit, often measured through the use of validated measures. For example, particular tools can be used to look at the impact of a service on service user well-being. Such tools can be administered to service users prior to and following service implementation, and comparisons are made which allow the researchers to draw conclusions about the impact of the service on well-being.

In this book, we discuss the different types of research in detail, identifying the strengths and limitations of each (see Chapters 11, 14–19 and 21). In doing this, we introduce you to the range of research methods that might be used either independently or as part of a mixed methods approach.

Given the complex nature of nursing research, finding one definition that achieves consensus is difficult. However, in most definitions of research there are some core elements:

- a systematic process
- a search for new knowledge or deepening understanding
- activities that are planned and logical
- a search for an answer to a question
- collection of new data.

We use the following basic definition for the purposes of this book:

> A systematic approach to gathering information for the purposes of answering questions and solving problems in the pursuit of creating new knowledge about nursing practice, education and policy. (Moule, 2015: 10)

WHO DOES RESEARCH IN NURSING?

As mentioned previously, researchers from other disciplines carried out much of the early nursing research in the 1950s, 1960s and early 1970s, including sociologists, psychologists, social and welfare policy researchers, and historians. Research was undertaken from a discipline perspective and nurse researchers at the time learned about a wide range of research approaches and methods. Nurse researchers developed their research skills from social scientists and health researchers, who included them on research teams. Historians, economists, statisticians, epidemiologists, geographers and anthropologists also brought their own approaches and techniques to nursing research.

This position has changed in the last 30 years or so, with many nurses now leading and undertaking their own research as well as being involved in multi-disciplinary research teams. Increasingly, health services research involves multi-disciplinary teams including health professionals, statisticians and health economists. Nurses can lead or be part of these teams, directly employed on a specific project – for example, a clinical trial examining the effectiveness of a particular drug treatment or practice, or an evaluation looking at what works in family support or child protection. Whilst a number of nurses are employed as 'research nurses' who work as part of a team with responsibility for recruitment and data collection, nurse researchers increasingly have a larger input into studies than in the past. Nurses can undertake principle investigator roles, leading in project design and management, as well as data collection and analysis. We could think about local examples of research that might provide further evidence of this change, for example: Are you aware of research projects in practice that involve nurses? What are the roles of nurses in these projects?

As mentioned at the beginning of this chapter, all nurses need to become 'research literate'. Nurses studying at undergraduate level are most likely to undertake activities such as designing a **questionnaire** or interviewing colleagues as exercises to help them understand research methods and the research process. Most commonly, nursing students will practise skills to enable them to find and critically appraise research literature. All nursing students are likely to write essays using research findings and evidence, and all these activities are important and necessary in helping nurses to become 'research literate'. Some nurses at undergraduate level may undertake their own literature-based review or research study. This may be a small individual research project as part of a pre- or post-qualifying degree course or can involve being a member of a project team, exploring an aspect of practice.

More and more nurses are educated to Master's level, with the number aspiring to doctoral-level education increasing both in higher education institutions and clinical practice settings. This is a major change from 30 years ago when those studying to Master's and doctoral level were less common. There are also opportunities for those successfully completing doctoral programmes to undertake funded research Fellowships and postdoctoral opportunities with universities and other research institutions. These opportunities are often made available through the UKCRC (2007) as part of the National Institute for Health Research (NIHR) Clinical Doctoral Research

Fellowship programme and by organisations such as The Leverhulme Trust, who provide funded fellowships for periods of 3 to 24 months, secured through a competitive tendering process. These posts are part of a research career pathway and researchers can work either as independent investigators or with the support of a principal investigator. This means that nurses have undertaken major pieces of research to a high level, and as nurses improve their capabilities as researchers they are more likely to lead research projects and teams and secure external funding through competitive tendering from major sources such as the National Institute for Health Research and Research Councils. There are many more Chairs in Nursing (professors) than ever before and nurses are holding senior board level positions in higher education, the NHS and other healthcare organisations. This all signals a healthy situation for nursing research, with nurses becoming more deeply involved in research. We can probably find evidence to support these changes in the local setting, for example: Are there nurses studying for Master's degrees and doctorates in the locality? Are professors of nursing employed in the hospitals or local universities? Do professors and those completing doctorates and higher studies publish nursing literature?

WHAT IS EVIDENCE-BASED PRACTICE?

Making decisions about the type of nursing care to give to service users is not easy. It may mean making choices between a number of alternative actions that involve treatment choices, provision of services or efficiency.

Evidence-based practice promotes quality and cost-effective outcomes of healthcare, with Schmidt and Brown suggesting it is 'practice based on the best available evidence, patient preference and clinical judgement' (2011: 5). From this definition, we can see that the decision should be made explicit and based on the current best evidence, as well as using the practitioner's own expertise, and taking account of patient views.

These days, the input of the service user is seen as paramount to any decision that is made about the provision of healthcare for an individual. The Health and Social Care Act (DH, 2012) gave patients a greater voice in the commissioning of services, with Healthwatch England and local Healthwatch organisations ensuring patient and carer views are an integral part of service commissioning being led by GPs. Therefore, it is reasonable to say that there are three clear key components to evidence-based practice. When making an 'evidence-based' decision about the care of a particular patient, the nurse should:

- use the best available current evidence
- consider the preferences of the individual service user
- use their own expertise and experience to make decisions.

In making decisions about how to care for a patient, the nurse should search for and use the best available evidence in their practice, they should consider the requirements, values, circumstances and preferences of the patient and they should integrate their own professional experience, expertise and judgement. All three elements need to be used together, although the importance of each may vary in different situations. The over-riding principle is that of giving the most effective care to maximise the quality of life for an individual.

Evidence-based practice is seen as comprising five explicit steps:

1. Identify a problem from practice and turn it into a specific question. This might be about the most effective intervention for a particular patient, or about the most appropriate test, or about the best method for delivering nursing care.
2. Find the best available evidence that relates to the specific question, usually through a thorough and systematic search of the literature.
3. Critically appraise the evidence for its validity (closeness to the truth), usefulness (practical application) and methodological rigour.
4. Identify and use the current best evidence, and together with the patient or client's preferences and the practitioner's expertise and experience, apply it to the situation.
5. Evaluate the effect on the patient or client, and reflect on the nurse's own performance.

Current pre-qualifying nurse education helps students address all these stages, but specifically practitioners need to learn how to search effectively for appropriate evidence and research through a range of literature sources (see Chapters 4 and 5) and how to critically appraise research (Chapters 4, 5 and 6).

Evidence-based practice emerged in the 1990s, starting with evidence-based medicine, and has impacted on health service delivery including nursing practice (Ellis, 2013). The successful emergence of evidence-based practice has been argued by those within the movement as being due to the obvious, simple, sensible and rational idea 'that practice should be based on the most up-to-date, valid and reliable research' (Melnyk and Fineout-Overholt, 2014). The context in which it has developed may go some way to explain why the movement has flourished in many areas of healthcare practice. Within recent years there has been a cultural shift within the healthcare professions from one of trusted professional judgement-based practice to that of evidence-based practice.

Glicken (2005) suggests that there are a number of contributing factors including: growth in an increasingly well-educated and well-informed public; increasing awareness of the limitations of science; growth in consumer and self-help groups; intensive media scrutiny; explosion of the availability of different types of information and data; developments in information technology; increasing emphasis on productivity and competitiveness; emphasis on 'value-for-money' and audit; increase in scrutiny, accountability and regulation of professional groups; lawsuits and compensation; and major adverse events within the health services.

This cultural shift has resulted in an explosion of evidence-based initiatives and new terminology within the health services since the mid-1990s. These include initiatives such as evidence-based child health and evidence-based mental health; specialist 'evidence-based' journals, websites and web-based discussion lists. It also includes the Centre for Reviews and Dissemination at York that undertakes the review and dissemination of research results to the NHS, and the UK Cochrane Centre that collaborates with others to build, maintain and disseminate a database of systematic, up-to-date reviews of randomised controlled trials of healthcare. This has had an effect on how research and evidence is considered and used by nurses and how evidence and practice drives (and is driven by) practice and policy more than ever before.

The growth of evidence-based practice is not without its critics. They point out that it constrains professional decision making and autonomy; that it is too simple and is 'cookbook' practice; that it is a covert method of rationing resources; that it exalts certain types of research evidence over other types of knowledge and evidence; and that research trials are usually not directly transferable (Jenicek, 2006). There are concerns that the effective implementation of evidence-based practice has been hindered by the hierarchy of evidence that promotes randomised controlled trials as the highest form of evidence and neglects to recognise the value of reflection in developing best practice (Mantzoukas, 2008).

There are limitations with evidence-based practice in all aspects of healthcare but particularly with nursing. For example, in mental health nursing there is less research evidence to support the development of effective nursing care. There are a number of reasons for this, including lack of time and resources to undertake the type of research needed such as controlled trials, and cultural barriers in health organisations and the organisation of nursing education, which has not equipped all nurses with literature searching and critical appraisal skills.

It is possible to overcome some of these barriers, particularly through education and training. There is also research examining the barriers to evidence-based practice, and ways to overcome them. Finally, there are ways of finding evidence that has already been reviewed and appraised. These include evidence-based clinical guidelines from the Cochrane Reviews (systematic reviews of healthcare interventions which promote the search for evidence in the form of clinical trials and other studies of interventions), National Institute for Health and Care Excellence, (formerly the National Institute for Clinical Excellence [NICE] – an independent organisation responsible for providing national guidance on promoting good health and preventing and treating ill health), which includes the Centre for Reviews and Dissemination based at York University. The Centre provides research-based information on the effects of health and social care interventions in a database and undertakes and publishes systematic reviews.

WHAT IS THE HIERARCHY OF EVIDENCE AND RESEARCH?

The idea of a hierarchy of evidence has evolved as a response to the notion that some research designs, particularly those using quantitative methods, are more able than others to provide robust evidence of effectiveness, that is, what works. The most common type of hierarchy therefore places evidence gathered through research at the top, with a systematic review of evidence from multiple randomised controlled trials (RCTs) being the pinnacle:

1. Evidence from a systematic review of multiple well-designed RCTs.
2. Evidence from one or more well-designed RCTs.
3. Evidence from experiments without randomisation or from single before-and-after studies, cohort, time series or matched case-controlled studies or observational studies.
4. Evidence from well-designed descriptive studies or qualitative research.
5. Opinions from expert committees or respected authorities based on practice-based evidence.
6. Personal, professional and peer expertise and experience.

This hierarchy of evidence is only appropriate for research questions that are seeking an answer about what works. For example, if a nurse wanted to know the best way to cover a particular type of wound, say a burn, then the above would help in making decisions about the best type of evidence. This would be well-designed RCT, or even better, a systematic review of RCTs. However, if nurses wanted to develop understanding about what it feels like to have severe burns, so that they could develop their communication and empathetic skills, then qualitative research would be more informative.

The importance of nursing research for practice was reiterated in the Francis Inquiry (2013) into the care delivered in one NHS hospital. The report made a number of recommendations and reinforced the need for the National Institute for Health and Care Excellence (NICE) evidence to inform evidence-based procedures and practice. Research provides evidence used in the development of NICE guidance, it improves nursing knowledge and practice, it can help reduce unnecessary costs and it can aid decision making.

Reflective exercise

Let's think about a possible practice situation where you are caring for a patient who has just been told he has prostate cancer. How would you know what was the best care to deliver for your patient and his family? Think about the steps you might take. One of the things you may need to do is source information that will help your patient understand more about prostate cancer. You could ask more senior staff for advice and what information they might use. It is also important to remember the need to deliver evidence-based care and use the best evidence available. You can use published evidence for healthcare professionals and patients and families, available from the Prostate Cancer UK charity (www.prostatecancer.org). You could read the current NICE guidance available on their website (www.nice.org.uk). This provides a robust evidence base for practice, which can give you both scientific and economic information to work with. The evidence covers what kinds of information might be provided; where to find this information; and what treatments might be considered. These guidelines are based on a range of research findings and evidence, and provide guidance for a range of healthcare professionals to help deliver best care.

HOW TO INVOLVE THE PUBLIC IN RESEARCH

Patient and public involvement in health and social care research (PPI) has increased in recent years. Developments have placed greater emphasis on the meaningful engagement of service users and carers in research, moving away from limited public participation to embrace public involvement. The public were encouraged to participate in research through their recruitment to clinical trials or the completion of interviews and question-naires. Whilst public participation remains vital, PPI takes a broader view and includes research undertaken with and by patients, rather than for, to or about them (Involve, 2012). This approach recognises the importance and relevance of involving patients in all stages of the research process, so that the public can influence research questions and design.

Different levels of involvement are seen within projects, often reflecting the nature of the research question being explored. Most funders of health and social care research include criteria for PPI in tender documents and assess the level of proposed public involvement as part of the process of reviewing funding applications. The National Institute for Health Research, for example, looks for active and meaningful PPI within all stages of the research process. The UKCRC has a strategic plan to support public involvement in its work, recruiting the public to advisory groups and providing informa-tion through its 'People in research' website (www.ukcrc.org).

The ways in which the patients and public can be involved in research are sum-marised in Table 1.2. The degree of involvement will vary according to a number of

Table 1.2 Involving patients and the public in research

Identifying and prioritising	Identifying research problems and questions and agreeing the research priorities.
Design	Informing/commenting on the research design for a study.
Development of a proposal	Involvement in developing and reviewing a research proposal to submit to a funder.
Grant holders and co-applicants	Involvement as a co-applicant or lead applicant for a grant means taking a leadership role in the research.
Steering group	Membership of a project steering group or advisory board, offering advice from their perspective on the ongoing progress and activities of the project.
Design of materials	Input into the development of data collection tools, research information sheets and assist in the development of materials for ethical approval, such as patient consent forms.
Data collection and analysis	Input into the development and implementation of a sampling strategy and help access the sample group. They can also undertake data collection such as interviews, and/or analyse research data.
Dissemination	Part of writing teams, leading or inputting into the development of academic papers. Can lead or be part of a conference presentation. Can help develop leaflets/information advising the public of the research outcomes.
Implementation	May have a role in implementing the research findings in practice, working with local networks and groups.
Evaluation	Can support the evaluation of new service developments resulting from the implementation of research findings and outcomes.

factors, such as the research question being asked, the skills of the patients and public involved and their preferred level of involvement, funder requirements, the skills and experience of the researchers and the level of research funding available for PPI. Involve, funded by the NIHR, provides detailed information, knowledge and understanding on how to involve the public in research and aims to share new learning of PPI with researchers. A review of PPI in research found impact in relation to developing research questions, prioritising topics and developing commissioning briefs. There was also evidence of impact in undertaking research, in particular the development of protocols, data collection tools and associated consent forms and research information sheets (Brett et al., 2010).

Researchers often require support with PPI, especially if new to working with the public in research. They need to recognise that whilst involvement will bring a range of potential benefits to the project, there are also additional considerations to be made and costed if PPI is to succeed. University of the West of England (UWE, 2011) guidelines (Pollard et al., 2015) highlight some of the areas for consideration:

- Researchers will need education and preparation to work with the public in research.
- The project plan must include time for meaningful involvement.
- Involvement should start as early as possible, preferably as part of the project planning/proposal stage, if not before.
- The researchers should be clear about what is involved in the project and what the expectations of the public/patient members are.
- Ongoing support should be provided for the public/patients and may necessitate a specific liaison/support role in the project.
- Communication between the researchers and public needs to be clear.
- All project materials should be accessible to the public, with care taken in presentation and the use of language.
- The public/patients should be involved in the dissemination of the project outcomes.

WHAT IS THE RELATIONSHIP BETWEEN RESEARCH AND NURSE EDUCATION?

The Commission on the future of nursing and midwifery in England (Commission on Nursing and Midwifery, 2010) suggested all pre-registration education should be offered at undergraduate level only (NMC, 2010). This brought England in line with the current graduate only pre-registration provision in Scotland and Wales. The change reflects a desire to ensure graduate nurses have the knowledge and skills to undertake complex assessments, use evidence to make decisions and agree interventions in a number of complex and changing healthcare environments. It affirms the importance of educating nurses to degree level and equipping them with the ability to critically review and implement research and evidence in practice. This is essential to ensure best care delivery, which uses the best available evidence. It also strengthens the integration of nursing practice, education and research. It is hoped that this integration will achieve excellence in education that will support research and innovative practice.

The ongoing development of research capacity and capability in nursing will also provide the nurse researchers of the future. Offering opportunities to engage with research and evidence-based practice at undergraduate level and beyond can inspire the next generation of nurse researchers who will address key nursing research questions from a nursing perspective. The ultimate aim of this is the development of best practice and quality patient care across a range of environments.

CHAPTER SUMMARY

- Nursing research today has been shaped by its historical roots, and political, economic and organisation influences.
- Defining research is not easy, and debates surround the nature of nursing and health services research.
- The development of evidence-based practice has been rapid and influential.
- All nurses must become 'research literate' and learn the essentials of evidence-based practice.
- Some nurses will become researchers as part of their role in practice, or through a career in teaching, policy development or leadership.
- There is recognition of the importance of involving the public in research.
- There is strengthening of the integration of nursing practice, education and research.

SUGGESTED FURTHER READING

Barker, J. (2013) *Evidence-based Practice for Nurses*. London: Sage. Introduces key information to help nurses understand and evaluate different types of evidence. It covers how to identify and critically appraise evidence.

Brett, J., Staniszewska, S., Mockford, C., Seers, K., Herron-Marx, S. and Bayliss, H. (2010) *The PIRCOM Study: A Systematic Review of the Conceptualisation, Measurement, Impact and Outcomes of Patient and Public Involvement in Health and Social Care Research*. London: UKCRC.

Schmidt, N. and Brown, J. (2011) *Evidence Based Practice for Nurses*, 2nd edn. Massachusetts, USA: Jones and Bartlett Publishers. This text defines evidence-based nursing practice and considers its implementation. It guides the reader in the appraisal of EBP through a series of chapters.

WEBSITES

Centre for Evidence Based Medicine: www.cebm.net – based at the University of Oxford, the centre provides courses and workshops for healthcare staff wanting to develop evidence-based medicine skills.

Centre for Reviews and Dissemination: www.york.ac.uk/inst/crd – part of the National Institute for Health Research, which provides a database of the effectiveness of health and social care interventions and systematic reviews.

Cochrane Reviews: www.cochrane.org/ – systematic reviews of primary research in healthcare and health policy, which address specific research questions. The reviews are internationally recognised and published on The Cochrane Library.

Foundation of Nursing Studies Centre for Nursing Innovation: www.fons.org/ – the FoNS is a registered charity that works with nurses and healthcare professionals to develop and share innovative practice with an aim of delivering high quality and evidence-based patient care.

Involve: www.invo.org.uk – provides information on the involvement of the public in health research.

National Institute for Health and Care Excellence (NICE): www.nice.org.uk/ – provides advice on best care developed from the best available evidence to health and social care professionals.

Royal College of Nursing Research Society: www2.rcn.org.uk/development/research_and_innovation/rs – provides information on the RCN research society and its activities, which include an annual international research conference.

UK Clinical Research Collaboration: www.ukcrc.org/ – aims to establish the UK as a world leader in clinical research through identifying the barriers to research and working to overcome them. One particular initiative is the support of clinical academic careers for nurses and allied health professionals.

University of the West of England, Bristol: http://hls.uwe.ac.uk/suci/Default.aspx?pageid¼49 – provides guidance on how to involve patients and members of the public in health research.

 To access further resources related to this chapter, visit the companion website at https://study.sagepub.com/mouleaveyard3e.

REFERENCES

Ball, J. and Pike, G. (2009) *Past Imperfect, Future Tense. Nurses' Employment and Morale in 2009*. London: Royal College of Nursing.

Bowling, A. (2014) *Research Methods in Health: Investigating Health and Health Services*, 4th edn. Berkshire: Open University Press.

Brett, J., Staniszewska, S., Mockford, C., Seers, K., Herron-Marx, S. and Bayliss, H. (2010) *The PIRCOM Study: A Systematic Review of the Conceptualisation, Measurement, Impact and Outcomes of Patient and Public Involvement in Health and Social Care Research*. London: UKCRC.

Commission on Nursing and Midwifery (2010) *Frontline Care: Report by the Prime Minister's Commission on the Future of Nursing and Midwifery in England*. London: Prime Minister's Commission on Nursing and Midwifery.

Committee on Nursing (1972) *Report of the Committee on Nursing (Briggs report)*. Cmnd.5115. London: HMSO.

Council of Deans (2009) *Nursing and Midwifery Research Comes of Age*. Available at: www.rcn.org.uk (accessed 9 July 2015).

Department of Health (1993) *Report of the Taskforce on the Strategy for Research in Nursing, Midwifery and Health Visiting*. London: Department of Health.

Department of Health (1999) *Making a Difference: Strengthening the Nursing, Midwifery and Health Visiting Contribution to Health and Healthcare*. London: DH.

Department of Health (2000) *Towards a Strategy for Nursing Research and Development*. London: DH.

Department of Health (2006) *Best Research for Best Health: A National Health Service Research Strategy*. London: DH

Department of Health (2006) *Modernising Nursing Careers: Setting the Direction*. London: Department of Health.

Department of Health (2012) *Health and Social Care Act*. Available at: http://services.parliament.uk/bills/2010-12/healthandsocialcare/documents.html. (accessed 30 July 2015).

Ellis, P. (2013) *Evidence-based Practice in Nursing*, 2nd edn. London: Sage.

Francis, R. (2013) *Report of the Mid-Staffordshire NHS Trust: Public Inquiry*. London: The Stationery Office.

Glicken, M. (2005) *Improving the Effectiveness of the Helping Professions: An Evidence-based Approach to Practice*. Thousand Oaks, CA: Sage.

Guba, E. and Lincoln, Y. (1982) 'Epistemological and methodological bases of naturalistic enquiry', *Educational Communication and Technology*, 30 (4): 233–52.

Higher Education Funding Council for England (HEFCE) (2001) *Promoting Research in Nursing and the Allied Health Professions*. Bristol: HEFCE.

Hopps, L.C. (1994) 'The development of research in nursing in the United Kingdom', *Journal of Clinical Nursing*, 3: 199–204.

Hunt, J. (1981) 'Indicators for nursing practice: The use of research findings', *Journal of Advanced Nursing*, 6 (3): 189–94.

Involve (2012) *Involve Strategy 2012–2015*, NHS National Institute for Health Research. Available at: www.invo.org.uk (accessed 12 July 2015).

Jenicek, M. (2006) 'The art of soft science: Evidence-based medicine, reasoned medicine or both?', *Journal of Education in Clinical Practice*, 12: 410–19.

Kirby, S. (2004) 'A historical perspective on the contrasting experiences of nurses as research subjects and research activists', *International Journal of Nursing Practice*, 10: 272–9.

Mantzoukas, S. (2008) 'A review of evidence-based practice, nursing research and reflection: Levelling the hierarchy', *Journal of Clinical Nursing*, 17: 214–23.

Melnyk, B. and Fineout-Overholt, E. (2014) *Evidence-based Practice in Nursing and Healthcare: A Guide to Best Practice*. London: Wolters Kluwer.

Moule, P. (2015) *Making Sense of Research in Nursing, Health and Social Care*, 5th edn. London: Sage.

NHS Education for Scotland (2011) *National Guidance for Clinical Academic Research Careers for Nursing, Midwifery and allied Health Professions in Scotland*. Available at: www.nes.scot.nhs.uk/ (accessed 10 May 2016).

Nursing and Midwifery Council (2010) *Pre-registration Education in the UK*. Available at: www.nmc.uk.org (accessed 9 July 2015).

Pollard, K., Donskoy, A-L., Moule, P., Donald, C., Lima, M. and Rice, C. (2015) 'Developing and evaluating guidelines for patient and public involvement (PPI) in research', *International Journal of Health Care Quality Assurance*, 28 (2): 141–55.

Rafferty, A. (1997) 'Writing, researching and reflexivity in nursing history', *Nurse Researcher*, 5 (2): 5–16.

Research and Development Office (2007) *Health and Social Care Research and Development Strategy 2007–2012*. Available at: www.publichealth.hscni.net (accessed 10 May 2016).

Schmidt, N. and Brown, J. (2011) *Evidence Based Practice for Nurses*, 2nd edn. Massachusetts, USA: Jones and Bartlett Publishers.

Thomas, E. (1985) 'Attitudes towards nursing research among trained nurses', *Nurse Education Today*, 5 (1): 18–21.

Tierney, A. (1997) 'Organization report: The development of nursing research in Europe', *European Nurse*, 2 (2): 73–84.

Tierney, A. (1998) 'Nursing research in Europe', *International Nursing Review*, 45 (1): 15–19.

UK Clinical Research Collaboration (UKCRC) (2007) *Developing the Best Research Professionals. Qualified Graduate Nurses: Recommendations for Preparing and Supporting Clinical Academic Nurses of the Future*. London: UKCRC.

United Kingdom Central Council (UKCC) (1986) *Project 2000: A New Preparation for Practice*. London: United Kingdom Central Council for Nursing, Midwifery and Health Visiting.

United Kingdom Central Council (UKCC) (1994) *The Future of Professional Practice: The Council's Standards for Education and Practice Following Registration*. London: United Kingdom Central Council for Nursing, Midwifery and Health Visiting.

University of the West of England (2011) *Public Involvement in Research: Guidelines for Good Practice*. Bristol: UWE. Available at: http://hls.uwe.ac.uk/suci/Default.aspx?pageid¼49 (accessed 29 September 2015).

Webb, C. and MacKenzie, J. (1993) 'Where are we now? Research-mindedness in the 1990s', *Journal of Clinical Nursing*, 2 (3): 129–33.

2
SOURCES OF NURSING KNOWLEDGE

Learning outcomes

This chapter will enable you to:

- Identify the sources of knowledge available to inform nursing and healthcare practice
- Understand the complex nature of nursing research
- Appreciate the importance of research and evidence-based knowledge in informing practice, theory and policy

Nursing knowledge is drawn from a multifaceted base and includes evidence that comes from science (research and evaluation), experience and personally derived understanding. Scientific knowledge is developed through enquiry and can use the research approaches discussed throughout this book. It is, however, not the only form of evidence used by nurses in their practice. Nurses also use experience gained from practice itself and their own personal learning. The relationship between research and the generation of scientific knowledge is understood and accepted by many. In contrast, a number of writers have proposed frameworks that describe knowledge as being generated through experience and personal understanding. Carper (1975, 1978) discusses the four fundamental patterns of knowing: empirics (know what), aesthetic (know-how), personal knowledge (do I know myself and others?) and ethics (know why I should). This work draws together a range of essential knowledge that can be used to inform nursing practice, acknowledging the importance not just of scientific knowledge, but of knowledge developed through experience, personal understanding and interpretation, and of moral and ethical reasoning. Schon (1987) developed the concept 'knowing how' as part of 'knowing-in-action'. This supports the generation of personal and tacit knowledge that Rolfe (1998) suggests we all possess but are unable to articulate.

This chapter considers the range of knowledge available to inform practice decisions. First, we review scientific knowledge and consider how it is generated. Second, we consider other sources of knowledge developed through experience that include tradition, intuition and tacit understanding. Third, personal knowledge is presented as individual knowledge used to support care delivery on an individual basis. Liaschenko and Fisher (1999) describe this as person knowledge, that of knowing the patient as an individual person.

It should be noted that, in making decisions to deliver care and using evidence to support practice delivery, nurses might draw on a range of sources of knowledge. None exists exclusively and nurses may use scientific knowledge, personal knowledge and experience in making judgements. Having considered the complexities of nursing knowledge, we will review the development of policy to support nursing research. The chapter will end by conceptualising nursing research, defining it and considering how it informs nursing practice as part of a range of evidence that supports care development and delivery.

SCIENTIFIC KNOWLEDGE

Scientific knowledge is positioned at level one through to four of the hierarchy of evidence (see Chapter 1) and makes a significant contribution to the development and application of nursing practice. Scientific evidence also informs nursing education, policy development and management. This form of knowledge is generated through research activity, where a rigorous approach is followed to obtain findings that will be used to inform nursing practice. We discuss the process that researchers use to generate scientific knowledge in Chapter 3, and within this book we explore a number of approaches that can be used to support scientific knowledge generation (see Chapters 14–19). Whereas many forms of knowledge can be based on individual experience, gained through trial and error and based on traditions, scientific knowledge results from a methodological process that is laid open for scrutiny and critical review.

Research activity can be classified as being part of inductive and deductive approaches. Generally, a deductive approach implies that there is a theory or knowledge in existence, which will be tested through the research process, whereas an inductive approach suggests that research will try to develop theory. Deductive and inductive positions in research are often described as being part of positivist and interpretivist research. Positivists emphasise the positive sciences, developing knowledge through testing and systematic experience. They employ quantitative methods to answer research questions and use scientific methods to test theory in a rigorous and controlled way. They aim to establish 'truth' that will allow the generalisation or wider use of the results (Polit and Beck, 2014).

The 'gold standard' randomised controlled trial is often employed in quantitative research to evaluate the effectiveness of interventions (Centre for Reviews and Dissemination, 2009), such as to see whether one approach to hip replacement works better than another. Elements of randomisation (selecting patients for either the control or research groups randomly), control (having the control group receiving the usual hip to compare with the research group) and manipulation (the research and control groups having different hips) are used (Polit and Beck, 2014) (see Chapter 14). Evidence from randomised controlled trials contributes to levels one and two of the hierarchy of evidence (see Chapter 1), whilst evidence at level three would come from experimental designs without randomisation (see Chapters 14). There are likely to be examples of care delivery based on scientific knowledge in practice settings.

Reflective exercise

Consider examples of care delivery you have seen in practice: Where has a randomised controlled trial or experimental design led to changes in practice? Think about the care you have delivered recently – is there an aspect of this which might be based on the research findings, for example, why might you administer a particular drug over another? Why do you encourage patients to change their position regularly?

Whilst positivist scientific approaches to knowledge generation have been important to the development of healthcare practice, especially medical practice, it is recognised that not all research questions can be addressed through such designs. Nursing and healthcare have a number of research questions related to the social aspects of life, wanting to explore the lived experience of patients, carers and staff. Research conducted in the interpretivist paradigm through qualitative approaches is employed to answer such questions and forms level four of the hierarchy of evidence (see Chapter 1). Interpretivists believe that in order to understand and make sense of the world, researchers must interpret human behaviour in natural settings. Qualitative researchers are therefore interested in gaining understanding of complex phenomena rather than testing for cause-and-effect relationships seen in positivist approaches (Burns et al., 2014). Qualitative methods involve listening to and observing people's interactions and patterns of behaviour. The types of designs used include ethnography, phenomenology, grounded theory, but may also encompass feminist and action research (see Chapters 15 and 19). Data collection is likely to include interviews, focus groups, diary recording and observations. This research approach, rather than seeking to control and measure, avoids exerting any influence on data collection and aims to describe reality and draw understanding from this.

Many studies use a mixed method approach that includes both qualitative and quantitative research (Bryman, 2001) (see Chapter 21). The use of mixed methods in social research allows the researcher to employ a number of methods to investigate research problems (Denzin, 2009). For example, when exploring the effectiveness of pain control, quantitative measures might include recording of physiological signs, with qualitative approaches gaining the patient's views on pain control. Measuring pain relief outcomes would draw on both qualitative and quantitative methods to provide a picture of patient experience and effectiveness of pain control.

Scientific evidence is not the only form of knowledge employed to support decision making in practice. It should be remembered that a range of sources informs nursing decision making and care delivery.

OTHER SOURCES OF KNOWLEDGE

Tradition

Knowledge passed down through generations of nurses forms the basis of traditional understanding. Traditional practices can be conveyed through observed practice, role modelling, written documents, books, journal articles and often from 'experienced' practitioners. These practices can be imposed: 'This is the way it should be done because this is the way it has always been done.' Such an approach can lead to the development of a nursing culture that accepts practices as being right, without questioning their foundation and evidence base. Examples from current practice can include the daily washing or bathing of patients before mid-morning, and recording observations of temperature, respirations, blood pressure and pulse on a regular basis. Some traditional practices can have a useful place in today's nursing, though the format in which they are delivered can be changed. For example, team handovers serve a useful purpose in ensuring the transfer of patient and other ward-related information from the outgoing to the incoming nursing team. The practice can also facilitate learning for student nurses and new staff members and offers an opportunity for socialisation of the team. However, the practice of handover can vary from the traditional office-based discussion, some being recorded, for the incoming team to listen to and some taking place at the patient's bedside. We can see evidence of tradition informing other areas of practice. Consider the following questions, for example: Which practices are informed by tradition? Why might this be the case?

As new evidence emerges there is often a need to challenge and change traditional and ritualistic practices. The need to practise using current evidence is expressed as part of the Nurses' Code of Professional Conduct (Nursing and Midwifery Council, 2015; www.nmc-uk.org), which requires all practitioners to 'Always practise in line with the best available evidence' (NMC, 2015: 7).

One major example of such challenge to traditional knowledge, through the development of new evidence, came in the 1990s. Manual handling practices underwent change, using risk assessment and equipment to encourage patients to move themselves. These guidelines replaced traditional lifting practices and improved the safety of staff and patients and have subsequently been updated based on new evidence and understanding.

Intuition and tacit knowledge

Any experienced practising nurse would probably be able to provide examples of employing **intuition** and **tacit knowledge** in practice situations. The use of intuition and tacit knowledge can include anticipating cardiac arrest, the need for pain relief or belief that a patient's life is near its end. Burnard (1989) has described intuition as an acute sensitivity or 'sixth sense', drawing on experience and knowledge to make a care judgement. Tacit knowledge is also developed through experience gained by engagement in practice. Gunilla et al. (2002) propose that tacit practice can be role modelled and displayed in practice delivery to future generations of nurses.

Benner (2001) has suggested that nurses evolve into expert practitioners, using experience to develop aesthetic knowledge (know-how). Expert nurses will use know-how to identify patients' needs, engaging in the delivery of holistic care as intuitive doers (Benner, 2001). Whilst Benner also acknowledges that the expert nurse will draw on scientific or 'know what' knowledge, she puts forward the idea that nurses' practice can be informed by intuition.

It is suggested that a lack of objectivity and ability to identify a rationale behind decisions taken using intuitive and tacit knowledge prevents it being viewed as a phenomenon for scientific study and adversely affects its recognition and standing as a knowledge base for practice (Moule, 2015). The use of tacit knowledge is not easily explained and providing a rationale for use is difficult. There are occasions, however, when such knowledge has been effectively employed to support decision making. Rew and Sparrow (1987) cite the use of intuition and tacit knowledge in situations where there may be limited information with which to interpret a possible behavioural response or in cases where ethical dilemmas are presented. Try to identify some examples of the use of intuition and tacit knowledge in practice. When is this type of knowledge used?

Dreyfus and Dreyfus (1985) offer a model of intuitive practice, described by Benner and Tanner (1987), which includes six elements of intuitive practice (see Table 2.1). The model provides a framework for the analysis of intuitive practice that includes know-how.

As debates surrounding the value and role of intuitive and tacit knowledge in nursing practice continue (Gunilla et al., 2002; Whitehead, 2005), it should be acknowledged

Table 2.1 Elements of intuition

Element	Form of intuition
Pattern recognition	The ability to recognise patterns of responses and changes of behaviour; for example, to recognise a rise in patient temperature through behaviour patterns.
Similarity recognition	Recognising patient characteristics seen previously and using these as part of interpreting a situation.
Common-sense understanding	Recognising and using commonly accepted practice
Skilled know-how	Making judgements about what seems to be the appropriate care for a patient.
Sense of salience	Recognising the importance of a particular information source, even though another may contradict this.
Deliberative rationality	Maintaining a broad view of the situation.

Source: Adapted from Benner and Tanner, 1987

that intuition and tacit knowledge can inform the development of **personal knowledge**. Such knowledge may ultimately, therefore, form part of the understanding that informs professional practice.

Personal knowledge

Personal knowledge is individual knowledge shaped through being personally involved in situations and events in practice. Liaschenko and Fisher (1999) refer to 'person knowledge', to knowing a person as an individual, understanding personal experience of illness and care delivery. Benner (2001) describes five levels of experience (see Table 2.2).

Often, experience is developed through observing role models in practice, and as such can be developed to include traditional and tacit knowledge. Trial and error can also play a part in the development of knowledge gained through experience, trying a different approach with unknown outcomes (Burns et al., 2014). Knowledge gained through this method becomes personal, often without formal documentation, sharing or research of the practice to confirm effectiveness for more general use. There are probably examples of drawing on trial and error to develop personal knowledge that we can identify. Consider an aspect of practice that may have been developed in this way.

Personal knowledge can be developed through the student reflecting on practice experiences. Personal expertise is therefore developed through a range of experiences and can be based on a number of sources of knowledge. Its status as a form of evidence on which to base practice is, however, subject to question. Closs (2003) suggests we should question expert knowledge that may be formed on limited experience and personal bias, without reliable foundation.

Table 2.2   Five levels of experience

Level	Type of experience
Novice	No personal experience of the activity. Preconceived ideas and expectations of practice that are refined and developed through experience.
Advanced beginner	Some experience to guide interpretation and intervention in recurrent situations.
Competent	Use personal knowledge gained through experience to undertake care that is deliberate and organised.
Proficient	Works with the individual patient and family, recognising the need to treat holistically and individually.
Expert	Extensive experience to analyse situations and deliver skilful care.

Source: Adapted from Benner, 2001

CONCEPTUALISING NURSING RESEARCH

In thinking about nursing research, a broad view of professional practice needs to be taken. Nursing research encompasses the practice of nursing, which is in itself complex. Practice-based research questions may try to test new practice or support care development. Additionally, they can measure the effectiveness of care, explore carer and family issues, or consider the interprofessional nature of care delivery.

Nurses do not work in isolation, but with a range of professionals in different healthcare environments. The research agenda needs to reflect this and consider questions where a multi-disciplinary approach to care is required.

Nursing research also explores the educational preparation of nurses, reviewing the pedagogy of nursing and how best to support learning and teaching of nurses and other healthcare professionals. Research will additionally review the management of nursing services, such as the development and effectiveness of new roles.

Nursing is an emerging profession and one that often draws on other disciplines in its execution of research. Psychology, the social sciences, physical sciences, environmental sciences and epidemiology can inform nursing research. Indeed, research teams may often reflect a number of disciplines in their make-up, utilising a range of professions and taking on board different discipline perspectives in the research design. For example, researching aspects of mental healthcare can take a pharmaceutical, psychological or sociological perspective. In Chapter 1, we discussed the developing research roles of nurses, engaging in nursing research within universities and practice settings. Attempts to increase the research capacity (number of nurses able to understand research) and capability of nurses (nurses able to research) through career mapping continue (UKCRC, 2007) and formally recognise the need for nurses to engage in researching their own professional practice, as highlighted in previous reports (HEFCE, 2001). Such drivers acknowledge the need to link practice, education and research within nursing in order to secure an evidence-based future (HEFCE, 2001).

Nurses should be involved not only in researching their practice but also in identifying the research agendas. In 2000, the Department of Health (DH, 2000) emphasised the need to identify research priorities within nursing to ensure that appropriate aspects of nursing delivery are considered. This aimed to engage nurses in developing the research priorities for practice and to ensure the focus of research activity.

In undertaking such research, a multitude of research methods will be employed, in both positivist and interpretivist paradigms. Depending on the research question(s), those exploring nursing issues will draw on qualitative and quantitative approaches and a range of methods of data collection. The social sciences play a key role in much nursing research activity as they are employed to consider issues related to the patient, carer and family that can be physiological, psychological or socially derived. These are not the limits of nursing research, however, which may need to test theory and practice developments through more rigorous positivist approaches. Given the scope and nature of nursing research, our definition offered in Chapter 1 reflects its complexity and recognises the need to employ a range of methods and methodologies to address the broad range of questions and create new knowledge for practice education and policy. As a reminder, our definition based on that within Moule (2015) is:

> A systematic approach to gathering information for the purposes of answering questions and solving problems in the pursuit of creating new knowledge about nursing practice, education and policy. (2015: 10)

The remaining chapters of the book consider more fully the complexities of developing, undertaking and implementing nursing research to support decision making and practice. Whilst we should acknowledge that a range of evidence could inform practice, that derived through scientific approaches is significant to the support of evidence-based practice.

CHAPTER SUMMARY

- Nursing knowledge is multifaceted and is developed through science and experience.
- Nurses can draw on a range of sources of knowledge to support decision making and care delivery.
- Scientific knowledge is constructed through methodological processes and is open to scrutiny.
- Scientific knowledge can be developed through deductive and inductive research approaches.
- Tradition, intuition and tacit understanding can underpin nursing care delivery.
- Personal knowledge is knowing the patient as an individual.
- The knowledge base for practice should be questioned.
- Nurses need to be involved in developing research agendas and in researching practice.
- Nurses are still developing research skills and expertise.

SUGGESTED FURTHER READING

Benner, P., Tanner, C. and Chesla, C. (2009) *Expertise in Nursing Practice: Caring, Clinical Judgement and Ethics*, 2nd edn. NY: Springer. This book is a report of a research study which investigated skill acquisition and the development of knowledge in expert practice.
Rolfe, G. (1998) *Expanding Nursing Knowledge*, 2nd edn. Oxford: Butterworth Heinemann. This book discusses different types of knowledge and explores how nurses can use and develop personal knowledge through reflective practice.

WEBSITES

Department of Health: www.dh.gov.uk – Provides strategic leadership for public health, the NHS and social care. Is responsible for improving health and well-being in England.

Higher Education Funding Council for Higher Education: www.hefce.ac.uk – Promotes and funds higher education teaching in England.

Nursing and Midwifery Council: www.nmc-uk.org – Regulatory body for the profession of nursing in the UK maintaining standards of care delivery.

UK Clinical Research Collaboration: www.ukcrc.org/ – Aim to establish the UK as a world leader in clinical research through identifying the barriers to research and working to overcome them. One particular initiative is the support of clinical academic careers for nurses and allied health professionals.

To access further resources related to this chapter, visit the companion website at https://study.sagepub.com/mouleaveyard3e

REFERENCES

Benner, P. (2001) *From Novice to Expert: Excellence and Power in Clinical Nursing Practice*, commemorative edn. Upper Saddle River, NJ: Prentice Hall.

Benner, P. and Tanner, C. (1987) 'How expert nurses use intuition', *American Journal of Nursing*, 87 (1): 23–31.

Bryman, A. (2001) *Social Research Methods*, 4th edn. Oxford: Oxford University Press.

Burnard, P. (1989) 'The sixth sense', *Nursing Times*, 85 (50): 52–3.

Burns, N., Grove, S. and Gray, J. (2014) *The Practice of Nursing Research: Appraisal, Synthesis and Generation of Evidence*, 7th edn. St. Louis, MO: Saunders Elsevier.

Carper, B. (1975) *Fundamental Patterns of Knowing in Nursing*. Dissertation for Degree of Doctor in Education, Columbia University, USA.

Carper, B. (1978) 'Fundamental patterns of knowing in nursing', *Advances in Nursing Science*, 1 (1): 13–23.

Centre for Reviews and Dissemination (2009) *Systematic Reviews: CRD's Guidance for Undertaking Reviews in Healthcare*, 3rd edn. University of York: CRD. Available at: www.york.ac.uk/crd/guidance (accessed 31 July 2015).

Closs, S.J. (2003) 'Evidence and community-based nursing practice', in R. Bryer and J. Griffiths (eds), *Practice Development in Community Nursing*. London: Arnold. pp. 33–56.

Denzin, N. (2009) *The Research Act: A Theoretical Introduction to Sociological Methods*. New Brunswick, USA: Aldine Transaction.

Department of Health (2000) *Towards a Strategy for Nursing Research and Development: Proposals for Action*. London: Department of Health.

Dreyfus, H. and Dreyfus, S. (1985) *Mind over Machine: The Power of Human Intuition and Expertise in the Era of the Computer*. New York: Free Press.

Gunilla, C., Drew, N., Dahlberg, K. and Lutzen, K. (2002) 'Uncovering tacit caring knowledge', *Nursing Philosophy*, 3 (20): 144–51.

Higher Education Funding Council for England (HEFCE) (2001) *Promoting Research in Nursing and the Allied Health Professions. Research Report 01/64*. Bristol: HEFCE.

Liaschenko, J. and Fisher, A. (1999) 'Theorising the knowledge that nurses use in the conduct of their work', *Scholarly Inquiry for Nursing Practice: An International Journal*, 13: 29–40.

Moule, P. (2015) *Making Sense of Research in Nursing, Health and Social Care*, 5th edn. London: Sage.

Nursing and Midwifery Council (2015) *The Code: Professional Standards of Practice and Behaviour for Nurses and Midwives*. London: NMC.

Polit, D. and Beck, C. (2014) *Essentials of Nursing Research: Appraising Evidence for Nursing Practice*, 8th edn. Philadelphia, PA: Lippincott Williams & Wilkins.

Rew, L. and Sparrow, E. (1987) 'Intuition: A neglected hallmark of nursing knowledge', *Advances in Nursing Science*, 10 (10): 49–62.

Rolfe, G. (1998) *Expanding Nursing Knowledge*. Oxford: Butterworth Heinemann.

Schon, D.A. (1987) *Educating the Reflective Practitioner*. San Francisco, CA: Jossey-Bass.

United Kingdom Clinical Research Collaboration (2007) *Developing the Best Research Professionals*. London: UKCRC.

Whitehead, D. (2005) 'Empirical or tacit knowledge as a basis for theory development?', *Journal of Clinical Nursing*, 14 (2): 299–305.

3
THE RESEARCH PROCESS

Learning outcomes

The chapter will enable you to:

- Identify the stages of the research process
- Understand how the research process guides research activity

The research process provides a structured approach used by researchers to generate evidence and guide research activity. It includes a series of steps or stages undertaken by researchers as they consider questions arising from practice and education. The process, though presented in a linear framework below, is not necessarily implemented in this way. Researchers can move backwards and forwards through the stages, often being involved in them consecutively rather than sequentially. An understanding of the research process is needed to identify published research, with knowledge of the processes involved in each stage being required to support critical appraisal and evaluation of research papers. The research process is closely aligned to the headings used to present research in reports and journals (see Figure 3.1). A comparison between the two shows distinct similarity between the process of research and its presentation to readers. Within this book, our aim is to provide readers with the knowledge and skills to critically read research (see Chapter 5) and we also provide insight into the stages and processes of research activity that might support the development of a research proposal. Additionally, theoretical guidance in the text will support those engaged in research activity, where research skills will be developed under supervision.

Introduction

Background (literature review)

The Study

    Aims (research questions/ hypothesis)
    Design/methodology
    Sample/participants
    Data collection
    Validity and reliability/rigour of the study
    Ethical considerations
    Data analysis

Results/findings

Discussion

Conclusions

Figure 3.1 *Journal of Advanced Nursing*: Research paper headings

Source: Onlinelibrary.wiley.com/journal/10.1111/(ISSN)1365-2648/issues (accessed 13 May 2015)

THE STAGES OF THE RESEARCH PROCESS

1. Developing research questions (Chapter 9).
2. Literature searching (Chapter 4).
3. Literature reviewing (Chapters 6 and 20).
4. Choosing a research design (Chapters 11 and 14–19).
5. Ethical considerations (Chapters 7 and 8).
6. Sampling (Chapter 12).
7. Data collection (Chapters 22–25).
8. Data analysis (Chapters 26 and 27).
9. Interpretation and implications of the research (Chapter 28).
10. Using research in practice (Chapter 29).

Developing research questions

Research questions are often developed from nursing practice, emerging from issues or problems in care delivery, or a desire to enhance practice. Questions can also emerge from educational and other settings. Key questions can be proposed at government or individual level. Government research agendas are often linked to changes in policy, for example, addressing a major healthcare concern such as diabetes or mental health. Individual professionals in the workplace can identify local research questions. These questions arise from experiences of immediate practice delivery, and can include questions about patient experience or the effectiveness of care or treatment. Examples might include:

'What are patients' experiences of cancer care treatment?'

'How does the Early Stroke Discharge Team impact on patient care?'

Members of the public and patients can also be involved in shaping research agendas.

Further details on problem identification and the formulation of research aims, questions or the development of research hypotheses, are reviewed later in the book (see Chapter 9). Researchers need to complete detailed literature searching and review to ensure the initial thinking about the research problem area is well founded. This process should provide a review of the existing research evidence in the field, confirming whether and what further research is needed. Thus, the stage of finalising the research question will overlap with the steps of literature searching and literature review, with the formulation of a question being guided by practice experience and critical review of the existing literature.

Literature searching

This stage of the research process is not only important in developing the research question, but also potentially links to all other stages of the research process. A successful search strategy is the key to identifying the existing literature in the field of study and will determine the current knowledge base. It should be ongoing throughout the period of research study, enabling the researcher to draw on any new thinking in the research field which might impact on their study.

The literature search can inform the development of the research design, sample, data collection and data analysis and is referred to when drawing research interpretations and implications for practice. The process of literature searching is discussed in Chapter 4, which suggests the need for a systematic approach to ensure all relevant literature is accessed. Given the importance of adopting a rigorous approach to searching, the chapter includes a number of strategies that can be employed, including the identification of key terms, sources and development of inclusion and exclusion criteria. The chapter also includes information on a number of organisations and key personnel with advanced searching skills whose expertise can be drawn on.

Researchers undertaking literature-based studies complete a systematic critical appraisal of existing research literature (see Chapter 20), a crucial component of the research methodology.

Literature review

A review of the literature follows the literature search, though in practice researchers might begin this process whilst still collecting papers and can use the review process to identify further literature. A review can be guided by a critical review framework and conducted following an appraisal process, as discussed in Chapters 5 and 6. The critical review framework (see Chapter 5) is based on the stages of the research process and includes a number of questions that allow the reader to interrogate the published research paper. A review framework will include questions on both research presentation and content, and when applied through an appraisal process will enable the reviewer to analyse the strengths and weaknesses of the paper. The process of review aims to support evaluation of the quality of the published literature identified in the search.

The advent of the Internet has facilitated access to a wider range of literature than previously available. Not all papers found on the Internet have been subjected to a formal peer-review process and some Internet-based literature can present personal opinion. Those reviewing any material will therefore need to appreciate the different levels of evidence available. To assist readers in this, Chapter 1 provides an introduction to the sorts of information and evidence accessible to support research, whilst Chapter 2 reviews the different sources of nursing knowledge.

Choosing a research design

There are a range of research designs available for use in answering research questions. Their function is to ensure that the evidence collected should be able to answer the research questions posed. The chosen design should enable the researcher to collect the evidence needed to answer the research question. The design is a plan of how the research will answer the research question and should include the overall research approach taken, ethical considerations, sampling, methods of data collection and analysis. Chapter 11 presents further discussions on selecting a research design. Often research designs and approaches can be presented as either part of qualitative or quantitative research, as a dichotomy, which polarises the approaches. This position isn't necessarily helpful as some designs, such as case studies (see Chapter 19) might include elements of both qualitative and quantitative approaches within them.

Quantitative research, in the crudest sense, is research that tends to be driven by a positivist or scientific approach, but more latterly by a post-positivist approach. It is often described as being part of deduction or **deductive reasoning** that starts with a general theory about something and moves to test a theory through undertaking further observations or by developing tests. Quantitative research is seen as attempting to answer questions and hypotheses through generating research data, often involving numerical data collection that can be analysed through statistical techniques. There is often an aim to generalise to a wider population, applying the results to a broader group of people.

Qualitative research is most commonly viewed as inductivist, where the aim is to develop concepts and themes from the interpretation of observations and interviews. **Inductive reasoning** is a process of starting with the details of an experience or our observation of something and using these to develop a general understanding of phenomena. Specific observations and descriptions are made and used to develop a hypothesis and theory of a more general situation that can be tested.

In its simplest form, qualitative research aims to generate data that comprises words and pictures. Qualitative researchers often focus on language, perceptions and experiences in order to understand and explain behaviour. They believe that the social world needs to be interpreted to be understood. Qualitative research may be used to explore beliefs and experiences. Evidence is analysed to identify key themes and issues. The results often describe the local context and can be open to transferability to other contexts.

Chapters 11 and 14 to 19 include more in-depth discussions on a range of research designs, including those that might be employed in quantitative research such as experimental and survey design and those drawn on within qualitative approaches, phenomenology, ethnography and grounded theory.

Crucially, the researcher needs to adopt the most suitable research approach to answer the research question. The approach selected should take account of the existing literature base and subject of the study. In some cases, adopting a qualitative approach might be reasonable and in others a combined approach might afford better answers. For example, if research aimed to review nurses' learning and skill development, a combined approach would offer scope to both test knowledge and skill attainment, measuring specific criteria and eliciting experiences of learning. Data collection in this case would include a range of methods such as pre- and post-tests of knowledge, testing skill attainment against specific criteria and interviewing nurses about their learning experiences.

The selection of a research design will also be influenced by a number of practical issues. In designing a study, researchers will think about their own research skills, the expertise of the research team and preferred working methods. The team also need to consider the amount of time for the study and the resources to support it. For example, it may be that there is a limited amount of time and resources available, in which case selecting a **longitudinal study** with the need for participant observations would not be sustainable. It may be more practical to arrange to collect interview data for analysis, though obviously the design selected must enable the researcher to collect the evidence needed to address the research question.

Rigour and trustworthiness must also be apparent in the application of the research design. Chapter 13 reviews issues of rigour, validity and reliability in quantitative research, and considers how these key characteristics reflect the quality in research design. Though measures of rigour in qualitative research are less developed, it must establish trustworthiness through being auditable, checking that the interpretations of data are credible, transferable, dependable and confirmable.

Ethical considerations

Ethical considerations are discussed here at an early stage of the research process, as such issues should be considered prior to undertaking sampling and data collection. It is good practice to secure ethical approval prior to sampling and data collection, with some research funders requiring confirmation of ethical approval prior to grant submission.

Within healthcare research, there are clear guidelines for researchers to work with which provide guidance on best practice for researchers. The British Educational Research Association (BERA) provides guidelines (BERA, 2011) to support ethical practice in education settings such as schools, encouraging researchers to reflect on their practice. This operates at an individual researcher level, encouraging researchers to work to ethical principles. The Health Research Authority of the NHS (a Non-Departmental Public Body), came into existence in 2015 and took on responsibility for issuing guidance for research in England, in place of the Research Governance Framework. A UK Policy Framework for Health and Social Care is intended to guide the practice of anyone researching with patients, clients or health and social care staff, and applies to all those undertaking research, whether it is part of professional development or a large-scale project. Often, research undertaken with staff and service evaluations do not require NHS approval but the project will need to be registered with Research and Development Departments. Researchers working in universities often secure ethical approval for projects through their own institution if NHS ethics are not required (see Chapters 7 and 8).

Sampling

Data are collected from a sample drawn from a population that the researcher is interested in. Such populations may be composed of subjects or incidents. The size and scope of the selected sample will depend on the research design that is being used to answer the research question and the methods of data collection employed. For example, an experimental design might employ a statistician to compute a power calculation to estimate the sample size needed for the study. The research would then aim to recruit that number to support rigour and confidence in the data analysis. In general, qualitative approaches can include smaller samples based on the characteristics of the population. The researchers are interested in collecting detailed and quality data from a smaller number of participants, so that they can understand people's experiences or perceptions. Where phenomenological approaches are taken to explore the lived experience of a particular group, sample selection will be purposive and will aim to include members of that population in the study.

Sampling theory includes two main strategies or techniques. These are commonly referred to as probability and non-probability sampling. Probability-sampling techniques involve the use of random selection, where in theory every member of the population has a chance of being included in the final sample. In contrast, non-probability sampling does not attempt to include random selection processes and can be determined at researcher level. Within each technique there are a number of approaches to sampling. These are discussed in further detail as part of Chapter 12.

Data collection

Each research design can employ a number of data collection techniques or methods. A case study design, for example, might include documentary analysis, observations, interviews and diary collection. Each data collection tool affords the researcher access to different types of data relevant to addressing the research question. Interviews will allow the researcher to explore experiences of providing patient care, whereas observations facilitate insight into actual practice delivery, and documentation provides written accounts of practice provision. A number of data collection techniques are presented in Chapters 22 to 25, spanning those that might be employed within the range of research designs. Commonly used techniques include interviews, questionnaires, tests and measurement scales. These are discussed in Chapters 22 to 25, and reference is made to the use of life history, critical incident technique and emerging Internet and web-based approaches. The discussion will cover the main approaches to data collection identifying the potential strengths and weaknesses of each.

Data analysis

The approach to data analysis will depend on the type of data that has been collected. Quantitative data analysis techniques include the analysis of numerical data, using descriptive and inferential statistics. The management of data includes working with data sets, understanding levels of measurement, the application of statistical tests and generation of probability figures. These are discussed in Chapter 26 where there is also a review of the types of computer packages available to assist those analysing numerical data. The chapter will guide those interested to resources that cover the mechanics of calculation as it does not aim to equip readers with the skill to compute tests, but to appreciate how researchers work with data and present it.

A further chapter presents the key issues of qualitative data analysis, which involves the researcher describing and presenting findings through developing interpretations of text or observational data. Chapter 27 considers the preparation of qualitative data and processes of analysis. This includes the use of computer software to support analysis and the presentation of findings.

Interpretation and implications of the research

Healthcare research often addresses research questions that are specifically related to issues in practice. There is an expectation therefore that research findings will have direct relevance to practice and possibly to policy development. Research may also identify the need for ongoing study in a particular field and make recommendations regarding the need for further research, identifying questions and possible designs. Chapter 29 reviews the implications arising from research activity for practice, policy and further research. In doing so it considers the importance of recognising any limitations in the research design that might affect the strength of the findings and quality of the research.

Using research in practice

Historically, nursing has reported difficulties in applying research findings to practice, identifying key obstacles to its use. Chapter 29 considers potential barriers to research implementation, though also comments on the use of research in developing clinical guidelines, practice protocols and standards of care as part of clinical audit. Effective strategies used to increase research implementation are reviewed, including the dissemination of research through the provision of research reports, journal papers, online media and **conference presentation**. These dissemination activities should be a mandatory part of the research process for any researcher. Research proposals, whether developed as part of an application for funding, for professional development as part of private study or as part of a review for ethical approval, should include a strategy for the dissemination of research findings.

Reflective exercise

To check your learning, you could search for a research paper and a systematic review paper (see Chapters 4 and 20 for help with this). Is the research paper presented using headings that reflect the stages of the research process, or are the headings different and, if so, how? How do you know you are looking at a systematic literature review paper? What are the differences in these papers?

CHAPTER SUMMARY

- The research process is a series of steps or stages undertaken by researchers in order to address research questions.
- The research process includes stages of: developing the research question; literature searching; literature review; choosing a research design; ethical considerations; sampling; data collection; data analysis; interpretation and implications of the research; and using research in practice.
- These stages can be interrelated, as research activity does not always follow the process sequentially.
- An appreciation of the stages of the research process enables professionals to identify and critically appraise research.

SUGGESTED FURTHER READING

Bowling, A. (2014) *Research Methods in Health: Investigating Health and Health Services*, 4th edn. Berkshire: Open University Press.

LoBiondo-Wood, G. and Haber, J. (2014) (eds) *Nursing Research: Methods and Critical Appraisal for Evidence-based Practice*, 8th edn. St Louis: Mosby Elsevier.

Polit, D. and Beck, C. (2014) *Essentials of Nursing Research: Appraising Evidence for Nursing Practice*, 8th edn. Philadelphia: Wolters Kuwer Health/ Lippincott, Williams and Wilkins.

WEBSITES

BERA guidelines: www.bera.ac.uk
NHS Health Research Authority: www.hra.nhs.uk

 To access further resources related to this chapter, visit the companion website at https://study.sagepub.com/mouleaveyard3e

REFERENCE

British Educational Research Association (2011) *Ethical Guidelines for Educational Research*. Available at: www.bera.ac.uk/files/2011/08/BERA-Ethical-Guidelines-2011.pdf (accessed 13 May 2015).

4
LITERATURE SEARCHING

Learning outcomes

This chapter will enable you to:

- understand the steps involved in searching the literature
- identify appropriate information to be retrieved when searching the literature
- carry out a literature search of a topic in your area of research/practice interest
- understand how to locate the relevant literature for a research question/topic

Any research project starts from an idea, the identification of a problem or something that a researcher wants to find out more about. To get started, a researcher needs to gain more information before the idea, query or topic of interest can be refined into a project that is manageable and researchable. An understanding of the literature that already exists is usually one of the first steps in this process. Searching for the literature that is relevant to a topic helps to refine a research question and should also confirm that it has not already been answered. The use of electronic databases has made searching more convenient and faster. Even so, searching for relevant literature is a skill that has to be developed but it will be invaluable in keeping you up to date with any relevant newly published literature as the research progresses.

The purpose of a literature review is to bring together all the relevant publications (and sometimes unpublished work) so that all of the literature can be reviewed together, rather than viewing individual studies in isolation (Aveyard, 2014). If you regard individual studies as pieces of a jigsaw, it is easier to see the full picture of research when you have all of the pieces. We discuss this again in the chapter on Literature Reviewing (Chapter 6) and in more detail in the chapter on Systematic Reviews (Chapter 20). This overview of existing research provides a platform from which to develop an actual research project. The literature review is an important section of all research projects. When researchers write up their research, the literature review is usually a formal section of the final project, in which the methods for searching for literature are fully documented.

A literature review can be divided into two sections:

- Searching for literature that is appropriate to a specific topic.
- Appraising and reviewing the literature.

This chapter introduces the practicalities of searching the literature and outlines some strategies for successful searching.

THE PURPOSE OF SEARCHING FOR LITERATURE

Deciding where to begin searching the literature on a specific topic can be daunting. What must be remembered is that a **literature review**, whether as background for a research project or as a standalone project in its own right, is *not* an attempt to identify every existing resource related to the topic of the research. Rather, the aim is to identify the research and other evidence that is truly *relevant* to the review (Aveyard, 2014). This means that you have to use judgement in deciding whether or not a particular resource is relevant to your review, as well as having some familiarity with the general area of the research and research methods typically used in the topic being reviewed.

Therefore, you, as the researcher, need to have a basic understanding of the specific research topic *before* embarking on the actual searching. This may sound contradictory, but without some insight into the research topic it will be very difficult to develop a research question, identify the terms for a search or make reasonable judgements about what to use or discard from the results of a search. A nurse researcher or group of nurses planning to undertake a research project are likely to have a grasp of the key issues relating to the topic; others may require a lot of discussion and prior reading before the process of transferring an idea for research into an actual project can commence. This may include discussions with relevant and interested colleagues who can help to find the focus of the topic, which helps lead to the development of a clear research question. Such informal discussions can assist, particularly, in refining search terms, and may even generate specific articles, references or contacts. Colleagues may have been involved in research on a related topic and be able to put you in touch with other researchers in the same area of interest or be willing to share papers and/or results. Others may have attended courses or conferences where the topic has been discussed and, again, may be willing to share notes and conference proceedings. In addition, teachers and supervisors frequently have access to a wide variety of resources and/or individuals that can provide assistance in gaining more understanding of a topic. This type of discussion should really be undertaken before starting a **literature search** but it can also be useful in the later stages of a search, particularly if the searching produces too few or far too many citations.

These initial discussions may also be able to stop you progressing too far with a topic that has already been very well researched or one that will be very difficult to research within the resources available, or where ethical considerations may make researching the topic impracticable.

STAGES IN THE LITERATURE SEARCHING PROCESS

The main stages of the search are discussed below:

1. Confirming the research topic or question.
2. Identifying which literature to include.
3. Identifying inclusion and exclusion criteria.
4. Identifying key terms.
5. Performing a search.
6. Revising the search, as necessary, and replicating it in other sources.

Confirming the research topic or question

As already suggested, before starting a search of the literature you need to determine what you are trying to find out about and what level of information is needed. It is important to remember that the aim of searching the literature for a research project is not to retrieve as many general references as possible. The reason for searching the literature is to identify what is relevant to the research question and, by extension, to identify the *main gaps* in knowledge. The search should also give some guidance on the general patterns of findings from multiple examples of research in the same area, and the types of research method that have been used by other researchers in the area. To do this, a clearly defined topic or research question is essential, otherwise there is a risk of not finding relevant information (that is, citations) or of wasting a considerable amount of time. For example, you could be interested in the management of constipation. Constipation is a very large topic with a myriad of causes, treatments and groups of patients affected. To avoid wasted time and effort, you should, before starting on your search, decide which group of patients you are interested in; whether you want to consider causation and/or treatment; and maybe even decide whether you want to limit the types of treatment option or include all options.

Identifying which literature to include

Once you have identified your research question, you need to consider what literature is most important for your review. Deciding on appropriate sources of information is important for the credibility of your review. Essentially, there are two sources of information: *primary* and *secondary* sources.

Researchers who carry out original work on a topic produce *primary sources*. For example, researchers who undertake empirical research collect first-hand accounts, observations and experiments to analyse data and draw conclusions. Primary sources do not have to be empirical research however; for example, an eye witness account of an incident is a primary source. Primary sources are usually preferred over secondary sources because the account of the work comes directly from those who authored it and there is decreased potential for bias and distortion beyond the control of the researcher (Powers and Knapp, 2010). Primary sources are usually published as journal articles or abstracts from conferences.

Secondary sources make reference to the original research by someone other than the researcher. The source of data consists of summarisation of, or commentary about, primary data, such as in a literature review. Secondary sources are usually found within journal articles or textbooks. As with primary sources, secondary sources will be of variable quality, for example a literature review of empirical research published in a journal is likely to be of better quality than reference to a research report in a newspaper.

It is very useful to become adept at recognising what is a primary and what is a secondary source. It is also useful to become adept at recognising what is empirical research and what is not. This might sound straightforward, but research in healthcare can be complex and it is not always as easy as you might think (Aveyard et al., 2016).

Relevant articles and information can be obtained from many sources; some of these are shown in Figure 4.1.

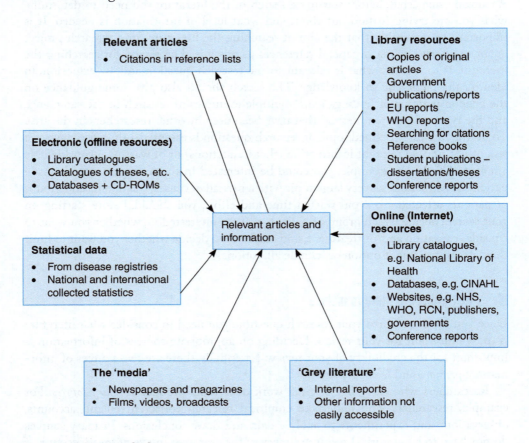

Figure 4.1 Sources of information

Books generally represent the acceptance of an idea or method into the mainstream thought of that discipline. They often make reference to empirical research but rarely report the whole study directly. The time it takes to publish a book means that the information contained in it may be older than that found in journals, reports and so on.

Journal articles vary in their content – most empirical research is published in journals, but you will also find editorials, discussion and opinion pieces, book reviews and so on so it is not possible to assume that everything published in a journal is research. Journal articles will be relevant when they are up to date (this is usually regarded as being within 10 years of publication), although it is possible to trace how trends have changed by reviewing older articles. It is also important to remember that not all articles meet academic standards. Most journal articles are now peer reviewed, which gives a degree of quality assurance, but this does not take away from the need for you as a reader to make your own judgement about the quality of the research being described (Aveyard et al., 2015).

Papers in the form of conference proceedings have the advantage of being timely and present the very latest thinking on a particular topic. However quality control may not be as rigorous as that of peer-reviewed journals, though it is now usual for there to have been some peer review prior to a paper being accepted for presentation at a conference.

Reports – research reports, technical reports, development reports, government reports – present details of research from a specific project. This is a growing body of literature that provides a good source of current tabular, graphic and statistical material. However, not all reports will be in the public domain and it may be difficult to obtain the full report; reports also tend to be confined to science and technology although this may be changing.

Dissertations and theses – undergraduate, Master's, MPhil, PhD – are an important source of primary material because they should contain original work and meet a minimum academic standard. It can be difficult to obtain copies and you may have to consult them in the library where the dissertation/thesis is held. However, it is possible to use the British Library EThOS service to search for PhD theses (http://ethos.bl.uk/Home.do;jsessionid=F1B71681C608651DF56FFB8A4B1D1B35).

Exactly which sources to use will depend on your research question, the time you have available to perform a search and review the literature retrieved, and what search resources you can access. You should, however, always remember that the quality of the information you obtain will vary. The next chapter discusses how to assess the quality of the articles you retrieve.

Inclusion and exclusion criteria

Once you have established which information is most likely to be useful to your review, you can refine this further by setting specific inclusion and exclusion criteria to help you set boundaries for the search and enable you to identify at a glance whether the literature you find is relevant for your review.

Inclusion and exclusion criteria are written specifically for each individual literature review and are used *after* the search has been undertaken to help check the relevance of each potential source to the review. However these criteria might also be used to influence the search. For example, it is common for literature reviews to focus on the primary empirical research that has been undertaken and to exclude more general discussions in books and journals. In this case, this would be stated in the inclusion and exclusion criteria.

Identifying key terms

The next step is to begin to consider how you will search for the literature. The main component of any literature search is the use of electronic databases. These are huge bibliographic files that can be accessed electronically, usually via an online search (using the Internet). In order to start searching using a database, you need to create a set of key terms in order to identify the key concepts you are interested in. There are likely to be two or three per research question.

Once these key terms are established, think about the alternative words that might have been used by researchers instead of the key term you have identified. To continue the example from above, you decide on the treatment of constipation in older people. The keywords in this example are *older people* and *constipation*. There are likely to be several ways of expressing these keywords – using alternative words, spelling variations and abbreviations. Below are some suggested search terms; these are the words or search terms that you will use to search the databases (though this is not a definitive list):

- older people/patient(s)
- elderly people/patient(s)
- geriatric(s)
- older adult(s)/patient(s)
- constipation
- defaecation/defecation
- bowel function(s)
- bowel habit(s)
- bowel movement(s).

Another way that is often used to generate search terms is to refer to one of the acronyms that can be used to develop research questions. We discuss these in Chapter 9. These can also be used to trigger ideas about possible key terms. For example, if you are interested in 'the effectiveness of nicotine patches in helping adults to stop smoking', you can use the quantitative version of the PICO tool formula to help you identify key terms:

What is the Problem?

= adults; cigarette smokers for at least three years' duration (you will have to decide if you are including pipe and/or cigar smokers).

What is the Intervention (or treatment)?

= application of nicotine patch or educational leaflet.

What is the Comparison (if any)?

= nicotine patch versus educational leaflet.

What is the Outcome measure?

= participants not smoking for at least one year.

You may identify some additional key terms from working through the key concepts in your research question. Once you have identified your key terms and their alternative words, you are ready to start searching.

Reflective exercise

Try using PICO yourself with the earlier example of the management of constipation in the elderly.

Performing a search

Once you have identified your key terms and your inclusion and exclusion criteria, you are ready to start searching the electronic databases.

There are many bibliographic (electronic) databases, the majority of which have user-friendly programmes that are menu-driven with on-screen support, making retrieving a reference relatively easy. Furthermore, most university and NHS libraries also offer training sessions on using the most popular electronic databases; it is very useful to learn your way around these search resources. It is generally advisable to take up the offer of support sessions to facilitate this.

The main electronic search resources that hold references on nursing studies include:

- CINAHL (Cumulative Index to Nursing and Allied Health Literature).
- British Nursing Index.
- Allied and Complementary Medicine.
- MEDLINE (Medical Literature Online).
- Cochrane Database of Systematic Reviews.
- EMBASE (the Excerpta Medical database).
- PsychoINFO (Psychology Information).
- National Research Register.
- ReFeR (Department of Health Research Findings Register).
- CancerLit (Cancer Literature).
- Dissertation Abstracts online.

All of the above databases can be accessed via the National Library for Health at www.evidence.nhs.uk. The most useful databases for nurses are probably CINAHL, British Nursing Index and MEDLINE.

There are a number of features used in databases that are worth understanding to make searching easier and more effective. These allow you to find references with:

- different spellings – for example, leukaemia or leukemia
- different terminology – for example, pavement or sidewalk
- prefixes – for example, prenatal, pre natal or pre-natal.

Wildcards (*, ?) are used to search for spelling variations and plurals. For example:

leuk?emia to find leukaemia or leukemia

p*ediatrics will retrieve paediatrics or pediatrics

child* will retrieve children and child, as well as childhood and childish.

You can also truncate (for example, *, $) words to search for different word stems and word endings. The truncation symbol is usually an asterisk (*), but this may vary from one database to another. For example:

use comput* to find computer, computers, computing, computed, and so on (comp* would also find compost!).

The search terms for the constipation example would look like this to cope with spelling and plurals, etc.:

- Constip*
- Defaecation/defecation
- Bowel function$
- Bowel habit$
- Bowel movement$
- Older people/patient$
- Elderly people/patient$
- Geriatric$
- Older adult$/patient$

Once you have established your key terms, you need to specify how your keywords or search terms relate to each other. This is usually done by using what are known as Boolean operators, that is, using the linking words AND, OR, NOT:

- **AND**: linking keywords with AND means that all keywords must appear in the search results.
- **OR**: combining terms with OR means that any of the keywords must appear in the search results. This will generate a larger set of results. You would use OR for

linking alternative ways of describing the same subject – for example, older people OR elderly OR geriatric.
- **NOT**: this is used to *exclude* search terms; use with caution as you may remove too many results, including those that are relevant!

Additionally, setting date limits for your search will make it more practical and ensure that you retrieve only citations that are up to date. It is important that the date range you set is realistic; a common convention is to set a 10-year limit to a search. However, you may wish to modify this if there are either an overwhelming number of citations or very few. Take care to check that it is your date range that is at fault rather than your search terms; your librarian will help you if this problem occurs.

It is also usual to limit your search to English-language publications for the purely practical reason of needing to be able to read the citations retrieved. Ordinarily, this will not be a problem (unless you are doing a systematic literature review – see Chapter 20). However, if your research is in an area where most of the literature has not been published in English, then it could be a disadvantage; for example, if the topic is about acupuncture, then using only English for a search will exclude the large body of Chinese literature.

Searching and retrieving citations using CINAHL

The Cumulative Index to Nursing and Allied Health Literature or CINAHL covers references to hundreds of English (and other languages) nursing journals, as well as book chapters, nursing dissertations and some conference proceedings for nursing and allied health fields. Abstracts are available for many of the journals and, depending on your access rights, you may also be able to download the full text of some articles.

You can access the CINAHL database via the National Library for Health website at www.library.nhs.uk. The website will give you a list of databases.

To use CINAHL, simply click on it in order to start searching.

- Step 1: Starting the search – for this example, the search is going to be for information about 'the use of laxatives in the management of constipation in elderly patients'. The logical way of searching is to search for one subject at a time: type 'constipation' into the search box. You also need to make sure that 'Thesaurus mapping' is ticked, and then click on it.
- Step 2: Thesaurus mapping – this will take you to a list of subject headings. Locate the subject heading closest to what you typed – here there is likely to be a 'constipation' subject heading, so just click on the word *CONSTIPATION*.
- Step 3: Thesaurus Tree – here you will see subject headings or descriptors related to the word ('constipation') you selected. This gives you an opportunity to broaden your search or narrow it down to more specific subjects if need be.

Explode offers you the chance to get all citations on 'constipation' and any narrower subjects associated with the main subject.

Major descriptors means that you will get citations where constipation is *one* of the major subjects, and if you do not tick this box you will also get citations where constipation is a minor subject in the article.

Subheadings relate to specific aspects of a subject that will help you to focus on your subject, such as diagnosis or aetiology. When you want to do a focused search, simply tick the box in the subheadings column next to 'constipation' to view what subheadings are available, make your choice and click to continue. This will return you to the opening screen and the result of your search.

For our example, because we are interested in the management of constipation, we want citations where constipation is the major subject, so tick the major descriptor box for 'constipation' and click on *SEARCH* which will take you back to the opening screen and you will see the result of your search.

- Step 4: Repeating the steps – the next step is to repeat the process, this time using the term *laxative*. Because the search is about the use of laxatives for the management of constipation, this time a subheading needs to be used, so tick the *drug therapy* subheading.

When you have completed these steps, you will have a set of results.

- Step 5: Combining – the results will be presented for each subject separately, which is not very useful for our review. So the next step is to combine the searches to give the citations applicable to our search question.

To combine the results of these searches, simply type the numbers that refer to the different search terms, i.e. constipation and laxative. At this time, you can also un-tick the box for Thesaurus mapping and then click.

- Step 6: Refining your search – if you recall, the search question was about 'the use of laxatives in the management of constipation in elderly patients'. So far, the retrieved citations are only about constipation and laxatives and not related to elderly patients. This can be done by using *special search terms*, which you can find in the section below your search results. To select *elderly patients*, click on *AGE GROUPS* and a pop-up box appears. Select the age groups that apply – here you have to decide the age ranges for the search, that is, whether to include the 'middle age' group in order to capture those between 60 and 64 years. Once you have selected the age groups, click on *SEARCH* to add these to your search list.

At this stage, you may also wish to set limits to the years of publication and limit your search to English-language publications. To limit your search to English, just click the box and set the limits for year of publication. Follow the same procedure that you used to select the age groups once you have decided how far back you wish to go for your review, for example 2006–2016.

These will all appear as additional lines on your search results. To complete the search, combine the lines as before to give you a final search result for English-language publications between 2006 and 2016 on 'the use of laxatives in the management of constipation in elderly patients'. The number of citations is shown in the results list, and you have finished your initial search!

Exercise

Try doing the above search for yourself.

Clicking on 'show titles' in the final line of your search will show you a list of citations, and you can start to decide which articles are really relevant to your research topic.

You can at this stage save the whole list of citations by clicking on *SAVE ALL*. When you are at this initial stage of your search, it is always a good idea to save the complete list as a reference – you may never need to refer back to this list, but it will avoid having to repeat the same search at a later stage.

Alternatively, you could review the full list and highlight those citations that appear to be relevant by ticking the box next to them on the left-hand side. To display the citations you highlighted once you have finished reviewing the complete list, scroll down to the bottom of the page, choose your display format ('medium' is the default setting) and click on the *DISPLAY* button. This will allow you to review your choices and to save in a variety of formats. Using the FULL display format will give you the abstract and references (and, if available, access to a full-text copy of the article). Using the box at the bottom of your screen gives you a variety of options for saving your search with or without your search strategy.

Revising the search, as necessary, and replicating it in other sources

You can save your search as you go along or alternatively you can email your results by clicking on the email button and following the instructions given, making sure that you select the delivery format (same as the display format) and output format *before* you click on *DELIVER*! Note:

- When you access CINAHL (or any of the other databases) via the National Evidence website, details of where you can retrieve the abstract (usually online) or article are included.
- There are more detailed guides available for each of the databases when you go online.

By now you should have a list of citations that appear relevant to your topic, that is, a list of titles. The next stage of the process is to review the abstracts of these articles against your inclusion and exclusion criteria to check that they really do relate to the topic you are researching, and then obtain copies of these articles. This is the main way of ensuring that you retrieve only those articles pertinent to your topic and hence your literature review. This process should narrow down the number of articles that you need to appraise in order for your literature review to be comprehensive.

However, for your search to be as comprehensive as possible you need to search more than one database, using the same search strategy for each database. This may yield some of the same information but it also ensures that you are less likely to miss an article that is relevant to your research topic.

Too many or too few results from a search

What you actually get from your search in numbers of citations and relevant articles is dependent on you having chosen appropriate search terms and on whether there is published literature that is relevant to your question.

Too many results are not uncommon when you first start searching, and this is often because you are afraid of missing something. However, getting too many results can be overwhelming, so you need to set some limits in order to make the information you retrieve more manageable. As indicated earlier, you can do this by setting publication date limits, using the thesaurus and combing searches using Boolean operators. If there are still too many results, you may want to consider selecting publications that review only higher-quality research studies.

Obtaining *too few results* is very frustrating, and there can be a number of reasons for this. The first step is to ask a specialist librarian or a tutor for advice. However, it may be that there is very little published literature relating to your topic. If this is what you suspect, then it is worth checking to see if you can find out about 'research in progress' that may be relevant. This may influence whether you start your own research and may guide you to potential collaborators and/or advisers.

Two useful databases that you can search for details of ongoing research are:

- *The National Research Register (NRR)*: this holds details of all research projects approved by the NHS and includes records of ongoing and recently completed projects (see www.nihr.ac.uk/Pages/NRRArchive.aspx).
- *The Health Technology Assessment (HTA) programme*: the HTA is a national pro-gramme of research funded by the Department of Health R&D unit. It makes available to all NHS staff high-quality research evidence about the effectiveness and cost-effectiveness of all types of healthcare interventions (details of reports in progress are included at www.ncchta.org).

Also, some older published research may not yet have been entered onto electronic databases, and you will only find this by trawling through the journal stacks in a bio-medical library. It is also worthwhile reviewing the references in any of the articles you have retrieved. This may reveal additional articles/research studies on the topic which have not been identified by your electronic search.

Alternatively, it may be that your search terms are inappropriate or that you have set limits that are too strict for your search. You should consider revising these and then redoing your search.

Getting unexpectedly few results can be worse than getting no results at all. It may appear satisfactory, but have you really done a *good* search? Once you are happy that you have done a good search, you need to review the abstracts and decide which articles you wish to retrieve in full so that you can start the next stage in the literature review process. This is considered in the next chapter.

Additional searches

It should be remembered that electronic database searching is never 100 per cent efficient and it is always useful to supplement your search with other methods, for example, by reading through the reference lists of journal articles and the content pages of journals. You can also arrange for papers that are potentially relevant to you to be sent to you using RSS feeds (Rich Site Summary) from many journals and databases. RSS feeds are automated links that you can set up from blogs, news websites and journals which can alert you to newly published articles and other information on your literature review topic.

CHAPTER SUMMARY

- A literature review helps to provide background information for a research topic and assists the development of an actual research project.
- A literature review can be divided into two sections:
  - looking for literature that is appropriate to a specific topic
  - a balanced review of differing viewpoints or findings.
- The purpose of a literature review is to find the resources most relevant to the topic.
- Having a clear idea of what you are looking for before you start searching is cost-effective in terms of time and effort.
- You need to devise a search strategy that accurately reflects your research topic/question before you start searching the databases.
- Searching electronically can increase the speed and convenience of literature searching.
- Primary sources of evidence come from researchers who carried out the original work on the topic.
- Secondary sources consist of summarisation of or commentary about primary data and refer to the original research.
- There is a range of different sources that can provide access to relevant articles.
- Always search the literature in a systematic way and keep a record of the searches you have conducted.
- The abstracts of articles identified by a search need to be reviewed to ensure that only articles pertinent to the topic are retrieved.
- Searching for articles is only one stage of the literature reviewing process.

SUGGESTED FURTHER READING

Aveyard, H., Payne, S. and Preston, N. (2016) *A Postgraduate's Guide to Doing a Literature Review*. Maidenhead: Open University Press. This book provides a detailed guide to searching in the context of doing a literature review.

Battany-Saltikov, J. (2012) *How to do a Systematic Review in Nursing: A Step-by-Step Guide*. Milton Keynes: RCN Publishing and Open University Press. This book provides a step-by-step guide to searching in relation to doing a literature review. It is presented in a straightforward way and is readily accessible.

Ridley, D. (2012) *The Literature Review: A Step-by-Step Guide for Students*, 2nd edn. London: Sage. This step-by-step guide provides a comprehensive overview to conducting a literature search and review. The budding researcher who lacks literature review skills should find it useful.

WEBSITES

Health Technology Assessment (HTA) programme: www.ncchta.org

National Library for Health: www.evidence.nhs.uk

National Research Register: http://webarchive.nationalarchives.gov.uk/+/www.dh.gov.uk/en/Aboutus/Researchanddevelopment/AtoZ/DH_4002357

 To access further resources related to this chapter, visit the companion website at https://study.sagepub.com/mouleaveyard3e

REFERENCES

Aveyard, H. (2014) *Doing a Literature Review in Health and Social Care*. Maidenhead: Open University Press.

Aveyard, H., Sharp, P. and Woolliams, M (2015) *A Beginner's Guide to Critical Thinking and Writing*. Maidenhead: Open University Press.

Aveyard, H., Payne, S. and Preston, N.J. (2016) *A Post-graduate's Guide to Doing a Literature Review in Health and Social Care*. Maidenhead: Open University Press.

Powers, B. and Knapp, T. (2010) *A Dictionary of Nursing Theory and Research*, 4th edn. London: Sage.

5
CRITICAL
APPRAISAL

Learning outcomes

This chapter will enable you to:

- recognise what is involved in reading analytically
- identify the findings of a research study that will be relevant to a specific topic of enquiry
- recognise the different questions that need to be asked when critically appraising qualitative and quantitative research and literature reviews
- appreciate researchers' interpretations of the data presented in published reports
- understand the role of critical analysis in research and evidence-based practice
- carry out a critical appraisal of a peer-reviewed paper

Reviewing research that has already been conducted is an important skill for all professionals. This is because it is vital not to take the results of the research at face value but to consider the methods used and the applicability of the findings to your own practice. The effect of the small case series which triggered the debate about the MMR vaccination is a clear example of this (Aveyard, 2014). Every time you use a piece of research as an assignment or professional practice, you are advised to assess the research through a process of critical analysis and evaluation, so that you can consider the strengths and weaknesses of the study. This is known as critical appraisal.

When research is reviewed formally as part of a literature review, critical appraisal is also part of the research process. The first step of this process – searching for the literature or assembling the evidence – was discussed in Chapter 4. The next stages in the preparation of a literature review are to start to draw some conclusions about the body of research that has been reported and make judgements about the quality of that original research.

Critical appraisal of the evidence, or analytical evaluation of the research relating to a topic, is the process of carefully and systematically examining research to judge its trustworthiness, value and relevance in a particular context (Burls, 2009). This involves examining the methods used in research and the way in which the data has been analysed and conclusions drawn. Critical appraisal requires a careful reading of the paper followed by the asking of directed questions about the paper. This chapter describes what reading analytically entails and offers guidance on how to critically appraise or evaluate different types of research study.

WHY IS A CRITICAL APPRAISAL NEEDED?

Critical appraisal is a structured process of identifying and evaluating the merits and/ or value of research. No research study will be perfect; therefore, all research may be critically evaluated. However, the critical approach must be thoughtful and thorough. It is important to be realistic about our ability to evaluate research, and recognise that research is ongoing and cumulative in the sense that it can always be improved, refined and expanded on. By being critical of the research of others, we can learn to discriminate between 'good' and 'bad' research. This will also help the development of our own ideas about what and how we research. Being critical involves making decisions about the merit or value of a piece of research, and by applying 'careful judgement', both the good and bad points of the research can be considered or appraised.

There are a number of reasons why a critical appraisal of published research is necessary:

- Researchers may make unjustified claims about what can be done or changed on the basis of their findings. There may be alternative ways of interpreting the results of a study that may not have been considered by the researcher(s).
- The process of peer review of published papers acts as a procedure of quality control in many academic journals. This may be a very rigorous process, with papers being scrutinised by independent reviewers as well as the editorial team. Independent reviewers will usually be specialists in the subject area and, when appropriate, include statisticians. However, the peer-review process is not infallible and readers/researchers should be able to make their own judgements about the quality of research. Just because a paper has been published does not guarantee that the findings are 'correct'; mistakes can be made and there will always be a risk of researcher bias. Bias in this context refers to a tendency to misrepresent (intentionally or unintentionally) any influence or action in a study that might distort the results of a research study.
- Most experienced researchers will be aware of the limitations of their research and hence will discuss these when they publish reports. This awareness should enable them to demonstrate their own critical appraisal skills by using them to refine their understanding of the research question or methods or potential practical application of their research.
- Appraising how other researchers have approached a topic should help your own thinking about it and what may be appropriate methods of investigation.

- Research is of little value unless it somehow influences practice. This means that nurses need to be able to evaluate effectively in order to determine whether findings should be implemented. There should also be dialogue between practitioners and researchers so that practice changes happen in response to available evidence, rather than simply because it seems like a good idea and/or is fashionable.

Critical appraisal is an evaluation of the strengths and limitations of the research report being reviewed. It should reflect an objective, balanced and thoughtful consideration of the validity and significance of the research in question. Critical appraisal is not a denigration of the study or the ability of the researcher(s), and the focus should be on the study itself rather than on the individual(s) who carried out the research and published the findings. Any implications arising from the identification of strengths and limitations should be discussed with reference to research literature. The first step of critical appraisal is to read the research analytically.

WHAT IS READING ANALYTICALLY?

Reading analytically is an active process concerned with learning to think, and hence read; that means using mental processes such as attention, categorisation, selection and judgement (Cottrell, 2011). This type of reading is often seen as moving from the general to the particular by skim-reading first and then re-reading to build up more understanding of what is being reported. It is a very different technique from reading a novel or a textbook where the aim, for the latter, is the acquisition of knowledge and learning. Reading analytically has the purpose of producing an evaluation of the research on a topic. A researcher should expect to be regularly reading and reviewing the literature throughout any research project. This will not only increase understanding of the topic, but will also help the researcher to develop and maintain analytical reading skills.

The focus for analytical reading is being able to identify the arguments presented, and good analytical reading is associated with an ability to recognise good or well-presented arguments (even if you disagree with them) and poor arguments (even if they support your own perspective). Effectively, to read analytically a sceptical approach has to be taken, that is, one that politely doubts the perspective being reported. This will include recognising that a research report does not give the full picture of the study and should prompt you to highlight the elements of a study that are concerning or problematic, as well as those aspects that have been done well. What the analytical reader, and critical appraiser, wants is evidence that the research is substantive and that methodological decisions are appropriate (Polit and Beck, 2014).

Deciding on an appropriate search strategy was discussed in Chapter 4, but it is still likely to give what may be a daunting number of articles/texts to read. However, in order to produce a proper review it is necessary to evaluate each research paper separately. What a reviewer has to do is develop a way of being selective so that it is possible to get the essence or general idea of the arguments and be able to pull out the main points quickly. Maslin-Prothero (2010) suggests that there are three different levels of reading – scanning, in-depth reading and inferring:

- *Scanning/skimming* is used to help decide whether an article is relevant to the specific topic being investigated. This can also serve to identify which sections of a text or article require more careful reading and can be done as part of searching the literature. By scanning you should also be able to reduce the amount of reading you have to do. But do be careful not to reject an article, or section of it, without good reason or you will be at risk of missing important aspects of the topic being investigated.
- *In-depth reading/re-reading* and *inferring* are necessary to achieve understanding and consideration of possible application of the literature to the 'real world', that is, clinical practice. Again, there is a need to be selective. Your concentration should be on the sections that take an argument forward or summarise.

Being selective about what is read, that is, not reading a whole article or chapter in a book, is not taking a short-cut. As a researcher and reviewer, you still need to gain enough understanding about your topic and related research to be able to criticise and summarise intelligently. This means being able to give a broad picture as well as focusing on those parts of the research literature that are of particular significance.

The reasoning or arguments presented in any research report, including the adoption of a research design, interpretation of data and recommendations, should lead towards the end point or conclusion. There is a need, however, to consider what the argument is predicated on, or what the underlying point of view is, and how this may impact on the conclusions reached. It is possible for the basis of an argument to be true or false, and a reader needs to be able to determine whether the arguments or reasoning actually support the conclusions. Flaws in reasoning can arise in a number of ways – for example, misinterpretation of results by using an inappropriate statistical test or assuming that one thing must be the cause of another when not all of the relevant variables have been considered (an inappropriate linking of cause and effect). Researchers may not always recognise their own flaws or that their arguments are predicated on erroneous or out-of-date assumptions – for example, 'the research was predicated on the assumption that all registered midwives are also registered nurses'.

The aim of analytical reading is to understand all the elements in a research paper; the methods, results and conclusions and to make a judgement about the extent to which the conclusions drawn are logical.

SYNTHESIS

Being able to recognise arguments is central to any **critical analysis**. Integral to this is the unpacking of the constituent parts of what the author(s) has presented in order to be able to infer or determine the relationship between them. **Synthesis** is about putting all your data together or combining it in order to identify the relationships between the different elements. A research report attempts to convince others of the **reliability**, **validity**, **trustworthiness** or **rigour** (depending on the methodology used) of a study, and critical analysis draws on the reader's knowledge and experiences to integrate these with other types of evidence to determine whether the arguments are convincing. Synthesis means being able to assess the arguments set out in the text, give reasons for beliefs and actions, analyse and evaluate one's own and other people's reasoning and devise and construct better reasoning.

This process of synthesis can be achieved by using the following technique as you read in depth after scanning:

1. Highlight any inference indicators (keywords to look for are: thus, therefore, so, hence, should).
2. Look for and underline any conclusions that follow on from these inference indicators.
3. Place in brackets any stated reasons for these (keywords to look for are: because, for, since).
4. Attempt to summarise the author's arguments at this stage. If there is no clear argument, ask what point(s) the author(s) is trying to make and why.
5. Look at the conclusions again – remember there may be interim as well as final conclusions. Typical indications of a conclusion are the use of the following words: therefore, thus, hence, consequently, and so on. Take care not to confuse a summary provided by the author of their argument so far with a conclusion.
6. Taking the main conclusion, ask what reasons are presented in the text for believing this conclusion or why you are being asked to accept this conclusion. Typical indications of reasons are words and phrases such as: because, since, it follows, and so on.
7. The reasons provided for the argument can be ranked into a **structure**. Go through each reason (R) and ask whether it is essential or secondary backing for the argument. From this you will be left with the core reasons for the argument. You should then be able to construct an argument diagram with the following structures:

    i.   R1 + R2 = (therefore) conclusion [for joint reasons]
    ii.   R1 or R2 = (therefore) conclusion [for independent reasons]. Variations on these structures are common. For example, a main conclusion may be supported by an interim conclusion and several basic reasons. This would give an equation something like this:
    iii. R1 + R2 = (therefore) interim conclusion
    iv.   R1 or R2 = (therefore) main conclusion. (Adapted from Hart, 1998)

This stage is analysis rather than evaluation but should, with practice, enable you, as a reviewer, to extract the details of any argument. At this stage, you do not need to consider whether the reasons are sound.

> **Reflective exercise**
>
> Read a research article that interests you and identify the inference indicators, conclusions and reasoning for the conclusions as outlined above. Then ask a colleague or tutor to check whether they agree with your analysis.

READING RETRIEVED ARTICLES

Alongside identification of the arguments being presented, there is also a need to ask questions about the research and its context. These questions should be systematically asked of each article being reviewed as you read.

Exactly how and what questions should be asked is down to personal choice. However, before starting to read and ask questions about the paper, you as a reviewer need to consider whether you have sufficient grasp of the research paper to be able to evaluate the study. Unfamiliarity with specific research methods is acceptable, but a basic understanding of research methodology is necessary in order to be able to identify the good and bad points used in a particular study. It is also important to have an understanding of the terms used in the report. Background reading prior to starting a literature review on a topic will help to develop a broader understanding and enhance your ability to evaluate a paper. When reading a research report, it is essential to ensure familiarity with the terms being used, otherwise there is a real risk of gaining only a superficial understanding of the study, which gives an inadequate basis for evaluation.

CRITICAL APPRAISAL TOOLS

There are numerous guides or tools available to help reviewers to **critique** research studies and these generally provide a set of critiquing questions that can be used to help evaluate published reports. These are often referred to as **critical appraisal tools**. There are many critical appraisal tools in the research literature, available in textbooks, journals and online. There are some tools that are generalisable to all research reports; others are specific to a type of research design. Questions focus on the different elements of the research process and usually follow the structure of research reports:

- title
- abstract
- literature review
- method
- results
- discussion and interpretation
- recommendations.

The questions will often be worded in a way that prompts a simple 'yes' or 'no' answer. The expectation is that a 'yes' response demonstrates a strength and a 'no' is indicative of a limitation. Ideally, the answer in all cases will be 'yes', and a study that has a large number of 'yeses' is likely to be stronger than or superior to one that has only a few 'yeses' (Polit and Beck, 2014).

Table 5.1 provides an example of a generic critical appraisal tool that can be used to critique any type of research study.

Table 5.1 Generic questions to ask about each section of a research paper

Section	Questions
1 Title	• Does the title provide a clear and unambiguous statement of the topic under investigation? • Is it concise and informative? • Is the type of approach used in the title, e.g. a comparative study of; an ethnographic approach to; a double-blind cross-over; a pilot study?
2 Author/researcher	• Does the author have the appropriate background to enable him or her to conduct the study successfully? • Look for qualifications, role/specialty and place of employment associated with good research. • Multiple authors may indicate a need for specialist expertise or team led by an experienced researcher who may have attracted funding. • An awareness of the researcher's background should improve understanding of the approach used and any assumptions that have been made but not necessarily stated in the report. For example, researchers with a clinical background are likely to have a different approach from that of researchers from an academic background investigating a ward-based problem.
3 Abstract	• Does this provide a clear summary of the research, i.e. problem being researched, methodology, significant results and conclusions? • This section is very helpful in confirming the relevance of the articles found by your search.
4 Introduction	• Clearly identified problem? If the research problem is not clearly set out, it will be difficult to interpret any findings. It is helpful if the actual research question is stated, but it does not always appear. Often, the aims and objectives of the study are given and sometimes these do not really explain what question the researchers were trying to answer. • Is the problem researchable or have the researchers been unrealistic in their expectations of the outcomes from the study? For example, 'Does preparation of the ward prior to meals being served improve patient nutrition?' is a very interesting topic which could yield much useful data. However, it is very broad and inevitably there will be many factors other than ward environment that impact on patients' nutritional status. This would not be a realistic research question for a single study. • Rationale for choice of topic described? • Rationale for methodology described? • Depending on the approach, research aims and objectives or the hypothesis/null hypothesis stated, is this consistent with the topic under investigation?

(Continued)

Table 5.1 (Continued)

Section	Questions
5 Literature review	Not all research papers will have a literature review section/heading. Sometimes the review is included in the introduction or background. Whatever it is called, it should come before any detailed information about how the research was conducted and the results section. Specific questions to ask about the review include: ● Does this indicate the author's familiarity with the topic under investigation? ● Is it pertinent to the research topic? ● Does it cover all the important aspects about the topic or have key references been omitted or ignored? ● Does the review inform the theoretical origins as well as previous articles on the topic? ● Are the references up to date? ● Is it easy to follow or is there a lack of structure, making it difficult to understand the arguments? ● Is there a summary of the key points that highlight the gaps the research aimed to fill?
6 Methodology/ design/methods	● Methodology = approach taken, e.g. action research: is the approach clearly stated with an identifiable underpinning theory? ● Research methods = the tools by which data is collected, e.g. pre- and post-intervention questionnaires, focus group interviews: are these described clearly? ● Design = how the whole study hangs together: is it justifiable and is there a logical description of what the researcher planned to do and how it was actually done? ● Is sufficient detail given to make it possible to repeat the study? ● Are technical terms used, and if so are they defined or is it assumed that the reader will understand them? Some level of expertise has to be assumed, but authors should explain any very specialist terms or when there could be more than one interpretation of a term.
7 Sample selection	● Who or what makes up the study population, and are they appropriate? ● Are the participants clearly defined? For example, if elderly people or children participated, are the age ranges explained and justified? ● Are the inclusion and exclusion criteria stated and justified? ● How was the sample selected, e.g. self-selection, convenience sample, randomly? ● Does the author justify the selection? ● Is the sample size explained and was the sample size appropriate? A comprehensive understanding of statistics is not required for this but rather an understanding of how sample sizes can be calculated and the sort of numbers of participants you would expect to see in different types of studies. (These issues are discussed in Chapter 12 of this book.) ● Qualitative studies can use quite small samples, whereas quantitative studies usually require larger samples, and statistical advice may be needed for the results to be statistically significant.

Section	Questions
8 Data collection	<ul><li>Is the way the data were collected described and discussed in enough detail? This should include justification for the choice of how data were collected which is robust enough to stand up to criticism. For example, if reminders were not sent to participants who failed to return questionnaires, were the reasons for this non-action explained?</li><li>Are the advantages and disadvantages of the method(s) discussed?</li><li>Are details given about the instruments or tools used, e.g. questionnaires, interview schedules and measurement scales? These details do not have to be comprehensive or necessarily include copies of the actual questionnaires. There should be just sufficient detail for the reader to understand the type of data being sought. For example:</li></ul> *The questionnaire comprised two parts. To evaluate the patients' constipation status, a constipation visual analogue scale (CVAS) was constructed. This was an 8-point scale, where a score of 0–1 indicates no constipation, 2–4 indicates constipation and 5–7 indicates severe constipation … For the management of patients' constipation, four further questions were asked to determine the advice provided, satisfaction with treatment, explanation of need for laxatives and patient preferences for laxatives.* *Patients' use of medication, specifically laxatives, opioids and other constipating medication, was collected from the patient records. (Goodman et al., 2005: 239)* <ul><li>This section should also include some reference to the reliability and validity of results for quantitative studies and plausibility and trustworthiness of findings for qualitative studies.</li><li>If justification of the research methods was not given in the methodology section, then it should be covered here, with reason(s) for choice of method(s) stated.</li></ul>
9 Ethics	<ul><li>Is there evidence of approval from the appropriate ethics committee?</li><li>Are any ethical issues around the conduct of the research discussed? For example, if the research involved vulnerable groups, how were they protected?</li><li>Are the methods of participants' consent and how confidentiality was protected explained?</li></ul>
10 Results/findings	<ul><li>Were the methods of data analysis appropriate for the research methods?</li><li>Is some raw data presented as well as the findings?</li><li>Are the results presented in a clear, concise, precise and logical manner?</li><li>Are the results sufficiently complete and detailed to answer the questions posed?</li></ul>

(Continued)

Table 5.1   (Continued)

Section	Questions
11 Discussion	• Are all the results discussed in relation to the original question/hypothesis? • Is it balanced and objective? • Does it draw on previous research findings and/or the literature review to explain, compare and contrast other results obtained? • Are any weaknesses and limitations in the study identified and, if possible, suggestions made as to how they might be overcome in the future?
12 Conclusions	• Do the results and discussion support these? • Are they confined to the original purpose of the study?
13 Recommendations	• Are these practical, accurate and appropriate?
14 References	• Are they complete and searchable?
15 Appendices	• Are they arranged in either a numerical or alphabetical order? • Are they clearly marked and appropriate?

A wide selection – but by no means exhaustive – of critical appraisal tools is currently available at The University of South Australia website at www.unisa.edu.au/Research/Sansom-Institute-for-Health-Research/Research/Allied-Health-Evidence/Resources/CAT/. It is important to remember that not all appraisal tools have been rigorously evaluated (Crowe and Sheppard, 2011); however they can be a useful aide to trigger critical thinking about a paper (Aveyard et al., 2015). The questions are posed to stimulate a reviewer into considering the implications of what the researcher has done. The critique will identify more than the strengths or limitations of the study. Relevant issues will have to be discussed – for example, if you answered 'no' to the question about whether participants were fully informed about the nature of the research, you should consider (and then discuss in the actual review) what impact this may have had on recruitment and results obtained.

QUANTITATIVE RESEARCH CRITIQUE QUESTIONS

Table 5.2 presents guidelines for use when appraising **quantitative research** reports. The questions suggested are basic and broadly applicable to quantitative research and so not all of them will be relevant to each study being reviewed. Some of the questions will not permit wholly objective responses – for example, there may be disagreement about the best research design for a study or which statistical test is most appropriate. This requires a reviewer to express an opinion which should be based on sound principles gained from an understanding of research and reading about research. An effective appraisal involves asking questions about all aspects of a published report.

Table 5.2   General guidelines for critiquing a quantitative research study

Element of the report	Questions
Global issues	
Writing style	• Was the report well written – grammatically correct, jargon use avoided and well organised?
	• Was the report written in a way that enables you or a practising nurse to understand the study and its findings?
Author(s)	• Was there sufficient detail to enable critical appraisal?
	• Do the researcher(s') qualifications/position indicate a degree of knowledge/experience in this particular field?
Title	• Was the title clear, accurate, unambiguous and did it indicate the research question?
Abstract	• Does the abstract give a clear overview of the study and summarise the main features of the findings and recommendations?
Introduction	
Purpose/research problem	• Was the purpose of the study/research problem clearly stated?
	• Was a quantitative approach an appropriate way of answering the problem?
Logical consistency	• Does the research report follow the steps of the research process in a logical manner?
Literature review	• Does the review give a balanced critical appraisal of the literature?
	• Was the literature up to date, original and mainly from primary sources and of an empirical nature?
Theoretical framework	• Does the literature review identify a firm foundation for the new study?
Research question or hypothesis	• Was the research question or hypothesis clearly stated? If not, is the absence justified?
Objectives	• Does the question reflect the information presented in the literature review and conceptual framework?
	• Are the objectives clearly stated?
Method	
Research design	• Was the design clearly identified and sufficiently rigorous, given the study purpose?
	• Were appropriate comparisons made to enhance the interpretability of the findings?
	• Were any threats to the internal and external validity minimised by the choice of design?
	• Does the design offer the most accurate, unbiased, interpretable and replicable evidence possible?
Population and sample	• Was the target population clearly identified?
	• Were there major differences between the target and accessible population?
	• How was the sample selected, and was it representative?
	• Were the inclusion/exclusion criteria clearly identified? Does the sample reflect these?
	• Was a sampling frame employed?

(Continued)

Table 5.2   (Continued)

Element of the report	Questions
	• Are there any concerns about the integrity of the sampling frame? • How was the sample size determined, and was it appropriate for the study? • What sample size was achieved? Did it achieve the numbers recommended by a power calculation? • How was the sample selected? • Was the method of sampling appropriate to the design? • Were there any biases in the method of selection and were these acknowledged? • Were there any limits of generalisation of the findings from the sample to the population?
Ethical considerations	• Were the participants fully informed about the nature of the research? • Was the autonomy/confidentiality of the participants guaranteed? • Was ethical approval given for the study?
Data collection and measurement	• Were the data collection strategies described? • Were the methods of data collection appropriate? • Were sufficient data gathered? • Were the data collection and recording procedures adequately described? • Did the researcher describe and discuss how rigour was assured? • Were data collected by appropriately trained staff in a way that minimised bias?
Data analysis/results	• Did the researcher follow the steps of the data analysis method described? • Were the strategies of data analysis described and compatible with the type of quantitative research utilised? • Were the findings presented appropriately? • Did the analysis provide insight into the phenomenon being investigated?
Discussion	• Were all major findings interpreted and discussed? • Were the findings linked back to the literature review and the study's conceptual framework? • Was the original purpose of the study adequately addressed? • Were the interpretations made within the limitations of the study?
Recommendations and implications	• Was a recommendation for further research made? • Were any implications for clinical practice discussed?
References	• Were all the books, journals and other media referred to in the study accurately referenced?

Global issues

Writing style

Research reports should be well written, that is, well organised, grammatically correct, concise and the use of jargon avoided where possible. Remember, though, that authors will often be restricted by word limits in any published report and expected to conform to the style of the journal publishing the report. This should not, however, result in a lack of information that makes comprehension of the report difficult. A report's style should encourage the reader to read the whole report (Polit and Beck, 2014).

Author(s)

You should judge each research report on its own merits and not assume validity and reliability on the basis of the author(s') qualifications and experience. However, the author(s') qualifications and job title(s) can give an indication of the researcher(s') knowledge and expertise in the topic being investigated.

Title

The title should unambiguously suggest the research problem/purpose of the study and its population. Titles can be confusing and make it difficult to recognise relevant research (Aveyard, 2014).

Abstract

The abstract should provide a concise overview of the research and a summary of the main findings, conclusions and recommendations. Ideally, the abstract will also include brief details of the study, method, sample size and selection, though this may not always be possible because of imposed word limits. The aim of any abstract is to provide the reader with sufficient information to be able to determine if the study is pertinent to their topic of enquiry and whether or not to continue reading. The abstract will give you a summary of the content of the article, in particular stating whether or not it is a research article (Aveyard et al., 2015). Abstracts are very important because they are usually the main section of a report that is read to determine whether the research is in fact relevant for a specific review.

Introduction

Purpose/research problem

The research problem, or purpose of the study, is frequently presented as part of the introduction of a research report. It should give a broad indication of what has been studied/investigated (Polit and Beck, 2014). Remember that broad problems often have many aspects that will need to become more focused before they can be researched.

Logical consistency

The reporting of a research study should follow the steps in the research process itself, and if this is done then a logical progression will be presented. This means that a reader will see clear links between the purpose of the study and what follows through all other sections of the report.

It is essential when reporting results to ensure that anyone reading the report understands the terms and concepts used for the research. To ensure this understanding, any concepts or terms referred to should be clearly defined in an introduction or background section (Aveyard, 2014).

Literature review

As described in the previous chapter, the aim of the literature review in a research report is to identify any gaps in the literature relating to the problem and to suggest how the study attempts to fill or partially fill those gaps. It should also assist in further defining the research question and can be very useful in explaining how a broad problem has evolved into the study that is being reported. The literature review should demonstrate an appropriate depth and breadth of reading around the topic being studied and assist in confirming the appropriateness of the study methodology.

Any studies included should be up to date, generally not more than 10 years old. Exceptions can be acceptable for topics where there is a paucity of research, or where there is a seminal or very significant study that remains relevant to current practice. Reference to some historical as well as contemporary literature is expected, as this will give a context to the topic. The majority of the literature in the review should usually be empirical data from the original source rather than from a secondary source or anecdotal evidence.

A good review will identify the keywords and details of databases used to conduct the search, with the themes that emerged from the literature then being presented and discussed (Aveyard, 2014). The data from previous research should be presented to demonstrate that it has been reviewed critically. The strengths and limitations of the studies should be highlighted, and the findings of the different studies also compared and contrasted (Aveyard, 2014).

Theoretical framework

Theoretical frameworks are a concept that both novice and experienced researchers find confusing. In many quantitative research studies, the research problem is not linked to a specific theory or concept (Polit and Beck, 2014). This means that a reviewer has to first determine whether the study actually has a theoretical or conceptual framework. If there is no framework, consideration of the level of contribution to knowledge by the study has to be made. Nursing can be criticised for its lack of theoretical foundations. However, it has to be acknowledged that much of the research is so pragmatic that the adoption of a theory will not enhance its usefulness (Polit and Beck, 2014). If a theoretical framework is presented, then it should be clearly identified and explained to the reader.

Research question or hypothesis and objectives

The research question and/or the research hypothesis should link with the initially stated purpose of the study or research problem. There might also be aims and objectives.

The aim of the study will relate to the research question and the objectives will explain in more detail what the study is expected to achieve.

The use of research questions, hypotheses and objectives is dependent on the type of research being reported. Some descriptive studies may not identify any of these items but simply refer to the purpose of the study or the research problem; others will include either aims and objectives or research questions and studies of relationships that exist between two or more variables, and will use either a research question or hypothesis. A hypothesis and a null hypothesis, identifying the variables to be manipulated, should be clearly stated in reports of experimental and quasi-experimental studies.

Method

Research design

The most important consideration for evaluating a research design is whether the design enables the research question to be answered (Polit and Beck, 2014). Essentially, this means asking whether the design selected matches the aims of the research. You would not expect an experimental design to be used when the purpose of the study is to explore or describe a phenomenon. Similarly, when a study is aimed at identifying the extent or range of a problem, a non-structured or flexible design would raise the possibility of bias and lack of rigour. The main questions to ask relate to whether the design offers the most accurate, unbiased, interpretable and replicable evidence possible (see Chapter 11).

Population and sample

A decisive factor in determining the adequacy of a quantitative research study is the degree to which a sample represents the population it was drawn from (Polit and Beck, 2014). Critiquing questions are aimed at identifying how generalisable the findings are likely to be. This means that a reviewer needs to be able to clearly identify the target population and how the sample was selected. The size of the sample is also important, as small samples give rise to the possibility of over-representation of small subgroups within the target population. For example, if, in a sample of registered nurses, 40 per cent of the respondents were males, then males would appear to be over-represented in the sample, thereby creating a sampling error. In addition, the report should clearly identify what criteria were used to include or exclude participants, how the sample was selected and how many were invited to participate (see Chapter 12).

Ethical considerations

Any research involving human beings should be conducted ethically, and in health-care where research participants may be particularly vulnerable there is even more of an imperative for ethical conduct in research (for a full discussion of **research ethics**, please see the National Research Ethics Service website). The onus when critiquing a research report is on confirming that ethical principles have been applied. Essentially, the reviewer needs to ask whether participants were told what the research entailed, how their anonymity and confidentiality were protected and what arrangements were in place to avoid preventable harms.

Health and social care research has to be approved by an ethics committee and the institution where the research is to be conducted before research can be undertaken. Any research report requiring ethical approval should state that this was given, and ideally which committee gave the approval (see Chapters 7 and 8).

Data collection and measurement

There are a number of strategies that can be adopted when collecting data in a quantitative study. In order to be able to assess whether data collection was appropriate, sufficient detail has to be included in a report to enable judgements. Additionally, there should be an indication of how any data collection **instrument** was designed. Researchers usually have the choice of using an existing instrument or developing one specific to their study. It should be clearly stated whether a study-specific or an 'off-the-shelf' data collection instrument has been used. In either case, it is essential that the data collected actually will elicit accurate information to help achieve the goals of the research, and that this is demonstrated in the report. It should, however, be remembered that existing instruments are often in the form of standardised tests or scales that have been developed for a purpose other than that of the study being reported. This requires the researcher to provide appropriate evidence in relation to the validity and reliability of the instrument (Polit and Beck, 2014) and its appropriateness for the current study. Validity is described as the ability of the instrument to measure what it is supposed to measure, and reliability refers to the level of consistency of values measured under specified conditions (see Chapter 13). It is important to recognise that if an instrument has been modified or used with a different population, then previous validity and reliability will not be applicable, and details of how the reliability and validity of the adapted instrument were established should be explained (Polit and Beck, 2014). This may mean that details of a **pilot study** are included to clarify the validity and reliability of the chosen instrument. Any adjustment made following a pilot study should be explained and justified.

The report should also include an outline, in clear logical steps, of the process by which and by whom the data was collected and details of any intervention used.

Data analysis and results

Reviewing the data analysis section of quantitative research studies is often seen as a daunting process because it is associated with an apparently complex language and the notion of statistical tests. A report should state clearly what statistical tests were undertaken, why these tests were used and the results. Some studies use only descriptive statistics. This means that they describe the results as statistical terms. Other studies such as correlational studies, quasi-experimental and experimental studies, use inferential statistics. Inferential statistics, as the name suggests, determine the extent to which the results of the study are applicable to a wider context. Statistical significance helps to identify whether a result could be due to chance rather than to real differences in the population. The convention in quantitative studies is to identify the lowest level of significance as $p<0.05$ (see Chapter 26). The percentage of the sample of study participants is important to any consideration of the generalisability of the results, and participation of at least 50 per cent of the sample is required to avoid a response bias (Polit and Beck, 2014).

The results should be presented in a way that makes it easy for readers to interpret them for themselves. The use of tables, charts and graphs is an acceptable way of summarising results. These should be accurate, clear and link into the text appropriately.

Discussion

The discussion of the findings should have a logical link with the presentation of the results and should relate to the literature review and, where appropriate, the conceptual framework in order to put the study in context. If the hypothesis appeared to have been supported by the findings, this should be developed in the discussion. All major interpretations or inferences drawn should be clearly identified and discussed. The significance of any findings, particularly generalisability, should be stated and considered within the overall strengths and limitations of the study (Polit and Beck, 2014). Questions to consider are whether the evidence in the paper supports the reasoning in the discussion and whether there are any other explanations.

Recommendations and implications

Finally, the report should indicate opportunities for relevant and meaningful further research on the topic. It is expected that the discussion section will have explored some of the clinical significance and relevance of the study. However, implications of findings and recommendations for practice should be made with caution and will obviously depend on the nature and purpose of the study.

References

The research study should conclude with an accurate list of all the books, journal articles, reports and other media that were referred to in the report (Polit and Beck, 2014).

QUALITATIVE RESEARCH CRITIQUE QUESTIONS

As with a quantitative study, critical analysis of a qualitative study involves an in-depth review of how each step of the research was undertaken. **Qualitative research** is essentially an assortment of many research designs, including phenomenology, grounded theory and ethnography. However, although the different philosophical stances of the various qualitative research methods generate discrete ways of reasoning and distinct terminology, there are many similarities within these methods. This, alongside the subjective nature of qualitative research, gives rise to an assumption that it is more difficult to critique. Table 5.3 presents guidelines for use when appraising qualitative research reports.

Table 5.3   General guidelines for critiquing a qualitative research study

Element of the report	Questions
Global issues	
Writing style	• Was the report well written – grammatically correct, jargon use avoided and well organised?
	• Was the report written in a way that enables you or a practising nurse to understand the study and its findings?
	• Was there sufficient detail to enable critical appraisal?
Author	• Do the researcher(s') qualifications/position indicate a degree of knowledge/experience in this particular field?
Title	• Was the title clear, accurate, unambiguous and did it indicate the research question?
Abstract	• Does the abstract give a clear overview of the study and summarise the main features of the findings and recommendations?
Introduction	
Statement of the problem	• Was the phenomenon to be studied clearly identified?
	• Was the phenomenon of interest?
	• Was a qualitative approach an appropriate way of answering the problem?
Literature review	• Has a literature review been undertaken?
	• Does the review give a balanced critical appraisal of the existing body of knowledge relating to the phenomenon?
	• Does the literature review identify a firm foundation for the new study?
Theoretical framework	• Has a conceptual or theoretical framework been identified?
	• Was the framework adequately described and appropriate?
Methodological and philosophical underpinnings	• Has the philosophical approach been identified?
	• Has the philosophical basis and underlying tradition been explained?
Research question	• Was there an explicitly stated question? If not, has its absence been justified?
	• Was the question consistent with the study's philosophical basis, underlying tradition and conceptual or theoretical framework?
Method	
Research design and research tradition	• Does the research tradition (if there is one) harmonise with the method of data collection and analysis?
	• Was the time in the field adequate?
	• Was there an appropriate level of contact with participants?
	• Was there evidence of reflexivity in the design?
Sample	• Were the sampling method and sample size identified?
	• Was saturation of data achieved?
	• Was the sampling method appropriate?
	• Were the population and setting adequately described and appropriate for informing the research?

Element of the report	Questions
Ethical considerations	• Were the participants fully informed about the nature of the research?
	• Was the autonomy/confidentiality of the participants guaranteed?
	• Were the participants protected from harm?
	• Was ethical approval given for the study?
Data collection	• Were the methods of data gathering adequately described and appropriate?
	• Were the questions asked, and observations made and recorded in an appropriate way?
	• Were the data gathered of sufficient depth and richness?
	• Were data collected in a way that minimised bias by appropriately trained staff?
Data analysis/results	• Was there a description of the methods used to enhance trustworthiness of data?
	• Were the data management and analysis methods adequately described?
	• Was the strategy used for analysis consistent with the research tradition and appropriate for the type of data collected?
	• Was the original purpose of the research adequately addressed?
Conclusions/ implications and recommendations	• Were the themes or patterns logically connected to form an integrated picture of the phenomenon?
	• Were the importance and implications of the findings identified?
	• Are recommendations made to suggest how the research findings can be developed?
References	• Were all the books, journals and other media referred to in the study accurately referenced?

Global issues

The questions that need asking about writing style, author, title and abstract of a qualitative research study are the same as those asked about quantitative studies, as described in the previous section.

Introduction

Statement of the problem

Many qualitative research studies are characterised by the abstract nature of the topics examined, and hence the particular experience may be interpreted differently by another individual or by the same individual under different circumstances, such as when in pain. These abstract encounters or experiences are known as 'phenomena' (Polit and Beck, 2014), and the phenomenon being investigated needs to be clearly explained in a research report.

There should be an explanation of why the study needs to be undertaken and what information could be expected to arise from conducting it. This should also include a statement of how it will contribute to the general body of understanding of the phenomenon.

The use of a qualitative approach and the qualitative methodology to be used also need to be justified.

Literature review

The role of a literature review is to give an objective account of what has been written on a given topic. Qualitative methodologies vary with regard to the conduct of a literature review before the data collection period. Equally, there is debate about whether the conceptual framework should come before data collection and data analysis.

When critiquing qualitative studies, the reviewer has to decide whether the researcher has justified the chosen approach. For example, a major premise of grounded theory is that data are collected in isolation from any pre-determined theory or conceptual framework. This means that the literature review is undertaken once the data have been collected. The rationale behind this approach is that the data analysis is not influenced by pre-existing research and thus data analysis is truly inductive. A similar approach is often employed in phenomenological investigations where the literature review may not be undertaken until the data analysis is complete. The same principle here applies. Researchers aim to ensure that the findings actually reflect participants' experiences and are truly grounded in the data rather than being influenced by previous research.

Where it was appropriate for the literature review to be done only after data collection, the report should explain the processes involved and the way the literature was used to determine similarities with, or differences from, the research findings. A literature review carried out before data collection and analysis should follow the usual remit of giving a comprehensive and balanced account of previous work. This will include identification, where appropriate, of relevant themes, conceptual models and theoretical frameworks that give a sound background to the research.

Theoretical framework

Many qualitative studies are described as inductive or theory-generating research, meaning that the purpose is to develop theory rather than to test a theory, and is linked with grounded theory, ethnography and phenomenology. The adoption of such a stance should be justified, for example where little is known about the phenomenon under study or where existing theories do not seem to provide the answer (Polit and Beck, 2014). However, as in quantitative research, sometimes qualitative researchers use theories to 'frame' their research (Aveyard et al., 2016) (see Chapter 15).

Methodological and philosophical underpinnings

It is important to recognise that the major qualitative approaches differ in their disciplinary or philosophical origins that incorporate a set of beliefs about knowledge and in how this knowledge is developed. Thus, the focus and manner in which sampling, data collection and analysis are undertaken will vary in relation to the approach used. For a reviewer to be able to establish coherence and congruence, the chosen approach should be outlined and justified.

Research question

In qualitative research, the research question reflects the identified phenomenon of interest that is directing the progress of the research. It is important to recognise that a qualitative research study does have some limits – for example, if post-operative pain is being investigated, then it is essential to identify which aspect the research is focusing on, and details should be given of how the particular focus was determined.

Depending on the type of qualitative approach adopted, for example grounded theory, the research question may be modified as new data bring new direction to the phenomenon of interest. Any modifications should be explained and justified in the report.

Method

Research design and research traditions

Actually evaluating qualitative research design can be difficult (Polit and Beck, 2014). Some of this is because decisions about design will not always be documented. There are also a great many approaches to qualitative research and a fair amount of flexibility within each approach so that establishing the 'correct' way to undertake a project can be difficult. There should, however, be an indication of whether a study has been conducted within a particular research tradition, possibly allowing a reviewer to reach some conclusions about the study design. For example, in a grounded theory study, was the data analysed as the study progressed to permit constant comparisons? The report should also give details of reflexivity.

Reviewers also need to be able to identify whether the researcher(s) spent an adequate time in the field or with study participants to gain a true picture of the phenomenon under investigation.

Sample

Participants are usually recruited to a study because of their exposure to, or their experience of, the phenomenon in question. This approach to sampling is often referred to as **purposive** or **purposeful sampling**. **Theoretical sampling** is frequently used in grounded theory. This type of sampling involves determining the sample as a result of themes that emerge from the data analysis, and the researcher then explores these themes in more depth and/or develops a theory from these data (see Chapter 12).

Qualitative research is often criticised because the findings are not generalisable as a consequence of the use of small samples. Instead, data collected from participants builds on the information from earlier participants and the accumulated data can then offer a significant depth of information about the phenomenon. Data are usually collected until no new material is emerging, that is, data saturation has been reached, and at this stage data gathering is usually stopped. Whilst it is true that qualitative research is not generalisable, most researchers agree that the findings are transferable to other settings.

Ethical considerations

The onus when critiquing a research report is on identifying whether ethical principles have been applied. Essentially, the reviewer needs to ask whether participants were told what the research entailed, how their autonomy and confidentiality were protected and what arrangements were in place to avoid preventable harms. Health and social care research has to gain an ethical committee and institutional approval before the research can be undertaken. Any research report requiring ethical approval should state that this was given, and ideally which committee gave the approval.

In qualitative research, the commonly used data collection tools include interviews and participant observation, and as a result anonymity is not possible. There is, therefore, even more of an imperative to assure participants that their identities will not be revealed in any research report (National Research Ethics Service, www.hra.nhs.uk). The role of the interviewer is to encourage participants to 'open up' and discuss their experiences of the phenomenon. Because of this, there will always be the possibility of unintended disclosure of personal information by participants, or uncomfortable experiences relating to the topic being studied may be reawakened. Therefore, consent needs to be a process of continuous negotiation with participants to be assured of their agreement to continued participation (Polit and Beck, 2014). You should also recognise that in qualitative research, ethical issues often arise at different stages and may be discussed in a report when they arise, rather than under a specific heading.

Data collection and measurement

There are a number of strategies that can be adopted when collecting qualitative data, including interviews (semi-structured and unstructured), participant observation, written texts such as **diaries** or emails, and historical or contemporary documents. The rationale for the chosen method of data collection should be described in sufficient detail to give a reviewer an overview of the process. It should be evident from the discussion that the researcher has adhered to the processes inherent in the particular approach being used. If a semi-structured interview format is selected, there should be an explanation of how the themes or questions were derived. For unstructured interviews, the initial question should be clearly linked to the purpose of the study. The rationale for the decisions about the type of interview, such as a face-to-face or focus group, should be clearly presented and justified (see Chapter 23).

Data analysis/results

The process of data analysis is fundamental to determining the credibility of qualitative research findings. Essentially, it involves the transforming of raw data into a final description, narrative or identification of themes and categories. The way data are 'transformed' varies; some researchers use generic data analysis tools whereas others use less structured and more creative approaches. What is important is that the process is described in sufficient detail to enable a reader to judge whether the final outcome is rooted in the data generated (Holloway and Wheeler, 2009). The description should enable a reviewer to confirm the processes of concurrent data collection and analysis, organisation and retrieval of data, as well as the steps in coding and thematic analysis. Any verification strategies used should be presented, for example member checking, that is, verifying with participants (see Chapter 27).

Rigour or trustworthiness is the means of demonstrating the plausibility, credibility and integrity of the qualitative research process. A study's rigour may be established if the reviewer is able to audit the actions and developments of the researcher (Polit and Beck, 2014). Rigour in documentation ensures that there is a correlation between the research process steps and the study being reviewed. Procedural rigour refers to appropriate and precise data collection techniques and incorporates a reflective/critical component in order to reduce bias and misinterpretations. Ethical rigour refers to confirmation that the study has applied ethical principles throughout.

The issue of transferability of a study should also be considered part of the appraisal process. This is determining whether the findings can be deemed relevant outside of the context of the study situation. Transferability is enhanced when the results are meaningful to individuals not involved in the research study.

Findings/results from qualitative studies can be represented as a narrative (story), themes, a description of the phenomenon under study or an interpretive account of the understanding or meaning of an experience. However, the outcomes that are presented should be discussed in the context of what is already known. Care should be taken to ensure that exaggerated claims about the significance of the study and implications for practice are not made inappropriately.

Conclusions, implications and recommendations

The report should have a clear conclusion that places findings in a context that indicates how this new information is of interest, and its implications for nursing. These should assist in being able to contrast a reader's own interpretation of the findings with those of the researcher (Polit and Beck, 2014).

There should also be reference to any limitations of the study that will help put the research into context and enable judgements to be made about the need for, and viability of conducting, further research into the same phenomenon. Recommendations should include detail of how they may be developed in practice.

References

An accurate list of all the books, journal articles, reports and other media referred to in the study should be included in a reference list at the end of the study (Polit and Beck, 2014). This list can also be a good source of further reading and is very useful when undertaking a literature search on a related topic.

SYSTEMATIC REVIEW CRITIQUE QUESTIONS

Systematic reviews are generally considered to be the best available evidence on a topic. However this cannot be taken for granted. Many systematic reviews conclude that there was insufficient good quality evidence upon which to draw firm conclusions so a systematic review might not be as useful as you had hoped. Many systematic reviews have clear quality criteria for included studies. Hence it is often the case that evidence that might be relevant to a systematic review question is not included for reasons of quality. In principle, systematic reviews should include the literature that is appropriate to answering the question. In early systematic reviews, this was almost exclusively RCTs because reviews tended to focus on questions about the effectiveness of interventions or treatments. Whilst the systematic reviews undertaken by the Cochrane Collaboration retain this focus, there are many systematic reviews undertaken on a wide variety of topics, for example socially complex interventions, such as nursing care, that will often yield qualitative data or a mixture of quantitative and qualitative data. There is, therefore, just as much of a need to critically appraise a systematic review as any other research report.

Essentially, the appraisal of a systematic review is the same as for any other type of research, that is, you need to ask a series of questions. The following checklist is offered as a framework for appraising a systematic review.

1.   Did the systematic review address a clearly focused clinical question?

As in all research, the question should be clearly defined. For example 'What are the effects of massage therapy for people with low back pain?' (Furlan et al., 2015). However, it may be stated as a statement rather than a question, for example 'We evaluated the effect of immunisation with influenza vaccines on preventing influenza A or B infections (efficacy), influenza-like illness (ILI) and its consequences (effectiveness), and determined whether exposure to influenza vaccines is associated with serious or severe harms. The target populations were healthy adults, including pregnant women and newborns' (Demicheli et al., 2014).

2.   Were the terms or concepts used in the review defined?

As in all research, the terms used need to be clarified so that the interpretations placed on them by the reviewers are transparent. A systematic review report should also include details of the search terms and combinations of terms used.

3.   Were all the relevant databases identified and searched?

In a systematic review, the reviewer(s) are expected to be as comprehensive as possible in searching for studies (see Chapter 20). This search strategy should be explicitly stated in the paper.

4.   Were inclusion and exclusion criteria stated?

This gives an indication as to whether the review considered all types of research study or concentrated on particular designs, such as randomised controlled trials (RCTs) and other types of clinical trial or experimental research.

5.   Was the quality of the included studies assessed?

Part of the function of a systematic review is to objectively assess the quality of each study. There should be a clear description of a scoring system or strategy against which each study was assessed. There is no set standard for assessing the 'true' quality of a research study, and it is not uncommon for reviewers to devise their own scoring system. Such a system will be based on a mixture of generic (common to all research studies) and specific (to the field/area) aspects of quality. This is discussed in Chapter 20.

6.   How was the evidence combined or summarised?

Did the approach to the interpretation of the results appear sound and reflect the question in the review as well as the broader context of the question? If a meta-analysis was undertaken, was this a reasonable thing to have done?

7.   What were the conclusions of the review?

Do the conclusions of the review reflect the results? To what extent can the results of the studies included be applied to a wider setting?

8.   Overall, do the findings help or confuse, and is the evidence presented sufficient to change practice?

Understanding of the outcomes of a review is necessary for an assessment of its relevance for practice, or a research topic. As with any piece of research, a systematic review should include recommendations for further investigation and/or implications for practice.

CHAPTER SUMMARY

- Critical appraisal of the evidence or analytical evaluation of the research relating to your topic is the means by which the reasoning that informs the research and arguments can be unravelled.
- Critical appraisal involves reading analytically and synthesising the information gained from reading.
- Reading analytically requires the reader to attend, categorise, select and judge.
- Analytical reading is associated with an ability to recognise well-presented and poor arguments regardless of one's own perspective on the topic.

- Synthesis is rearranging the elements derived from analytical reading into the actual identification of the relationships between the different elements.
- Each study should be appraised in accordance with the type of research design used.

SUGGESTED FURTHER READING

Aveyard, H., Sharp, P. and Woolliams, M. (2015) *A Beginner's Guide to Critical Thinking and Writing*. Maidenhead: Open University Press. This book provides a basic guide to critical thinking generally in addition to the critical appraisal of research.

Cottrell, S. (2011) *Critical Thinking Skills*. Basingstoke: Palgrave Macmillan. This book provides another guide to critical thinking in a general context in addition to the critical appraisal of research.

WEBSITES

Critical Appraisal Skills Programme (CASP): www.casp-uk.net
National Library for Health: www.library.nhs.uk

To access further resources related to this chapter, visit the companion website at https://study.sagepub.com/mouleaveyard3e

REFERENCES

Aveyard, H. (2014) *Doing a Literature Review in Health and Social Care*. Maidenhead: Open University Press.

Aveyard, H., Payne, S. and Preston, N.J. (2016) *A Postgraduate's Guide to Doing a Literature Review in Health and Social Care*. Maidenhead: Open University Press.

Aveyard, H., Sharp, P. and Woolliams, M. (2015) *A Beginner's Guide to Critical Thinking and Writing*. Maidenhead: Open University Press.

Burls, A. (2009) *What is Critical Appraisal?* Available at: www.whatisseries.co.uk.

Cottrell, S. (2011) *Critical Thinking Skills*, 2nd edn. Basingstoke: Palgrave Macmillan.

Crowe, M. and Sheppard, I. (2011) 'A review of critical appraisal tools shows they lack rigor: Alternative tool structure is proposed', *Journal of Clinical Epidemiology*, 64 (1): 79–89.

Demicheli, V., Jefferson, T., Al-Ansary, L.A., Ferroni, E., Rivetta, A. and Di Pietrantong, C. (2014) *Vaccines to Prevent Influenza in Healthy Adults*. Cochrane Database of Systematic Reviews, 3.

Furlan, A.D., Giraldo, M., Baskwill, A., Irvin, E. and Imamura, M. (2015) *What are the Effects of Massage Therapy for People with Low Back Pain*. Cochrane Collaboration.

Hart, C. (1998) *Doing a Literature Review*. London: Sage.

Holloway, I. and Wheeler, S. (2009) *Qualitative Research in Nursing*. Oxford: Blackwell.

Maslin-Prothero, S. (2010) *Baillière's Study Skills for Nurses and Midwives*, 4th edn. London: Ballière Tindall.

Polit, D. and Beck, C. (2014) *Essentials of Nursing Research: Appraising Evidence for Nursing Practice*. Philadelphia, PA: Lippincott Williams & Wilkins.

6

LITERATURE REVIEWING

Learning outcomes

This chapter will enable you to:

- recognise the purpose of a literature review in a research project
- understand how to manage the information gained from reading effectively
- prepare a research literature review

The starting point for any research is finding a gap in knowledge that the study is aiming to fill. In order to be able to do this, researchers have to review and evaluate the research that has already been done on the topic. Reviewing the existing body of evidence is an important part of the research process and can be undertaken for a variety of different purposes. The main reasons to carry out a research literature review are: to support a research proposal; to introduce a research report; as part of a dissertation or thesis. In addition, a literature review can be undertaken as a study in its own right, as a standalone project in order to answer questions, for example about the effectiveness of different ways of delivering care, interventions and new products/procedures. The imperative driving these questions is the need to ensure that practice is evidence-based, and hence there is a need to examine research already conducted to be able to determine what best practice actually is. Standalone literature reviews are usually conducted as a form of systematic review which are discussed in Chapter 20. The principles for conducting a systematic review and reviewing the literature prior to a research project or proposal, as discussed in this chapter, are very similar.

Chapters 4 and 5 described how to search for relevant literature and critically appraise the evidence presented by the literature. In this chapter we will focus on reviewing the literature prior to a research project or proposal. We will describe the different stages involved in preparing a research literature review that could be used when writing a proposal or a research report.

WHAT IS A LITERATURE REVIEW?

A literature review is summary of previous research and other relevant evidence, which is reviewed collectively so that each piece of research is seen within the context of other research. This prevents one piece of research or other evidence being reviewed in isolation and therefore taken out of context. If each single piece of evidence is considered as a piece of a jigsaw, the review is the whole picture.

A literature review uses a systematic framework that includes a thorough **search strategy, critical appraisal** and **synthesis** of the evidence. It is structured and goes into sufficient detail to make it possible for the reader to be able to replicate the review. The literature review follows the same principles as a systematic review but is less detailed.

Table 6.1 gives an indication of some of the differences between **literature reviews** and **systematic reviews**.

A literature review helps to focus on a research topic and, by so doing, enables the progressive narrowing that turns a topic into a practical and doable research project. Doing a literature review may be seen as a laborious and difficult aspect of the research process and less interesting than the actual research study itself. However, there is a lot to be gained from a carefully conducted review. In addition to a thorough understanding of the research already undertaken in an area, researchers get ideas about possible

Table 6.1   Differences between literature reviews and systematic literature reviews

	Literature review	Systematic literature review
Focus	Provides an examination of recent or current literature. Can cover wide range of topics at various levels of completeness and comprehensiveness.	A comprehensive search process which addresses explicit questions to produce 'best evidence synthesis'.
Search strategy	Usually only published literature will be reviewed, and this can be subject to a selection bias. The search strategy is often stated in the review.	Draws together all known knowledge on a topic area, including unpublished 'grey' sources. Uses exhaustive methods. The search strategy is clearly stated.
Analysis	Chronological, conceptual or thematic.	Identifies what is known and makes recommendations for practice.
Synthesis methods	Typically thematic.	Either meta-analysis (a re-analysis of the statistics in each individual paper) or thematic approach.
Conclusions	Summative (does not re-analyse data collected).	Summative or analytical.

Source: Adapted from the work of Sim and Wright (2000: 283), Grant and Booth (2009: 94–95), and Aveyard et al. (2016)

research methods to use in their own research, what has worked well and not so well in previous projects (Aveyard et al., 2016). Care and attention to detail at this stage can reduce work and wasted effort at the later stages of a project.

WHAT IS THE PURPOSE OF A LITERATURE REVIEW?

A literature review sets out to provide answers to the following questions:

- What is currently known about the topic?
- What are the main questions and problems that have been addressed to date?
- What aspects of the topic have not been considered? What are the gaps?
- What are the major issues and debates about the topic?
- What research has previously been done?
- What are the origins of and definitions for the topic?
- What recommendations for further research have previously been made but not acted upon?
- What methods have other researchers used to investigate this topic? Were some of these methods better suited to investigating this topic than others?

Overall, a literature review will question how the approaches to the above questions have increased understanding and knowledge of the topic being researched. It should put the research question/problem into context and critically appraise the merits of the research. The results from a literature review can be written up to present a logical coherent case for pursuing the study or provide the informed introduction to a research study report. The task of asking all of the above questions may seem rather daunting, but if approached in a systematic way it will be possible to construct a review that actually provides the answers being sought.

HOW DO YOU CARRY OUT A LITERATURE REVIEW FOR A RESEARCH PROJECT?

A literature review starts by defining the exact topic to be explored or investigated. This is more or less the same as deciding on a research question, though, as discussed in Chapter 9, a literature review often helps to inform the development of a research question. Once the topic for the review has been decided upon, then the literature can be searched to find what research has already been undertaken on the topic. A search of the literature, as described in Chapter 4, enables articles relating to the topic to be retrieved. Each of the retrieved articles then needs to be read and critically appraised, as described in Chapter 5. These processes enable an account of the available research literature on a specified topic to be presented by providing an evaluation of the quality of the research and identification of the gaps in the existing research evidence. Chapter 5 gives suggestions for the type of question that should be asked of the different types of research. Some questions will be specific to quantitative research, some to qualitative but some will be generic to all and can be more appropriate when a diverse range of research methodologies are present in the literature found by the search. Essentially, the aim is to assess the value of the research that has already been done on your topic and confirm that there is a need for your proposed research study.

As discussed in Chapter 5, some degree of understanding of research, and particularly of research methodology, is necessary before you can properly appraise research papers. A critical appraisal tool will not assist this process unless researchers have an understanding of what they are assessing.

Author(s)

Year of publication

Title of article/book

Journal name   volume   issue   pages

Book publisher and edition

Website address   Date downloaded

Research problem/question

Type of study   Quantitative ❑   Qualitative ❑   Mixed ❑

Design   e.g. experimental, survey, grounded theory, phenomenology

Description of intervention   e.g. self-report questionnaire, observation, comparison of wound dressings

Sample   Size: Sampling method:

                                      Sample characteristics:

Key results/findings

Recommendations

Strengths

How does this advance our understanding of the subject?

Are the hypotheses, methods, sample sizes or types of control for variables, recommendations appropriate?

Were ethics considered?

Limitations:

In what ways is it limited?

When and where would it not apply? Are there any flaws in the research design and methods, sample size or type, conclusions not based on results?

Figure 6.1   Example of a critical appraisal record for a research article

There are some tips that can help researchers with the process of understanding the research papers. It can be helpful to make notes about what the research reports say as each paper is read. An example of a pro-forma (sometimes called a data extraction sheet) that could be used for compiling a record of what you gleaned from this reading is given in Figure 6.1. The important thing is to keep a record so that you can refer to what you found in the paper without having to re-read it as it is likely that you will have forgotten the details of the results etc.

What you actually decide to record will vary with each research project, but you should get into the habit of making detailed notes from the outset. The basic details that should be recorded are described in Chapter 5. As each article is read, it is useful to add comments to the basic information so that the evaluation and details of what has been read are all kept together. This is where storage on a reference database can be useful, but a paper-based system can be just as efficient. Whatever system is used, it is essential to keep a back-up copy – otherwise there is a real risk of having to repeat the search or re-read all of the articles.

Having completed a critical appraisal of the important papers relevant to the topic, you are ready to bring together the main themes that arise in the papers included in the review. This is the process that moves on from simply presenting an account, albeit critical, of each article to one that provides a comprehensive picture of the common themes that have been reported from the different research studies. This involves not taking things at face value but looking at different ways that the data in each paper could be interpreted, especially in the light of the other papers. It requires comparison between different papers and texts that indicates where there are differences, similarities, contradictions and deficiencies (or gaps in the research). This is an essential skill for a researcher and is best developed by adopting a systematic approach towards analysis of the arguments and then evaluation.

HOW DO YOU WRITE UP THE SUMMARY OF THE LITERATURE IN A REVIEW?

There are a variety of ways that you can write up your literature review, depending on the purpose of the review. The literature review may be for a proposal to support the need for a research project or in a research report to justify the conduct of the study. The difference between these literature reviews is usually in the length. A literature review used in a proposal may be regarded as a précis of what will be included in a literature review of the study report. The aim for this review is to provide supporting evidence to convince, say, grant-making bodies, ethics committees and supervisors of the need for the research study, whilst a literature review in a final report is expected to contain a detailed appraisal and be more up to date simply because it forms part of an actual study.

There is no recipe for writing a literature review, but there are certain principles to follow. The aim is to convince the reader that the research study is necessary and represents the next step in knowledge-building for the topic. In order to do this, the reader needs to be convinced that a thorough search has been undertaken so relevant literature has not been overlooked, as described in Chapter 4, and that the literature has been critically appraised, as described in Chapter 5. This should be documented in the review; the detail given will be dependent on the length of the review.

Once the method of undertaking the review has been described, the reviewer will discuss relevant findings, together, where appropriate, with a comment on the methods used and any strengths and limitations of the work. In this way, it will be possible to demonstrate that there has been a considered and justified examination of what others have discovered and written about a specific topic. It is unlikely that a chronological approach for reviewing the literature will be possible, say by starting with the earliest work on the topic and progressing through to the latest publication. Similarly, it is unusual to present an individual review of each paper in turn. Instead, many researchers present the common themes that arise in the included papers. This can be summarised in a tabular format where the themes arising in the different papers are charted so that the reader can see at a glance which papers gave rise to which themes and how common each theme was throughout the different included papers.

A literature review has to have a structure that follows a logical argument if gaps in the literature are to be highlighted. Therefore, the themes emerging from the literature should reflect the research questions or identified problems. It also means that, although each study will have been critically appraised, not all aspects of each study will necessarily need to be included when writing the literature review. Remember, it is a summary of work that has been done that is relevant to the needs of the review and not a comprehensive description of each research study. Suggested headings for a literature review are as follows:

1. Introduction – overview of what will be covered by the review.
2. Review of the search strategy.
3. Review of the approach to critical appraisal.
4. Overview of studies and types of research design used.
5. Themes identified from the literature with critical evaluation.
6. Critical summary of current knowledge and gaps in the literature.
7. Identification of research needs.
8. Rationale for the study design.
9. Overview and niche for proposed study.

There are also some conventions of language associated with writing a critical review of research literature. For example, authors suggest, assert, argue, state, conclude or contend. A good way of developing an understanding of these conventions is to read a few critical reviews before embarking on writing your own.

REFERENCING THE RESEARCH LITERATURE

In order to be able to discuss the research literature relevant to your project, you will need to refer to the actual papers: this is called 'referencing' or 'citing'. It demonstrates and attributes the source of the information used, lends authority to the claims made and allows readers to refer to full copies of articles of interest to them.

It is possible to use too many or too few references; the aim is to achieve a balance and arrive at what is felt to be the appropriate number of references necessary to support the arguments being presented. It may also be necessary, in a review for a proposal, to take account of guidelines from grant-making bodies (when applying for funding) or regulatory authorities that will be reviewing your proposal. Suggestions of how to use and not use references are given below.

Use and abuse of references

References should be used to:

- justify and support your arguments
- allow you to make comparisons with other research
- express matters better than you could yourself
- demonstrate your familiarity with your topic or field of research.

You should not use references to:

- impress your readers with the scope of your reading
- litter your writing with names and quotations
- replace the need for you to express your own thoughts
- misrepresent the authors of those works. (Blaxter et al., 2010)

There are several conventions available for referencing published work, and authors usually use one that they are familiar with and prefer, or follow the referencing style requested by a journal. Some electronic reference databases may be able to format your references in one of a range of different styles.

The two most commonly used conventions for referencing are by numbering (e.g. Vancouver) or by author and year (e.g. Harvard) in the text, with the full details of the reference only appearing in a list at the end of an article. Nursing journals such as *Nursing Times*, *Nursing Standard* and *Nurse Researcher* use the author and year style, whilst the *British Medical Journal* uses the numbering system.

> ### Exercise
> Review the last piece of written work you did and ask yourself whether your references match the guidelines given here.

CHAPTER SUMMARY

- A literature review provides an overview of the research available to support a research proposal and inform a research report.
- Literature reviews and systematic reviews share a similar method but the detail of a systematic review is greater.

- A literature review helps to focus on a research topic.
- Critical appraisal is a structured process of identifying and evaluating the merits and/or value of research.
- When reading a research study, questions should be asked about each section.
- Evaluation of the literature involves giving a critical account and comparison of the different studies to highlight similarities, contradictions and gaps in the literature.
- When writing a literature review, the aim is to convince the reader that the research study is necessary and represents the next step in knowledge-building for the topic.
- All the literature used should be referenced using a recognised system.

SUGGESTED FURTHER READING

Aveyard, H., Payne, S. and Preston, N. (2016) *A Postgraduate's Guide to Doing a Literature Review in Health and Social Care*. Maidenhead: Open University Press. This book provides an in-depth but accessible guide to doing a literature review.

Battany-Saltikov, J. (2012) *How to Do a Systematic Review in Nursing: A Step-by-Step Guide*. Maidenhead: RCN Publishing and Open University Press. Chapters 6–9. This book provides a step-by-step guide to doing a literature review. It is presented in a straightforward way and is readily accessible.

Ridley, D. (2012) *The Literature Review: A Step-by-Step Guide for Students*, 2nd edn. London: Sage. This step-by-step guide provides a comprehensive overview to conducting a literature search and review. The budding researcher who lacks literature review skills should find it useful.

WEBSITES

Critical Appraisal Skills Programme (CASP): www.casp-uk.net/
National Library for Health: www.library.nhs.uk

To access further resources related to this chapter, visit the companion website at https://study.sagepub.com/mouleaveyard3e

REFERENCES

Aveyard, H., Payne, S. and Preston, N.J. (2016) *A Postgraduate's Guide to Doing a Literature Review in Health and Social Care*. Maidenhead: Open University Press.

Blaxter, L., Hughes, C. and Tight, M. (2010) *How to Research*, 4th edn. Maidenhead: Open University Press.

Grant and Booth (2009) 'A typology of reviews: An analysis of 14 review types and associated methodologies', *Health Information and Libraries Journal*, 26(2): 91–108.

Sim, J. and Wright, C. (2000) *Research in Healthcare: Concepts, Designs and Methods*. Cheltenham: Nelson Thornes.

PART 2

PREPARING FOR RESEARCH

7

RESEARCH ETHICS AND GOVERNANCE

Learning outcomes

This chapter will enable you to:

- recognise the specific guidance and ethical codes for those involved in research
- recognise the important legislation that nurse researchers need to consider
- have an understanding of research governance
- have an understanding of research ethics committees and their role
- have an appreciation of the principles of Good Clinical Practice in research

Just as in clinical practice, ethical issues arise at all stages of the research process, commencing with decisions about whether or not the research should be conducted at all. For example, there may be some research so controversial that it may be unethical for it to be conducted. On the other hand, there may be some research that it would be unethical not to do, such as the evaluation of new services or the effectiveness or acceptability of new treatments to patients. There is also a strong argument that supports the idea that research should only be undertaken when it is apparent (usually based on findings from a comprehensive literature review) that there is no clear answer to a question or problem and that research will help to provide an answer.

The first ethical question is whether the research is worth doing. For most research, the intention should be to improve knowledge, whether it is about treatment and care, diagnosis and prophylactic procedures or gaining an understanding of people's experiences, perspectives and behaviours. Certainly, anyone funding research or giving permission for research to be conducted, such as a research ethics committee (REC), R&D department of a healthcare institution or grant-giving body, will want evidence and a justification for carrying out the research before giving funding or approval for a specific research project. This process will include researchers having their proposals subjected to independent scrutiny by research ethics committees established by, for example, universities, healthcare institutions and social care providers, to ensure that the research is ethical.

Once it is established that there is a research question that needs answering, we need to establish how we do this within an ethical and legal framework. This chapter concentrates on the ethical and legal processes that have been developed to guide research in nursing and multi-disciplinary and interdisciplinary studies. The next chapter (Chapter 8) discusses how we should conduct research in an ethical manner, with particular emphasis on the responsibilities that a researcher must consider in relation to gaining consent and avoiding harm to any potential and actual participants.

ADVANCING KNOWLEDGE, PROTECTING FROM HARM AND MAINTAINING PATIENT CHOICE

The imperative of any healthcare research is to balance the advancement of knowledge with the need to respect human integrity, protect from harm and maintain the right to self determination. Virtually all research has the potential to cause harm of some description. Harm in the research context refers to anything that 'disrupts a research participant'. Harm could be an unpleasant side-effect from a drug or simply the time taken by a participant to complete a questionnaire. Whilst harm can be a consequence of day to day clinical care, the difference is that when a patient participates in research he or she is contributing to the advancement of knowledge rather than receiving a direct clinical benefit (although in many instances, he or she will receive a direct clinical benefit from involvement in the research). Strict regulations are therefore in place to ensure that those involved in research are protected from harm and that procedures for obtaining informed consent are explicit.

There have been some well-documented, major blunders in our recent history which have demonstrated the need for the regulation of research. Probably the most well-known abuse of research participants was the use of human subjects in biomedical experiments in the Second World War. The subsequent Nuremberg War Crimes Trials resulted in the creation of the Nuremberg Code in the late 1940s. The Nuremberg Code set out the standards for judging physicians and scientists who had conducted biomedical experiments on concentration camp prisoners. This code became a prototype for many later regulations, particularly those relating to human experimentation, with voluntary consent being the central tenet.

The Nuremberg Code was superseded in 1964 by the Declaration of Helsinki when the World Medical Association adopted the code. It is regularly amended to take into account changing perspectives and remains a current reference point today (see WMA, 2008). The Declaration of Helsinki sets out principles to safeguard research participants. Fundamentally, the role of informed consent is at the centre of the principles and the declaration clearly states that the interests of society should never take precedence over the well-being of participants. The latest version emphasises the need to provide access to research for otherwise under-represented populations, the registration of clinical trials, post-study access and compensating participants with research-related injuries. It also highlights the need for continuing research into the safety of current interventions, which is particularly relevant for drugs and devices, as seen in the recent examples of Rofecoxib and the questions associated with the use of industrial-grade silicone for breast implants. These changes are important because they reflect developments in medical research and increasing recognition that clinical trials need to be conducted with populations that are likely to use the drug/device/intervention and not just a narrow group from within a population, such as those aged between 18 and 60, those not at risk of becoming pregnant or those having pre-existing medical conditions.

More recently, in Europe, including the UK, there has been a steady increase in the regulations, requirements and governance relating to the conduct of research in health and social services. These have been driven by highly publicised scandals such as research without consent using the organs of children who had died; malpractice and misconduct by health researchers which have been reported in the press; increased public interest in health and research issues; an increasingly litigious society; and increased public expectation of accountability, transparency and fairness within health and social services. Furthermore, in the past many health and social care organisations have not always had a comprehensive record of all the research being undertaken in their organisations, on their premises or involving their staff and patients/clients. All of these factors, together with legislation that relates to the protection of the rights of individuals, have contributed to new policies and practices that are designed to protect research participants and give greater confidence to the general public who are potential research participants.

In order to balance the aim of advancing knowledge with protecting the patient from harm and facilitating informed consent, there are a number of regulations and legislation to direct the conduct of ethical and legal research. Examples of specific legislation that has an impact on research are detailed below.

The Mental Capacity Act 2005

The principles of informed consent and the patient's right to self determination are clearly established in English law and most recently in the **Mental Capacity Act**. It is long established that patients have a right to give their informed consent prior to all treatment and research and subsequently have the right to refuse even life saving treatment; even if this risks the life of an unborn child (St. George's Healthcare NHS Trust v S [1998]). The patient therefore has a right to refuse to participate in research and it is not possible to undertake research unless the participant has given their informed consent, unless justification is made under the Mental Capacity Act (2005). For consent to be valid, research participants need to have full information about the research, have the capacity to understand the information and not be coerced into making a decision to participate, for example, by the researcher who is leading the study and who also might be responsible for their clinical care.

The principles of informed consent prior to research require specific consideration when research is planned with vulnerable participants or those who lack the capacity to give consent. The Mental Capacity Act (MCA) 2005 provides guidance on this.

Of specific interest are sections 30 to 34 of the MCA. These go into detail about undertaking research with individuals who lack the capacity to consent, and what is required by law. This includes approval of a research project involving people who lack the capacity to consent by an appropriate body who need to be satisfied that the research is connected to the impairing condition affecting such people or its treatment. There must be justification that the research cannot be carried out on individuals who have the capacity to consent, and the study must have the potential to benefit participants without imposing a burden disproportionate to the benefit, or an intention to provide knowledge of the causes or care and treatment of people affected by the same or similar condition.

Researchers who involve individuals who lack the capacity to consent must have reasonable grounds for believing that participating carries negligible risk to the individual, is not unduly invasive or restrictive and does not interfere with the participants' freedom of action or privacy. They must also do nothing to participants that participants appear to object to (unless this is to protect an individual from harm or reduce or prevent pain and discomfort). Researchers must also withdraw such individuals from the study if a participant indicates in *any way* that they wish to be withdrawn, or withdraw them from the study if the researcher believes there is a risk to the participant and, at all times, the interests of participants must be assumed to outweigh those of science and society.

As well as establishing whether an individual has the mental capacity to make a decision, such as whether to participate in a study or not, researchers must consider the likelihood of whether an individual will at some other time have capacity and, as far as is reasonably practical, encourage them to participate in any decision affecting them. This might also include considering the person's past and present wishes and feelings, their beliefs and values, and the views of anyone who has been named by the individual, cares for them or has a lasting power of attorney and would consider what was in the person's best interests.

The MCA provides a legal framework to protect people with impaired capacity and supports them so that they are given every opportunity to make decisions for themselves. It sets out a number of principles that should be used when determining whether a person has mental capacity. A person is defined as lacking capacity if *at the time* of the decision, or act, they are unable to make a decision for themselves because of impairment or disturbance of brain function. This disturbance can be temporary or permanent, and assessment of capacity should not be referenced to their age, appearance or any aspect of behaviour that might lead to unjustified assumptions about their mental capacity.

A person is deemed to be unable to make a decision for themselves if they are unable to understand the information relevant to that decision (the information must be given in a way appropriate to the individual's circumstances, such as simple language, visual aids); retain the information (even if it is only for a short period, it does not prevent them from making a decision); weigh up information and reasonably foresee the consequences of deciding one way or another as part of the decision-making process; and communicate the decision by talking, sign language or other means.

The MCA also contains a duty to consult, where practicable and appropriate, the next of kin of a person with impaired capacity, and has introduced new forms for proxy decision making and advocacy.

Data Protection Act 1998

This is an important Act for researchers, who must consider how they handle and process personal information and data. The **Data Protection Act** lays down the legal requirements for handling personal data to protect the confidentiality of the individual and the interests of those who have legitimate reasons for using personal information. Personal information includes both facts and opinions about the individual, including images, recordings and samples. It places obligations on those who process information (controllers), and rights on those, living or dead, who are the subject of the information (subjects/participants). There are eight principles of good practice and anyone processing (controllers) personal information (written or electronic) must comply with them. The Act requires that personal data must:

1. be fairly and lawfully processed
2. be processed for limited purposes; these purposes must be specified and lawful and must not be further processed in any way incompatible with the purpose
3. be adequate, relevant and not excessive for the purpose
4. be accurate and kept up to date
5. not be kept longer than is necessary for the purpose; for research purposes this can be an unspecified period providing it can be justified
6. be processed in accordance with the individual's rights (see below)
7. be kept secure
8. not be transferred to countries outside the European Economic Area (EEA) unless the country has adequate protection for the individual.

Some data are particularly sensitive and there are extra provisions for information about ethnic or racial origin, political opinions and religious beliefs, trade union membership, physical or mental health conditions, sex life, criminal proceedings and convictions. These conditions include having the explicit consent of the individual concerned or there are legal requirements or protection issues associated with the data.

The subjects of the information also have rights under the Data Protection Act. There is a right to find out what information is held about them on computer and some manual records. A data controller can be asked by an individual not to process information relating to them that causes substantial unwarranted damage or distress to them or anyone else, and not to process information for direct marketing purposes. Subjects of the information also have the right to compensation for damage or distress caused by breach of the Act and to apply for a court order to get rectification, blocking or destruction of data if it is inaccurate or based on opinions formed from inaccurate information.

In addition, all NHS providers of healthcare have someone appointed as a 'Caldicott Guardian' (named after the Caldicott Report of 1997). This is usually a senior manager who has responsibility for the safekeeping of patients' records and for ensuring that patient information is used appropriately by staff.

Freedom of Information Act 2000

This Act allows access to information regardless of when it was created or how long the public authority has held it. There are, however, a number of exemptions, such as information relating to national security and confidential information. Other exemptions also require a public authority to consider whether it is in the public interest to withhold information. If an individual wants to gain access to information about themselves, they should use their rights under the Data Protection Act. However, personal data about other individuals cannot be released, as it would breach the Data Protection Act.

The difference between the Freedom of Information Act and the Data Protection Act is essentially that the former is designed to allow access and the latter to restrict access to data. Both aim to protect the individual by making sure that access to data about them is only released under strict conditions, whilst also allowing free access to anonymised data to assist in improving services and research. For researchers, knowledge about what is available from public authorities under the Freedom of Information Act can be useful if background information is required. Furthermore, in some types of research, access to such public information may be an important stage in the research process and researchers should familiarise themselves with the guidelines available.

Public Interest Disclosure Act 1998

This act provides a mechanism for the disclosure of information, which *prima facie* should be considered as confidential. All healthcare staff owe a duty to the patient to maintain confidentiality and face serious implications if this is breached. However there are certain instances in which it is considered permissible to breach confidentiality. Decisions about breaking confidentiality 'in the public interest' are complex. Each case is considered on its merits as to whether the duty of confidentiality to the research participant should prevail over the disclosure of information. In terms of research, if confidentiality or anonymity cannot be guaranteed, participants must be warned in advance before they agree to participate. If information needs to be disclosed in the public interest without a participant's consent, there must be a benefit to the individual or society that outweighs the individual's right to confidentiality, for example, if the health and safety of anyone has been, is being or is likely to be endangered.

The Public Interest Disclosure Act is particularly important for nurse researchers who want to include work colleagues as participants.

Human Tissue Act 2004

For anyone involved in research with organs or tissue, the full legislation of the Human Tissue Act must be consulted and particular reference made to the consenting process.

The National Research Ethics Service gives specific guidance on this. The Human Tissues Authority (HTA) has a specific role in informing the public about **storage** and use of human bodies and tissues and the disposal of human tissue. They also license and inspect some activities, including research activities, and produce good practice guidelines.

The Human Tissue Act came about as a direct result of a number of enquiries into the retention and use of organs and tissues. The public enquiries showed that storage and use of organs and tissue without proper consent after people had died were commonplace. A legal review also found that the law on tissue retention was inadequate and, following public consultation, the Human Tissue Act 2004 replaced the 1989 Human Organ Transplant Act. This Act introduced a new offence of DNA theft and also includes a change that allows museums to move human remains out of their collections.

Human tissue is defined in the Act as material that has come from human body cells. Hair and nails from living people are excluded, as are live gametes and embryos, which are covered under the 1990 Human Fertilisation and Embryology Act.

The fundamental principle of the Human Tissue Act is consent. The Act lists the purposes for which consent is required and these include research, clinical audit and training, including training for research purposes. There are a few exceptions – for example, where 'residual' tissue from the living cannot be identified and can be used provided certain conditions apply, existing holdings of tissue, and where there is a case of extreme public health emergency.

Human Rights Act 1998

In terms of research, the Human Rights Act has no specific conditions other than requiring that researchers respect the basic human rights of participants and anyone connected with the research at all times.

Understandably, these recent developments have resulted in more formalised ethics procedures and additional bureaucracy for researchers in the fields of health and social care. Social science research, which often spans health and nursing research, has become more bureaucratised and this moves it away from its former reliance on self-regulation and professional codes. However, it must be recognised that the protection of participants, and researchers, is the prime reason for these procedures being put in place.

RESEARCH GOVERNANCE FRAMEWORK

In addition to the legislation that guides research, in the UK, the Research Governance Framework (DH, 2005) was developed with the overall aim of setting standards; defining mechanisms to deliver standards; describing monitoring and assessment arrangements; improving research quality; and safeguarding the public. Research governance is one of the core standards of all organisations delivering NHS care.

All research-active healthcare organisations must comply with the **Research Governance Framework**. There are five areas of responsibility in the Research Governance Framework, and different legislation and guidance apply to the different areas: science, information, health and safety, finance and intellectual property, and ethics.

Science

It is important that the proposal is a worthwhile scientific project. Proposals for research should be subjected to peer review, giving independent advice on quality, though this should be proportionate to the scale of the research and the risks involved. For example, a small-scale student project should not be subjected to the same level of review as a multi-centre randomised controlled trial. All research involving patients should apply the principles of **Good Clinical Practice** (MRC, 1998), and the Medicines and Healthcare Products Regulatory Agency (MHRA) must authorise any trials on people of medicines/devices. Good Clinical Practice (GCP) is an international ethical and scientific quality standard established to provide a unified standard for the European Union (EU), Japan, the USA, Australia, Canada and the Nordic countries, as well as the World Health Organisation (WHO). Although the principles were designed primarily for the conduct of drug trials, there is an expectation that all research studies comply with them to give assurance of the quality and safety of research.

Information

The Framework states that there should be free access to information on the research and its findings after appropriate critical scientific review. This information should be presented in a format understandable and accessible to those who have participated, those who have the potential to benefit and the general public.

Health and safety

The safety of participants and researcher should be given priority at all times, and health and safety regulations must be strictly observed.

Finance and intellectual property

There must be financial probity and compliance with the law and rules of HM Treasury for the use of public funds. This includes employers having in place arrangements for compensation if any of their staff harm anyone through negligence. Consideration of the exploitation of intellectual property should be part of the governance framework for any research study.

Ethics

For research involving patients, service users, healthcare professionals or volunteers or their organs, tissues or data, there must be an independent review to ensure that ethical standards are met. There must be appropriate arrangements for obtaining informed consent. This includes the provision of suitable material, such as written or pictorial information, so that participants, care-givers, parents or supporters have clear explanations that they can understand. When tissues and organs are to be used, the special arrangements specified under the Human Tissues Act 2004 must be applied.

Responsibilities of sponsors

The sponsor of the research is usually, but not always, the employer of the researcher or the supervisor of the student. They could also be the funder or the care organisation, or there could be joint sponsorship arrangements between a university and a care organisation, for example. Essentially, sponsors are responsible for ensuring that the research proposal respects the dignity, rights, safety and well-being of participants, and that the relationship with care professionals and arrangements for the conduct of the research are consistent with the Research Governance Framework. This will include confirming that an independent expert review and appropriate **research ethics committee** or independent ethics reviewer have given favourable opinions about the proposal.

It is also the responsibility of sponsors to ensure that the chief investigator and other key researchers, including those at collaborating sites, have the necessary expertise, experience and access to resources to conduct the proposed research successfully.

Responsibilities of researchers

Researchers also have detailed and specific responsibilities under the Research Governance Framework. These include the need to:

- follow the agreed research proposal or protocol
- select a means of communication which ensures that potential participants are fully informed before deciding whether to participate or not
- help healthcare professionals ensure that participants receive appropriate care whilst involved in the research
- report adverse events
- protect the confidentiality of records and data.

In addition, a senior individual with suitable experience and expertise must be designated as the chief investigator. The chief investigator has additional responsibilities, such as project design, conduct, analysis, reporting, gaining ethical approval and ensuring that the study adheres to the standards required in the Research Governance Framework. Nurse researchers, particularly those leading projects, must thoroughly familiarise themselves with the requirements of the Research Governance Framework if they are conducting research in health services.

RESEARCH ETHICS APPROVAL

There are essentially two processes for gaining approval to carry out research in health and (in some) social services:

- NHS Trust R&D department approval
- Research Ethics Committee (REC) approval.

However, if you are doing research as part of an educational qualification, you will also need to gain approval from your university.

NHS Trust Research and Development approval processes

There is a requirement, in the NHS, for any care provider research and development (R&D) department to be satisfied that a number of requirements as set out in the Research Governance Framework have been fulfilled. This means that all research undertaken within each organisation is notified to, and monitored by, the R&D department.

NHS R&D departments will also monitor and audit research that is within their sphere of responsibility, as well as giving approval for the research to begin once they are sure that the above conditions have been satisfied. Researchers are responsible for ensuring that the requirements of NHS R&D departments are met.

Research ethics committees

Before a research project can start, any researcher has to seek an independent ethical review of their proposed research. There are a number of different types of research ethics committees (RECs), and which committee(s) need to give approval depends on the nature of the proposed research. For NHS research which involves patients and/or clients, access to notes and records, access to staff within health and social services and access to health or social care premises, a researcher must apply to a local NHS REC. If the research is to be undertaken at more than five different NHS or social service premises, then the application for ethical approval needs to be made to a REC that can give approval for a multi-centre research study. For research by a student or member of staff of a university, a university research ethics committee (UREC) will need to be approached to approve the research; this will usually be required in addition to the NHS REC approval. In the social services, there may be a Social Services Ethics Committee but, more likely, a UREC or REC will provide this function. Similarly, research that falls outside the NHS and social services but is social science research will also require independent ethics scrutiny and approval. Again, this will usually be gained through a UREC or REC or a Social Services Ethics Committee.

Ethics committees are multi-professional, with members having experience across all types of research design. Lay people are included on these committees to provide an ordinary person's perspective. Ethical review involves completing an application form, providing a research proposal that gives details of the proposed research, providing copies of research instruments (for example, questionnaires, interview schedules) and, most importantly, producing participant information sheets and consent forms.

CHAPTER SUMMARY

- There is an expectation that any health and social service research is ethical, of good quality, safe and that data are credible.
- Ethical and governance issues must be considered at all stages of the research process.
- Individual researchers have a responsibility to abide by the regulations and legislation as they apply to research and their professional practice.
- All NHS research is subject to the Research Governance Framework (DH, 2005).
- Researchers are expected to follow Good Clinical Practice principles (ICR, 1997).
- Any health and (some) social service research has to be approved by:

  o one or more NHS Trust R&D department(s)
  o an REC.

- Approval processes, research governance, regulations and legislation are all designed to ensure that the integrity and safety of the research participant are respected and safeguarded.

SUGGESTED FURTHER READING

Di Iorio, C.T., Carinci, F. and Oderkirk, J. (2014) 'Health research and systems governance are at risk: Should the right to data protection override health?', *Journal of Medical Ethics*, 40 (7): 488–92. A critical look at research governance.

General Medical Council (2010) *Good Practice in Research and Consent to Research*. London: GMC. A document outlining the principles of good practice in ethical research.

Shaw, S.E., Petchey, R.P., Chapman, J. and Abbott, S. (2009) 'A double edged sword? Health research and research governance in UK primary care', *Social Science & Medicine*, 68 (5): 912–8. A critical look at research governance.

The NIHR HTA programme has published the following monographs (in depth reviews):

1. 'Ethical issues in the design and conduct of randomised controlled trials: A review' (Edwards), Vol. 2, No. 15.
2. 'Implications of socio-cultural contexts for the ethics of clinical trials: A review' (Ashcroft), Vol. 1, No. 9.

WEBSITES

Health Research Authority – National Research Service website: www.hra.nhs.uk.
Integrated Research Application System (IRAS): www.myresearchproject.org.uk.
NIHR HTA programme: www.hta.ac.uk/project/htapubs.asp.
Research Ethics Guidebook: www.ethicsguidebook.ac.uk/.

To access further resources related to this chapter, visit the companion website at https://study.sagepub.com/mouleaveyard3e

REFERENCES

Caldicott Committee (1997) *The Caldicott Report*. London: Department of Health.

Department of Health (DH) (2005) *Research Governance Framework for Health and Social Care*, 2nd edn. London: DH.

Institute of Clinical Research (ICR) (1997) *ICH Guidelines for Good Clinical Practice*. Bourne End: Institute of Clinical Research.

Medical Research Council (MRC) (1998) *Guidelines for Good Clinical Practice in Clinical Trials*. London: Medical Research Council.

St. George's Healthcare NHS Trust v S [1998] 3 WLR 936.

World Medical Association (WMA) (2008) *The Declaration of Helsinki: Ethical Principles for Medical Research Involving Human Subjects*, 6th revision. Seoul: WMA General Assembly.

8
RESEARCHING ETHICALLY

Learning outcomes

This chapter will enable you to:

- appreciate ethical principles and how they relate to research practice
- understand the needs of vulnerable research participants
- understand the nature of informed consent
- recognise what needs to be included when giving information to a participant
- understand how anonymity and confidentiality can be preserved in a research project
- appreciate and understand the need for data storage
- be able to identify the risks to researcher safety
- appreciate the issues raised when in a role of researcher and nurse

---

In the previous chapter, we examined the legal and statutory regulations that govern our approach to the research in nursing and healthcare more generally. We also explored some of the unethical research that has been undertaken which forms part of the rationale as to why these regulations are in place. The aim of this chapter is to explain the ethical principles that underpin the conduct of research and how these can be put into practice in developing a project and when actually carrying out a research study.

ETHICAL PRINCIPLES

Before embarking on a discussion of **ethical principles** in relation to research, it is important to understand the term *ethics*. Ethics is a generic term for various ways of understanding and examining the moral life. There are two types of ethical enquiry; normative and non-normative:

- Normative ethics attempt to answer the question 'Which general moral norms for the guidance and evaluation of conduct should we accept and why?' (Beauchamp and Childress, 2013). Practical or applied ethics is the attempt to implement general norms and theories for practical problems and contexts.
- Non-normative ethics fall into two categories: descriptive and meta-ethics. Descriptive ethics refer to the factual investigation of moral conduct and beliefs, and meta-ethics analyse language, concepts and methods of reasoning.

Morality refers to 'norms about right and wrong human conduct that are so widely shared that they form a stable (although usually incomplete) social consensus' (Beauchamp and Childress, 2013), such as not lying, stealing or killing, keeping promises and respecting the rights of others. Because most of us are comfortable with these 'rules', there is no debate about them and they are accepted as *common morality*. *Professional morality* again refers to commonly accepted norms of conduct, but specifically moral responsibilities applicable to a specific profession. From a healthcare professional perspective, it refers to things like ensuring **informed consent** and patient **confidentiality**.

The ethical principles that should guide nurse researchers, particularly in relation to protecting potential research participants, are essentially the same as those that guide nursing practice. These principles are set out in codes of conduct both nationally and internationally. In the UK, the Royal College of Nursing (RCN) provides specific guidance for research as it may relate to nurses involved in research in any way. Beauchamp and Childress (2013) identify four principles that guide ethical practice. Based on these, the ethical principles that are usually associated with research include: informed consent, **justice**, **non-maleficence**, **beneficence** and confidentiality.

- Informed consent: The researcher must be honest with participants and inform them about the study including the potential risks and benefits, as well as of their right to decide whether to participate or not, without any coercion, and to withdraw at any time.
- Veracity is the ethical principle of 'telling the truth'. This principle links to the need for researchers to consider how to establish a trusting relationship, and how they will respect the rights of participants. This includes a duty to **respect the autonomy** and dignity of participants.
- Justice: the principle of being 'fair' to participants and not giving preference to, or being discriminatory with, some participants over others. Being fair also means that the interests of participants must come before those of the researcher(s) and before the objectives of the study. Justice also requires that there is no abuse or exploitation of participants on the grounds of race, religion, sex, age, class or sexual orientation.
- Non-maleficence: the principle of 'doing no harm'. Essentially, it is a duty, wherever possible, to prevent physical, psychological, emotional, social and economic harms, though it is recognised that it will not always be possible to avoid harms and that some harms may be necessary to avoid other harms and promote an eventual good. The trauma associated with an operation, for example, is an acceptable harm provided that the anticipated outcome is recovery of health as far as this is possible.

There is also a duty to protect the weak, vulnerable and incompetent by adapting procedures and processes to take into account their vulnerabilities.

- Beneficence: the principle of 'doing good' for both research participants and society. The expectation is that research should aim to benefit the individual participants and society in general. The imperative of beneficence is to do good and prevent harm. Harm is defined as: whatever is bad for someone is harmful, and nothing is harmful unless it is bad for the one harmed. In healthcare, consideration must be given to patients' evaluation of the harmfulness of a proposed or actual intervention, irrespective of what is perceived to be the outcome of the intervention.

- Confidentiality: the ethical principle of 'safeguarding' the personal information which has been gathered in a study. This means that researchers should never report data about an individual without that individual's explicit permission. Additionally, researchers must explain to participants who will have access to their data and that sharing of data with others is only by an individual participant's explicit permission. Contained within this principle is also a duty to store data safely.

These principles can be used as a framework to critically appraise research and to examine the effects of research on the participants. You should, however, be aware that some research designs, as will be seen later, will need to have ethical issues considered in certain and more specific ways – for example, in some ethnographic studies, where crowd behaviour is being observed and the participants (i.e. members of the crowd) may not know they are being watched for the purposes of research and therefore have no choice about participating or not; in disseminating the research findings of **action research**, issues of confidentiality may be compromised; and in experimental research, a random selection might result in a voluntary group which is not representative of the target population, such as being better educated, of a higher social class or more socially involved.

In addition to the methods and procedures used in research, the topic being considered may also raise ethical concerns, such as research in the area of abuse or criminal activity, or with particularly vulnerable groups such as the very old, or people with a severe learning disability or severe mental illness. The challenge for readers of research or nurses undertaking research is to ensure that research evidence is produced ethically whilst at the same time employing good research practices.

INFORMED CONSENT TO PARTICIPATE

The first principle governing participation in research is informed consent. Consent is required prior to all involvement and this must be informed, voluntary and made by someone who has the capacity to consent. Some people who participate in research may be considered to be vulnerable for a variety of reasons. Some individuals may feel obligated to take part in a study because a researcher has power or perceived power, such as when the researcher is a member of the healthcare team. Others may have the capacity to give consent to participate, but find it difficult to withhold consent if they are put under implicit or explicit pressure. Individuals with learning disabilities or mental health problems, those who are frail and elderly or living in an institution such as a residential home or prison, may all be considered vulnerable, as may children and young people, and women who are pregnant. Furthermore, in theory at least, any individual can be considered to be vulnerable if they are in any way debilitated, and this means that any patient can be considered as being vulnerable in some respect.

Others may be vulnerable because they have limited ability to decide whether or not to participate in research due to difficulties in making a reasoned decision because they do not understand what is involved – for example, potential participants who do not speak the same language as the researcher, or have special language needs due to visual, hearing or learning impairments, or with concealed particular needs such as limited reading and writing ability. Some potential participants may be temporarily vulnerable, such as if they have just received bad news or are just about to receive treatment. Researchers must be sensitive to these issues and, when necessary, make specific arrangements when seeking to recruit such participants to ensure that they have appropriate and timely information, and in a medium that helps them understand what might be involved when deciding whether or not to participate.

Some adults may not have the capacity to give consent. There must be clear justification for researchers including such groups of participants in research, and they should never be asked to participate if the research could be equally undertaken with other adults. However, if a researcher wants to involve adults who lack the capacity to give consent, it should be limited to the areas of research related to their incapacity (see Chapter 7, Mental Capacity Act). A researcher will also need to demonstrate that the research could be of direct benefit to, or improve knowledge of, their health or that of people with the same state of health or the same incapacity. Furthermore, the researcher must establish that the individual has not expressed any objection, either verbally or physically, and that participation will not cause the participant emotional, physical or psychological harm. The risks to participants must be negligible and not interfere with their freedom of action or privacy.

Researchers may want to involve children and young people in research; however, as a potentially vulnerable group they must not be exploited. You need to remember that children will not always be able to express their own needs or protect themselves from harm, or make informed choices about being involved in research. Children are, however, capable of giving consent if they are deemed as 'Gillick' competent (also known as the principle of 'Fraser'). This means that children who are felt to be competent to understand the proposed research and make decisions on their own behalf can consent on their own behalf. A child may need extra time to understand what is involved and may need to be given an explanation of the research in a way that is appropriate to their level of understanding, such as by using pictures or video. If children and young people are not competent to give consent independently, then the consent of someone with parental responsibility must be obtained and, in addition, the child must not object to participation. The Children's Act 1989 sets out the legislation relating to consent and the responsibilities of parents when children are research participants.

Issues of vulnerability may apply when the researcher is in a position of power over potential participants. For example, nurses wanting to study care assistants they work with, or managers wanting to undertake research with their staff, will need to carefully consider whether their participants are in a potentially vulnerable position. Vulnerability in this context may be in terms of relationships with participants and issues of power and authority, or it may be because participants feel themselves to be in an obligatory position and, therefore, unable to make a fully autonomous decision whether to participate. There is also potential for coercion and, in some instances, peer pressure to participate. This can be particularly so when students want to research other students, or when staff undertake a course and want to research their work colleagues.

Including vulnerable individuals in research requires careful consideration, as excluding them from research may be a form of discrimination or may mean that some groups are not researched adequately. For example, excluding the elderly and/ or women of childbearing age from a drug trial may result in a lack of evidence about the drug's side-effects on these populations. This may be because of difficulties relating to consent or perceptions that specific groups should not be approached to participate because of their vulnerability, such as palliative care patients. It does, however, lead to a researcher having to justify why certain groups of people should be included in research. Consideration should be given to an individual's ability to comprehend the informa-tion given, but just as important are the form and nature of the explanation given, and the way that consent is obtained, particularly if participants are only intermittently competent to consent or have difficulty retaining information, such as individuals with dementia.

Nurse researchers must be fully aware of the issues of involving **vulnerable participants** and recognise that it is up to individual participants to decide whether or not to participate in research. The next section on informed consent considers how vulnerable participants can be included in research with due regard to their vulnerability.

Reflective exercise

Make a list of all the vulnerable groups you can think of. Are any of these likely to be involved with your research? How will you justify to a research ethics committee the need to include these vulnerable individuals in your proposed research?

OBTAINING INFORMED CONSENT

The consent of participants is accepted both legally and professionally *only* when a participant has been properly informed, has agreed without any coercion and is deemed competent to give consent.

Communicating clearly with potential participants in a form they can understand, and addressing their individual needs for receiving information, are key to the consent process. The information given to potential participants should either be written or in another appropriate format, such as an audio or video recording. Potential participants should be given the opportunity to ask questions, allowed adequate time to consider whether to take part, and given the opportunity to discuss with others if they wish. Only after this process should participants be asked to give written consent or another form of consent, such as video- or audio-recorded consent, if written consent is not possible. For some participants, ongoing consent is required. This applies particularly in longer studies, in research that has a number of stages or research that involves participants who may have difficulty retaining information. Figure 8.1 gives an indication of what research participants need to know before deciding to take part in a research project.

Preparing information that will enable potential participants to make an informed decision about whether to participate takes time and effort and should be built into the research process. Potential participants should be given information in the most suitable format to meet their individual needs, for example, written, audio/video recorded, using pictures or artwork, read aloud, using an interpreter and so on. The person discussing the information with the potential participant should not be in a position of power or authority where there could be coercion; if the researcher is in such a position, then someone else should be responsible for the information-giving and consent process. Wherever possible, an appropriate period of time, such as three to four days, should be allowed between giving the information and seeking written consent.

Participants should:

- know that they are being invited to take part in a research study
- have time to consider being involved and consult with family and friends if they want to
- be assured that they can decline to participate or withdraw at any time without giving a reason
- understand that their care, treatment, education or support will be unaffected whether they decide or not to participate, or if they withdraw at any point
- understand the purpose of the research
- know why they have been chosen
- understand what will happen to them if they agree to take part, for example: how long they will be involved, whether they need to do anything such as have an interview, keep a diary, give blood, complete a questionnaire, visit a clinic, take some medication, have a telephone interview, etc.
- understand any risks, costs, disadvantages and benefits
- know whether there will be any discomfort, or psychological or emotional distress
- understand how their confidentiality will be safeguarded, how their data will be collected and stored, e.g. anonymously, who will have access to the data, and how long it will be retained
- understand arrangements for any payments, expenses or benefits
- understand what will happen at the end of the study
- know who is organising and funding the study
- know who to contact for queries and for any complaints
- know the name of the Research Ethics Committee who reviewed the study
- have the opportunity to ask questions and receive full and honest answers

Figure 8.1   What research participants need to know before deciding to take part in a research project

Written information sheets should be non-technical and written in a language that is easily understood by a layperson. Short sentences and words should be used with clear subheadings and a font size that is easy to read. Bullet-point lists should be used when appropriate. The language should be appropriate to the intended audience, for example, patient, work colleague, student or manager. Where necessary, the information should be on appropriately headed paper such as that of the university or NHS Trust, and have a short self-explanatory title appropriate for a layperson. The tone of the information should be invitational and not overly persuasive or coercive. It should be clear that potential participants have free choice whether to accept or decline the invitation without any impact on their current or future care. The information sheet should be dated. An example of a participation information sheet for a nursing research study is given in Figure 8.2.

Participant information (this should be on headed notepaper)

1. **Study title:** Patient self-monitoring of bowel habits study

2. **Invitation paragraph**

   You are being invited to take part in a research study being conducted by the Practice Development Team at XXXX NHS Trust. Before you decide it is important for you to understand why the research is being done and what it will involve. Please take time to read the following information carefully and discuss it with others if you wish. Ask us if there is anything that is not clear or if you would like further information. Take time to decide whether or not you wish to take part. Thank you for reading this.

3. **What is the purpose of the study?**

   Constipation is a problem that can affect any individual at any time of life and ill health is likely to increase the risks of developing constipation.

   Although constipation is rarely life-threatening it can cause a variety of physical discomforts and have psychological and social consequences which may contribute to a reduction in a person's quality of life. The development of constipation and associated discomforts may also delay a patient's recovery leading to an increase in the associated risks, and for in-patients may result in longer hospitalisation.

   It is, however, known that there is often reluctance by some patients, and even some healthcare professionals, to discuss bowel function until it has become a significant problem. It has been suggested that an effective way of assessing patients' bowel function is by asking patients to self-record frequency, type of stool and whether there is any defecation discomfort. The idea is that self-recording is more likely to result in a more realistic record of bowel function and avoids patients having to discuss bowel function with a healthcare professional when there are no problems. It should also increase patients' understanding about what is considered 'normal' bowel function and act as a prompt for seeking advice when their bowel function is not normal.

   The aim of this study is to determine whether a patient-held bowel monitoring card is an effective way of monitoring bowel function for patients who are at risk of becoming constipated. We are doing this by asking some patients to use a Bowel Monitoring Card (BMC) to record their bowel movements for themselves. We will then compare the information on the BMC with that of the records of those patients who have not used the BMC.

   The study is being undertaken on a few wards at XXXX NHS Trust and with District Nursing Teams in XPCT.

(Continued)

Figure 8.2   (Continued)

4. **Why have I been chosen?**

You have been chosen because you are either a patient on one of the wards at XXXX NHS Trust or a patient of a District Nursing Team in XPCT taking part in the study.

5. **Do I have to take part in the research?**

It is up to you to decide whether or not to take part in the research. If you do decide to take part you will be given this information sheet to keep and be asked to sign a consent form. Even if you decide to take part you are free to withdraw at any time without giving a reason. A decision to withdraw at any time, or a decision not to take part, will not affect you in any way.

6. **What do I have to do?**

Complete and return a signed copy of the consent form. Then you just need to complete our questionnaire, put it in the addressed envelope provided, seal the envelope and give it back to a Ward Nurse or your District Nurse. Your Ward or District Nurse will then return your questionnaire with a copy of your bowel function record — this will be a bowel monitoring card or a copy of the part of your notes where your bowel function has been recorded. No other details will be taken from your healthcare records.

7. **What are the possible benefits of taking part?**

It is unlikely that you will gain any immediate benefit from taking part in this study; however, the information we get from this study may help us to improve the way patients' bowel function is recorded. This should help to improve the way patients' bowel function is monitored and help to highlight those patients who are at risk of developing constipation.

8. **Will my taking part in this study be kept confidential?**

All information received will be treated as confidential. Your name will not appear on the questionnaire; instead a code number will identify you. Questionnaire data will be input onto a datasheet that can be accessed via a password known only to the research team.

9. **What will happen to the results of the research study?**

The results of the study will be presented as a report to XPCT and XXXX and used to inform the development of effective bowel function monitoring. The findings will also be disseminated at conferences and in academic publications. As already mentioned, results will be reported in such a way that preserves confidentiality. It will be the responsibility of the research team to collect and analyse all data.

10. **What if I have any concerns?**

If you have any concerns or other questions about this study or the way it has been carried out you should contact the principal researchers:

MLG & EF — tel:.......................   or   email:.........................

Contact for further information:

MLG & EF

Governance Office, East Wing,

XXXX Hospital,

Thank you

MLG & EF

Figure 8.2   Example of a participant information sheet

For any researcher undertaking research with NHS patients, there is clear guidance for preparing information sheets on the Integrated Research Application System (IRAS), and the latest guidance should always be used. Even if your research does not involve patients, the IRAS website provides a good and readily understood guideline to follow when composing a participant information sheet.

Written consent should be obtained whenever possible, and if it is not possible there should be a justifiable reason. **Participant information** sheets and consent forms need to be prepared on separate sheets of paper, and participants should keep the information sheet and be given a copy of the consent form they signed.

Consent forms should record specific information on headed paper entitled 'Consent Form'; researchers are advised to use the format suggested by the IRAS, which includes the title of the project, the name and signature of the researcher and of the participant, and the date that consent is given. There should be tick-boxes for the participant to initial the following statements where appropriate:

- I have read the information sheet dated … and have had an opportunity to consider the information, ask questions and have had these answered satisfactorily.
- I understand that my participation is voluntary and that I am free to withdraw at any time without giving any reason, without my healthcare/education/work circumstances or legal rights being affected.
- I give permission for my medical records/work records/exam marks to be examined.
- I agree to my interview being audio-taped/video-taped.
- I understand that direct quotes may be used when the project is written up, although they will be anonymised.
- I agree to my doctor being informed of my participation.
- I agree to take part in the above study.

There are a few situations when implied consent can be used. This is most likely when a participant implies their consent by returning a questionnaire. In such cases, a letter of invitation to complete the questionnaire will be sent together with an information sheet to potential participants. It should be clear from the letter and the information sheet that returning the questionnaire implies consent and that a separate consent form is not required. The information sheet should contain all the information previously outlined. However, some ethics committees require researchers to obtain informed written consent prior to administration of a questionnaire.

ANONYMITY

Not using the names and addresses of participants and assigning each of them a unique study number can achieve **anonymity**. This process should be undertaken as close as possible to when data are collected. A list of the unique study numbers together with the individual's name should be kept separately and securely and not referred to unless there is specific need, such as a medical emergency, in order to ensure that the researcher cannot link data with a particular participant. This process is mainly for insurance purposes or for use in the case of a complaint where there may be a need to find out the study number of a particular participant. An ethics committee will expect an explanation about how data will be anonymised.

A common understanding in the NHS is that NHS-anonymised data are basically a 'free good'. For 'routine' uses of data, such as when conducting an audit, consent need not be 'explicit' under the Data Protection Act but can be 'implied'. However, obtaining data for research purposes is not usually considered a routine use and informed and explicit consent is nearly always required before researchers can access patient-identifiable records or data. Introducing anonymisation techniques before data are passed to a third-party researcher may be an option for some researchers, and this is allowable under the Data Protection Act. However, advice will be needed from an NHS Trust data protection officer and permission obtained from the R&D office.

In the UK, under Section 60 of the Health and Social Care Act 2001, the Secretary of State for Health is authorised to allow the processing of personal medical data for specific purposes without consent. This includes surveillance of communicable diseases, diagnosis and treatment of cancer and some limited research activity; however, support will be required from the Patient Information Advisory Group (PIAG) and researchers will need to discuss their project with them.

If a researcher wants direct access to patients' records to get names and addresses of patients to invite them to participate in a study, this can be a problem. Section 60 guidance makes it clear that either explicit informed consent is required to gain access or the researcher must apply to PIAG for Section 60 support. Alternatively, a clinician such as a doctor or nurse who is directly responsible for the patients could approach them to invite them to participate, thus avoiding the need for the researcher to have access to patients' confidential records.

Personal, fully non-reversible anonymised data should be used whenever possible by researchers, and it should be processed and stored appropriately for the purposes of a research project. In all other circumstances, explicit informed consent should be obtained at the very first stage, including consent to access the names and addresses of potential participants.

CONFIDENTIALITY

Participants in research have a right to expect that any information they provide will be treated confidentially and that any disclosure of information about them will only be done with their consent. There must be a clear understanding between the researcher and participant concerning the use that will be made of the data provided and how personal information will be stored. Participants must be given details, usually on the participant information sheet, of who will have access to their data other than the researcher, such as a supervisor or other research team members. Research participants should not be discussed beyond the needs of the project team and the data must be kept secure at all times. This is particularly important with data stored on a computer, and an ethics committee will normally expect electronic data to be password-protected. Access to the data should be restricted only to those people who have a legitimate reason to see it.

If confidentiality or anonymity cannot be guaranteed, participants must be told in advance before they agree to participate. For example, when interviewing nurses, a participant may reveal that they have made a drug error, or that they have a heavy drinking problem, or that they have witnessed another member of staff dealing in drugs, or have cheated in an exam. The researcher needs to make it clear on the information sheet that if, for example, criminal activity or issues of misconduct are revealed, then they will need to take some action. The action needs to be appropriate to the situation and risk, and could be, for example, encouraging them to speak to their line manager; encouraging them to phone a helpline; offering a counsellor; or reporting them to their line manager. This all needs to be made clear on the information sheet – although, of course, not everything a participant may reveal or be observed doing can be anticipated. If information needs to be disclosed in the public interest without a participant's consent (see Chapter 7), there must be a benefit to the individual or society that outweighs the individual's right to confidentiality.

DATA STORAGE, RETENTION AND SECURITY

Data collected during the process of research needs to be kept safely and with due regard to issues of confidentiality and anonymity as outlined above. Information on paper or disk/memory stick should be stored in locked, fireproof cabinets. Data entered and kept electronically should be password-protected, and have firewall, virus and spyware protection. Researchers need to consider how this will be achieved and if there are any cost implications for the project. Transporting data in cars and trains, for example, needs careful consideration not just to protect the confidentiality of participants' information, but also to protect the data collected in the research project and avoid the risk of having to repeat data collections.

The Data Protection Act (see Chapter 7) makes it clear that data must be fairly and lawfully processed, kept secure, accurate and up to date, adequate, relevant and not excessive. All this applies to research data; however, some types of data are exempt, such as data which has been anonymised and where the link between the data and the individual has been irreversibly broken so that the individual can never be identified, such as in the example of data that has been supplied by another organisation which has the code.

Data should be retained for the most appropriate time in which to facilitate realistic completion of a project, dissemination, any future analysis, and any potential claims for insurance purposes. Not all data needs to be retained; for example, once transcripts of audio-tapes are made, the original recording could be destroyed. Clinical research data used during clinical trials have to be kept for a specific length of time depending on the trial agreements. This is usually 15 years but can be longer. Other types of data should be stored for 5–10 years, but this is dependent on what data are to be kept, and is likely to be shorter for students on short courses such as Master's degrees, where the requirement may be to keep the data for only three years. Some forms of historical research may need to be kept much longer for justifiable reasons. The advice of the **research ethics committee** where the research is being reviewed is necessary to ensure that data are retained for an appropriate length of time, and provide for how it should be destroyed at the end of the project.

POTENTIAL HARM TO THE RESEARCHERS

Nurse researchers may be undertaking their research in unfamiliar environments or in private dwellings. This may put them in potentially risky situations, and requires some preparation to be done to reduce and control risks and minimise any anxieties that the researcher may have. Research managers may need to budget for the **safety of researchers** on a project, such as providing taxis, mobile phones, special training or counselling for staff researching difficult topics, or budgeting for extra time to allow researchers to work in pairs, or have overnight accommodation.

There may be potential risks in a research project that are more than the risks encountered in daily life. Clearly, each research project is different, but researchers need to consider whether there is a possibility, and the potential consequences, of causing physical or psychological harm to participants. For the researcher, risks of physical or psychological threats, abuse or trauma, increased risk of exposure to infections, accidents or harm and the possibility of researcher or participant being in a compromising position with a risk of accusation of inappropriate behaviour to either person must all be considered.

When interviews are to be conducted, then decisions about the site should reflect the need for the participant to feel comfortable and safe and whether a neutral area might be possible and safer for the researcher. For example, a researcher carrying a mobile phone and having arrangements in place to notify a colleague/office of their whereabouts can confirm safe arrival and departure from the interview site, as well as providing a reassuring 'lifeline' for a researcher. When appropriate, researchers should also work out how not to look 'out of place' and how best to keep valuables and equipment out of sight. It may also be worthwhile visiting unfamiliar environments before starting fieldwork to identify any specific risks. Researchers should not forget the tiring and emotional effects of interviewing and observing. Carrying identification related to the research and an employer which can be checked by participants may be necessary, and it is also worth considering whether local police should be informed if cold calling is involved.

During an interview, in particular, participants may become distressed or angry and researchers need to be able to spot the signs and be prepared to terminate an interview or take some other action; the health of the participants must come before the needs of the research. After interviewing, researchers, particularly inexperienced ones, may need a period of debriefing and, in some situations, counselling. There should certainly be a discussion and review of the fieldwork with a supervisor or other team member as to whether there were any safety issues or difficult situations to deal with, or things that needed to be done differently.

THE DUAL ROLE OF RESEARCHER AND NURSE

Nurses must always uphold the principles of their own code of conduct, as well as research-related codes and guidance. Nurses undertaking research should possess the relevant research skills and knowledge compatible with the demands of the proposed research, as with any other professional role, and this includes acknowledging any limitations of their ability.

All research is potentially exploitative and researchers' motives can be mixed with a blurring of roles. This is particularly so when the researcher is a healthcare professional such as a nurse, or is undertaking the research as part of career development. Nurses undertaking research may also feel that some of the tasks they perform, such as seeking consent and interviewing patients, are the same as in their normal nursing role, and this can lead to lack of thought and proper preparation for a research role.

Nurses must always make it clear to participants that they are undertaking a research project and that their role is that of a researcher, not a nurse/healthcare practitioner. This is particularly important when seeking consent, as patients could be easily coerced or misled into taking part in a research project by mistakenly thinking that it is all part of their nursing care. Furthermore, participants who see researchers as nurses may disclose too much, and this can create difficult situations for both the participant and researcher, particularly if the researcher is the 'normal' carer for the participant. Similarly, managers researching their own staff can get into difficult situations if participants are not fully aware of the role the manager is playing – researcher or manager – hence the importance of fully comprehensive participant information before seeking informed consent.

Reflective exercise

Make a list of the issues you could encounter when undertaking research in your own clinical area with either colleagues or patients/patient families.
A suggested list is given in Figure 8.3.

WHAT MEMBERS OF A RESEARCH ETHICS COMMITTEE ARE LOOKING FOR

This final section considers what an ethics committee will be looking for in an ethics application. All these points have been covered by earlier sections in this chapter and the list below could be used as an aide-memoire.

The application forms and associated papers such as research protocols, information sheets, consent forms, interview schedules and questionnaires should:

Researching colleagues

- Role becomes blurred – colleagues may assume that you are available to give advice/support when you are actually doing your research.
- Colleagues find it difficult to refuse to participate – this may be particularly the case if you are in a senior role.
- Colleagues may find it difficult to be completely honest/open with you – they may fear reprisals if they disclose 'data' that is controversial or puts others in a poor light.

Researching with patients

- Role becomes blurred – patients may find it difficult to separate your role as a researcher from that of their carer. Even if you are not a direct carer of the patients involved in your research, they will often find it difficult not to treat you as a nurse rather than a researcher and seek advice, etc.
- Patients find it difficult to refuse to participate:

  o they may feel an obligation to participate because you are part of their care team
  o they may even feel that they will receive inferior care if they refuse to participate.

- You may inadvertently coerce a patient to participate in your research by your actions/body language.
- Patients give you the answer that they think you want rather than being totally honest.

Figure 8.3   Suggested issues that may arise when researching in your own clinical area

- be written in language suitable for an intelligent layperson
- be free of grammatical and typographical errors
- provide a clear explanation about how the physical, psychological and emotional well-being of participants will be protected
- give clear descriptions of the potential health and safety issues for both participants and researchers, and what will be done about them
- give clear descriptions of how consent will be gained and how it will be recorded.

There should also be clear descriptions in the application and the participant information sheet of:

- how potential participants will be identified, approached and recruited
- any inclusion/exclusion criteria for participation
- any special groups that need justifying, which should include:

  o real and direct benefit to participants
  o foreseeable risks
  o foreseeable discomforts
  o others giving consent

- whether there will be any withholding of treatment or care from participants
- any procedures additional to normal care
- the length of time each individual will participate in the study
- any sensitive, embarrassing or upsetting questions

- any possibility of disclosures by participants and what will be done about this
- any risks and hazards, pain and discomfort to participants
- any benefit to participants
- any risks and hazards to researchers
- the length of time participants have to decide whether to take part
- what will happen if any information becomes available during the course of a project that may have an impact on the study
- whether a participant's general practitioner is being informed of their participation
- any payments or expenses due to participants and how they will claim them
- how results will be given to participants
- how data will be protected and stored, and for how long
- how the study is being funded
- who is sponsoring the study.

Information for participants should be provided in the most appropriate format, particularly for those who might not understand written or verbal explanations, or have special communication needs. This might be written, audio-taped or video-taped, for example, and for those participants unable to retain information it may need to be repeated. There may need to be accompanying letters of permission for access to organisations, and all information and interview schedules, questionnaires and research tools must be produced on headed notepaper.

CHAPTER SUMMARY

- All research should be undertaken ethically.
- Nurse researchers should be guided by ethical principles.
- Conducting research with vulnerable participants is ethically acceptable provided care and attention are given to their specific needs, particularly in respect of ensuring effective communication with them.
- Informed consent is a prerequisite for undertaking any research with human beings.
- Consent can only be informed if potential participants are given information in a form that they can understand and if it is prepared in a manner that meets their individual needs.
- NHS researchers should follow the guidelines from the National Research Ethics Service (NRES) in the content and format of information sheets and consent forms.
- Information/data given by participants to researchers should be anonymised as close as possible to when data are collected.
- Participants have a right to expect that any information they give to researchers will be treated confidentially and only disclosed with their full consent.
- Data must be stored safely and with due regard to issues of confidentiality and anonymity.
- Researchers and participants have an equal right to be protected from harm.

- Nurses must maintain awareness of the potential conflict of interests associated with the **dual role of practitioner and researcher**.
- Ethics committees are looking for evidence to confirm that any proposed research will be conducted ethically and have 'rules' about the information that researchers need to provide to them.

SUGGESTED FURTHER READING

Beauchamp, T.L. and Childress, J.F. (2013) *Principles of Biomedical Ethics*, 6th edn. Oxford: Oxford University Press. This is a detailed text and has become almost the prime book on biomedical ethics, including general ethical principals as well as research ethics. It is one for dipping in and out of on topics as they arise.

Acts (available on the HMSO website at: www.hmso.gov.uk/acts)

Children Act 1989
Data Protection Act 1998
Health and Social Care Act 2001
Human Rights Act 1998
Mental Capacity Act 2005
Public Interest Disclosure Act 1998

WEBSITES

British Educational Research Association: www.bera.ac.uk
British Psychological Association: www.bps.org.uk
British Sociological Association: www.britsoc.co.uk
Economic and Social Research Council: www.esrc.ac.uk
Integrated Research Application System (IRAS): www.myresearchproject.org.uk
International Council of Nurses: www.icn.ch
Medical Research Council: www.mrc.ac.uk
Royal College of Nursing: www.rcn.org.uk

To access further resources related to this chapter, visit the companion website at https://study.sagepub.com/mouleaveyard3e.

REFERENCES

Beauchamp, T.L. and Childress, J.F. (2013) *Principles of Biomedical Ethics*, 7th edn. Oxford: Oxford University Press.

9
DEVELOPING RESEARCH QUESTIONS

Learning outcomes

This chapter will enable you to:

- understand the importance of having a research question
- understand the origins of a good research question
- recognise the steps involved in developing a research question
- understand the differences between research questions, aims and objectives

Every research project begins with an idea or set of ideas. These ideas will generally arise from clinical practice and usually stem from situations or experiences which you would like to know more about or better understand. They may prompt you to ask questions such as:

- Why does this happen?
- Is it possible to stop or prevent this from happening?
- Does this happen anywhere else?
- Is the effect of this different from the effect of something else?

When reflecting on nursing practice, situations or experiences, the following types of question may be prompted:

- Is it possible to improve the way I/we do this?
- Is there a way I can do this more quickly/less expensively/less painfully?
- Are my/our patients satisfied with the care I/we give?
- Is what we do effective compared to other options?

Turning these broad ideas into a researchable focused question is the first stage of the research process. A common misconception is for novice researchers to equate the breadth of a research project with its value. In reality, research questions need to be very focused; a lack of focus often results in broad and unmanageable questions and, hence, over-ambitious research proposals which lack sufficient depth. The purpose of this chapter is to help guide you in how you can translate a broad query into a question that can be answered by undertaking a research study.

GETTING STARTED – GENERATING RESEARCH QUESTIONS

Research is about finding answers to questions, but where do these questions come from? The terms 'research problem' and 'research question' can be confusing:

- A **research problem** can be defined as a broad topic area of interest that has perplexing or troubling aspects which can be 'solved' by the accumulation of relevant information or evidence.
- A **research question** is more concise and is a description of exactly what issues the research intends to acquire information about.

For example, if a nurse is concerned about the healing of wounds in patients with burns, then this is the research problem. This is a very broad topic and needs to be narrowed down to a manageable focus. The following research questions could be developed from this research problem: 'Does patient mobility have an effect on the rate of healing in patients with lower-limb burns?' or 'To what extent does mobility affect the rate of wound healing in patients with lower-limb burns?' Alternatively, research around this topic could be expressed as a problem statement: 'The purpose of this study is to examine the effect of patient mobility on the rate of wound healing in patients with lower-limb burns.'

A good research question is one that is clearly expressed and focused on a researchable problem (key components of a research question are given in Figure 9.1). A research question or problem statement may be further amplified through an aim that serves to give a more direct focus to the significant and relevant issue which is to be researched. This may be necessary because a research question is expected to be short, precise and direct. In some types of research, a **hypothesis** is used, instead of a research question, to attempt to answer a question and predict an outcome. These terms will be discussed in more detail later in this chapter.

A **research aim** is, in effect, a description of exactly what issues the research intends to address. It is a broad statement that often uses words such as examine, describe, explore, and so on. Using the earlier example of wound healing, the aim might be: 'To investigate whether mobility promotes healing in patients with lower-limb burns.'

Research objectives are a way of breaking down a research aim into more manageable sections. It is likely that a research study will have an overall aim and a number of objectives which explain how the research question will be answered.

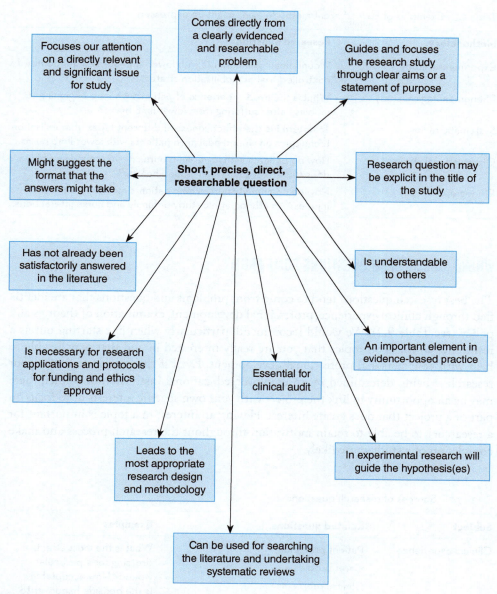

Comes directly from a clearly evidenced and researchable problem

Focuses our attention on a directly relevant and significant issue for study

Guides and focuses the research study through clear aims or a statement of purpose

Might suggest the format that the answers might take

Short, precise, direct, researchable question

Research question may be explicit in the title of the study

Has not already been satisfactorily answered in the literature

Is understandable to others

Is necessary for research applications and protocols for funding and ethics approval

Essential for clinical audit

An important element in evidence-based practice

Leads to the most appropriate research design and methodology

In experimental research will guide the hypothesis(es)

Can be used for searching the literature and undertaking systematic reviews

Figure 9.1 Key components of the research question

In addition, for some types of research, the research question can be expressed in a particular way so that it indicates the methodological approach being used. Table 9.1 shows how use of the different methodologies might be expressed for research on the wound healing topic:

Table 9.1   Examples of how different methodologies might be expressed

Methodology	Research question
Experimental study	Wound healing in patients with lower-limb burns: A randomised controlled trial of mobilisation strategies.
Phenomenological study	What is the lived experience of patients who are beginning to mobilise after suffering from lower-limb burns?
Systematic review	To determine the effectiveness of different types of mobilisation techniques on wound healing in patients with lower-limb burns.
Observational study	How do patients with lower-limb burns move around and how does this affect the rate of wound healing?
Ethnographic study	How do community nurses help patients mobilise after burn injuries? An ethnographic study of family and nurse interactions.

WHERE DO RESEARCH QUESTIONS COME FROM?

The best research questions tend to come from problems and questions that are identified through clinical experience, professional development, examination of theories and policy (see Table 9.2). We would recommend, particularly when just starting out as a researcher, to focus on topics that you are really interested in and that may be able to help with your personal professional development. Even if the general topic for your research is being determined by an employer, educational institution or funder, there may be an opportunity to link the project with your own specific interests or to focus on part of a project that does create interest. Having an interest in a topic is important for a researcher to be able to retain motivation throughout the research process and make completion of a study more likely.

Table 9.2   Sources of research questions

Subject	Related questions	Examples
Clinical experience	Patient problems Carer problems Clinical problems Patterns and trends Frequently occurring problems Effectiveness outcomes New roles High incidence Prevalence Costly procedures	What is the most effective dressing for a particular wound? How acceptable is the bedside handover to patients? Do nurses comply with infection control procedures?

Subject	Related questions	Examples
Professional development	New approaches, e.g. interprofessional learning Behavioural change Preparation for new roles Student problems Evaluation of courses, conferences and literature Identifying new areas for research Programmes of research identified by NHS Trusts	What is the best way of retaining student nurses? What are the educational needs of modern matrons? Are short intense full-time cardiac care courses better than longer part-time courses? What are the benefits of nurses learning together with doctors and social workers?
Policy imperatives	National initiatives Consensus activities National priorities Local service delivery National Service Frameworks Clinical guidelines Nursing policies Health and social care policies Public health policies	The effect of policy changes on the health needs of asylum seekers; the impact of a National Service Framework on staff training needs; the nature of school nursing following the new public health policies.
Theoretical frameworks	Theory testing Theory development Replication studies Validation of tools Methodological testing	Validation of a post-operative pain assessment tool for young children; testing a Finnish care dependency scale in British nursing homes; evaluating the validity, reliability and readability of a critical care family needs assessment tool.
Other sources	Unusual or unanticipated events, e.g. ebola crises; new phenomena; radiation leak; violent event; natural disasters such as floods and storms	The long-term health needs of survivors of an earthquake; the impact of contaminated food products on mothers' attitudes to breastfeeding; post-traumatic stress disorder in older victims of crime.

Clinical experience

Clinical experience could involve problems you face in clinical practice, such as why particular patients are reluctant to take their medication; concerns about how best to break bad news to carers; an observation that male surgical patients seem to mobilise more quickly than female patients, even though they have the same type of surgery; a concern that patients who complain appear to receive less attention from nurses than patients who don't complain; an interest in the difference between a specialist nurse and an advanced nurse practitioner; an observation that MRSA appears to be increasing in a particular area; wondering what happens to patients who are discharged early. Clinical experience is a key source of research questions that interest nurses because it is based on their everyday work experience.

Professional development

Professional development issues may also be a rich source of topics for nursing research, and these could lead to questions such as whether interprofessional learning leads to enhanced patient care, whether e-learning is as effective as more traditional learning styles in terms of student knowledge outcomes or whether degree entry to nursing impacts on student nurse recruitment. Professional development issues can be a key source of research questions but they are a step away from clinical practice issues.

Policy imperatives

Another rich source for research questions may come from policy imperatives. These might be associated with, for example, health policy, health and social care policy, nursing policy or even international policy. In these cases, an organisation such as the Department of Health or the Royal College of Nursing may advertise that they want research in particular areas, and they often identify problems or concerns that need to be answered through research. This is sometimes called 'an invitation to tender' and can be highly competitive. For example, Department of Health Research Programmes driven by policy imperatives have previously wanted research undertaken in the areas of in-patient discharge procedures; information needs of patients; urban community hospitals; the relationship between A&E and Primary Care; the outcomes and effectiveness of rehabilitation programmes for patients being looked after at home; and patients' and carers' social needs. The Research for Patient Benefit (RfPB) programme is intended to provide a real opportunity for projects to emerge out of healthcare practice and to be designed to improve that practice. Whilst it does not deliberately specify topics to be covered, applicants need to ensure that a clear case is made of the potential for patient and/or public benefit arising from the study. Alongside rigorous research designs and methodologies, they also look for dissemination strategies that will enhance the likelihood that the results can be rolled out within the NHS.

Clinical guidelines such as those produced by the National Institute for Health and Care Excellence (NICE) are likely to identify areas where further research is needed because they have found minimal evidence.

For novice researchers looking for a topic to research, clinical guidelines produce a rich source of ideas that are topical. Such guidelines are based on a systematic literature review of previous research on the topic and will identify where there are shortfalls in the evidence base and suggest where further research is needed.

Theoretical frameworks

Some researchers are interested in developing theory in a particular area. The research questions they seek to answer might be about testing an existing theory or developing a new theory. Such theories may have arisen from the work of other disciplines such as sociology or psychology, but may need to be tested in practice. Part of this might be about validating a particular data collection tool to ensure that it measures the phenomena accurately, reliably and without bias. Or it may be about examining the uses of different theoretical perspectives in practice. For example, Melendez-Torres et al. (2015) undertook a systematic review to explore the range of approaches to qualitative data synthesis in recently published systematic reviews.

Other sources

Research questions might also be developed from events that are unpredicted or accidental. The effects of a salmonella outbreak in a small community might interest school and public health nurses.

Conferences and networking

Attending a conference on a particular topic, such as cancer nursing, exposes nurses to cutting-edge research. Some presentations will conclude with new research questions that need to be answered, or areas/topics that need further research may become apparent in the course of the presentation. Likewise, many published research studies will identify further research questions that need to be addressed. This can be a very useful way of generating research questions as they come directly from research that is topical and has a good evidence foundation.

Discussion with experts and leaders in a particular field is also likely to lead to useful research questions. Healthcare professionals may be able to identify specific questions that need researching to help build up expertise in a particular area as well as support the research remit of an organisation.

Reflective exercise

Think of issues/problems that are currently impacting on your own practice and identify their source.

FINDING THE RESEARCH QUESTION IN PUBLISHED STUDIES

Despite the fact that all research studies have a research question, it can be difficult to find the question clearly expressed in published literature. In the literature, it is more common to find specified aims and objectives, or a hypothesis may be presented. This may be because the publisher has word limits for articles and the authors try to be succinct in their writing. Research studies, however, need a research question to guide the whole research process – it is the starting point. Furthermore, the research question will be one of the first things that need to be formulated in a research proposal, an application proposal for funding and an application to a research ethics committee.

A simple examination of recently published studies in high-quality research journals can indicate how authors describe their research problem and specify the focus of their research. In Table 9.3, some recently published studies have been identified to demonstrate the ways in which authors use research questions, research aims and research objectives. In all cases, the authors' exact words are used. In addition to the aims or objectives and research questions (when provided), the title of the article is given to demonstrate how they link together.

It can be seen from these examples that the range is large and that some studies clearly express what the research is trying to find, whilst in others it is not so obvious. For example, it is not clear in Allen et al.'s (2015) study which outcomes are considered in the research. Furthermore, some titles of published articles are nearly the same as the research questions, whereas in others they differ. In some cases, there is also an indication of the research methodology adopted, such as Jiang et al. (2015) include 'systematic review' and 'meta-analysis' in their title to indicate that the approach to analysis that they used in their systematic review. Allen et al. (2015) also refer to the use of a cohort study in the title of their paper. Bahorski et al. (2015) refer to a randomised factorial study.

Table 9.3   Examples of research questions in recently published literature

Title of published article	Research question, aim or objectives	Authors
Changes in use, knowledge, beliefs and attitudes relating to tobacco among nursing and physiotherapy students: A 10 year analysis.	**Research question**: not specifically identified **Aim**: To analyse changes in prevalence, knowledge, beliefs and attitudes relating to smoking among undergraduate nursing and physiotherapy students over a 10 year period.	Ordas et al. (2015)
Systematic review of decreased intracranial pressure with optimal head elevation in post-craniotomy patients: A meta-analysis	**Research question:** not specifically identified **Aim:** to determine an optimum head elevation degree to decrease intracranial pressure in post-cranial patients by meta-analysis	Jiang et al. (2015)

Title of published article	Research question, aim or objectives	Authors
Does the quality of life construct as illustrated in quantitative measurement tools reflect the perspective of people with dementia?	**Research question:** Does the quality of life construct as illustrated in quantitative measurement tools reflect the perspective of people with dementia? **Aim:** to discuss the extent to which people with dementia's perspectives on quality of life have been included in quantitative research.	Harding et al. (2015)
Are patient–nurse relationships in breast cancer linked to adult attachment style?	**Research question:** Are patient–nurse relationships in breast cancer linked to adult attachment style? **Aim:** to ascertain if patients with breast cancer who have positive attachment models of 'self' and 'other' perceive higher levels of support from nurses than do patients with negative attachment models.	O'Rourke et al. (2015)
Does the model of maternity care make a difference to birth outcomes for young women? A retrospective cohort study.	**Research question:** Does the model of maternity care make a difference to birth outcomes for young women? **Objective:** To determine if caseload midwifery or young women's clinics are associated with improved perinatal outcomes when compared with standard care.	Allen et al. (2015)
Mitigating procedural pain during venepuncture in a pediatric population: A randomised controlled factorial study.	**Research question:** not specifically identified. **Objectives:** To determine if there was a difference in the perceived pain associated with a venepuncture in a group of pediatric patients based on the preparatory intervention used during the procedure, and to determine if age, sex or ethnic group were associated with the effectiveness of the preparatory interventions used.	Bahorski et al. (2015)

DEVELOPING A RESEARCH QUESTION

As we have just seen, it can be difficult to find research questions clearly stated within published literature. However, researchers need to be able to clearly express the research question(s) and, usually, they will also identify aims and objectives, although as Table 9.3 indicates, sometimes the terms 'aims' and 'objectives' are used interchangeably.

A good research question is clear and focused and is based on a researchable problem. A common difficulty when trying to explain what problem is to be addressed is to

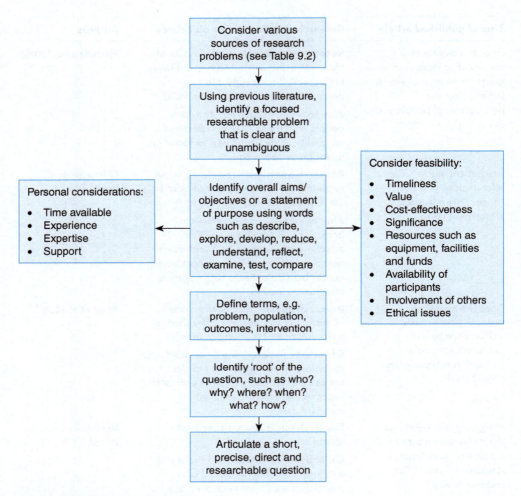

Figure 9.2　Building up a research question

think 'too big' and try to do too much in a single research study. The research question should be very narrow and 'small'. Consider the difference between the broader question: 'Does mobility influence wound healing in patients with lower-limb burns?' and the more focused question: 'In 12- to 16-year-old young people, what is the effect of a "supported walking" programme, of 30 minutes per day, on the rate of wound infection of lower-limb burns?'

Background information, brief details of previous research that identify the problem and an underlying rationale as to why it is an important question to answer, will all support the research question. However, actually formulating a question can be troublesome, and it can be quite difficult to get the length of the question right. There is a need to find a balance between being succinct and trying to get everything fully detailed in the question. Identifying the key elements and then moving them around so that they make sense can help the development of a research question. The example given earlier in this chapter includes 'rate of wound healing', 'mobility' and 'patients with lower-limb burns'. Focusing on these elements will assist in determining exactly what question the research is attempting to answer.

Figure 9.2 suggests a number of stages in developing both research questions and research aims and objectives. At this stage, it is also worth remembering that the research question and the title of the research will not necessarily be the same, and it is not unusual to have a short working title for headings on information sheets and so on, reserving the use of the full research question for the full research proposal.

Having identified what problem(s) the research will address, or focus on, the problem needs to be clearly articulated. When asked by an interested colleague, you, as a researcher, need to be able to succinctly answer the question 'What is the research problem?' If you cannot do this, then further background work needs to be undertaken by looking at the literature and other research.

When preparing research questions, and ultimately research aims, it helps to consider personal constraints, such as how much time is available, how much experience and expertise are needed and what support is available. At this stage, you should also think about:

- the feasibility of undertaking the study, that is, will it actually be possible to conduct this research study?
- the availability of participants
- what resources will be required
- the availability of necessary equipment and facilities
- how others will be involved, including service users
- ethical issues.

Remember that the significance of a research study may have an impact on the responses of others to the proposed research and may even determine whether it will be possible to get the necessary co-operation and resources required. It is also worth seeking advice from more experienced researchers at this early stage on any of the above aspects, as well as enlisting their help in devising the research question.

Tools to assist in the development of research questions

There are a variety of tools available that may help in the development of research questions. One of the most well known is the PICO framework: Problem, Intervention, Comparison, Outcomes (Straus et al., 2010). This framework is often used to frame questions when searching for evidence of a quantitative nature. If PICO were applied to the earlier example, we might end up with a question such as: 'For young people aged 12–16 with lower-limb burns (*problem*), does a supported walking programme of 30 minutes a day (*intervention*) when compared with bed rest (*comparison*) increase the rate of wound healing and reduce rates of infection (two *outcomes*)?'

Although PICO was originally designed as a tool to assist the development of questions of a quantitative nature, it has been adapted for use with qualitative research questions, where Intervention is replaced by Issue and Comparison is replaced by

Context. For example, 'What factors (*outcome*) contribute to the uptake of smoking (*issue*) in young people (*population*) looked after by the state (*context*)'

There are other frameworks that can be used to help formulate research questions (McKeon and McKeon, 2015). The important point to remember is that these frameworks are only a guide – they can help the researcher shape the question but will not provide ideas and justification for a good research question and are hence only useful in the later stages of research question development.

Another activity that can help with framing research questions is to consider words such as: who, why, where, when, how and what. These can be extended to phrases such as: To what extent …? How do …? What are …? This is particularly useful in qualitative research, which by its nature has a more open and 'holistic' approach in its methods.

Prioritising research questions

Sometimes research questions need to be prioritised. This can help in determining what is the most important thing to study and can be of benefit, particularly for the novice researcher, when undertaking a time-limited project. One way to prioritise is to consider the following:

1. level or degree of importance to patients', clients' or participants' well-being
2. most feasible question to answer in the time available
3. most interesting question
4. most likely to be a recurring problem in own practice
5. level or degree of importance to nursing
6. most likely to produce recommendations that can be implemented
7. there may be other aspects such as cost, ethical considerations, accessibility to facilities and/or participants or policy imperatives that need to be taken into consideration.

RESEARCH AIMS AND OBJECTIVES

Once the research question is explicit, it is possible to begin to specify research aims and objectives. Traditionally, the research aims describe the overall purpose of a project and research objectives describe the individual tasks that need to be carried out in order to meet the aims. However, as identified in Table 9.3, aims and objectives are often used interchangeably in research papers.

Research aims are usually quite broad and will summarise the overall goal of the research and maybe identify key variables (see later in this chapter). They are developed from the clearly articulated research problem or question.

Specifying overall aims can be aided by using words such as describe, explore, reduce, and so on. It is also useful to define specific terms such as the type of problem (lower-limb burns and healing), population or sample (young people aged 12–16 years), and outcome (rate of wound infection or increased healing rate). If the study is looking at a particular intervention, then this too will need to be defined (supported walking programme of 30 minutes per day).

Objectives are usually a way of giving detail based on a research aim or a 'statement of purpose'. Objectives are often statements that are more specific and broken down into smaller researchable chunks. These might be called objectives or they might be worded as smaller research questions. Rather than debate the difference between aims, objectives and questions, it is important to recognise that each research study should have a clear research question(s) that is short, precise, direct, researchable, and that drives the study.

HYPOTHESES

In some types of research, a hypothesis, or hypotheses, are used to drive the research. The main types of research using hypotheses will be deductive studies that are trying to test a theory. These are normally studies that take a quantitative approach and most commonly, but not exclusively, will be experimental studies.

A hypothesis attempts to answer a question which has emerged from a research problem. A hypothesis goes further than a research question and predicts an outcome. This can make it a very powerful tool, as will be seen in Chapter 14. As well as predicting an outcome, a hypothesis is a statement about the relationship between two or more variables. The hypothesis statement will go as far as predicting the relationship between variables and, through testing the hypothesis, may or may not support the theory. There are two types of variables used in hypotheses: independent and dependent variables. Independent variables are those seen as a 'cause', which might be an intervention or treatment, whilst dependent variables are seen as the 'effect' or outcome. This is commonly phrased as a 'cause-and-effect relationship'.

Using the earlier example, the independent variable would be 'supported walking for 30 minutes' and the dependent variable would be 'wound healing rate'. Because hypotheses are expressed clearly with all the variables identified explicitly, we might end up with a hypothesis such as:

> Young people, aged 12–16 years, with more than 20 per cent lower-limb burns who have a supported walking programme of 30 minutes per day will have a reduced wound size within 10 days of injury compared to those who are placed on bed rest for 10 days following injury.

In this example, the supported walking programme and bed rest are the independent variables (cause) and wound size (effect) is the dependent variable.

A hypothesis can also be stated as a 'null' hypothesis, which begins 'There is no difference …'. The null hypothesis states that there is no relationship between variables. It is used predominantly in research where there are to be tests of statistical significance (see Chapter 26). Hypotheses are never 'proved' or 'disproved'; rather they are supported or unsupported, accepted or rejected by the data.

Chapter 14 explains in more detail how hypotheses are used in experimental design studies but, for the purposes of thinking about the research question, it is important to note how hypotheses are much more detailed and specific, and how they will predict an outcome. The hypothesis is the bridge between the research problem, as identified from a review of the literature, the research question and an appropriate research design.

Defining the variables

A variable is a characteristic that varies between individuals and can be measured, such as weight, age and gender. Some of the examples given earlier are variables: young people aged 12–16, wound healing and bed rest. Variables can change or be changed depending on the design of the study. They can be studied in isolation or in combination, depending on the design of the study. During the course of a study, a new variable may arise which could affect the data collected. Variables are used in different types of research including experimental designs, surveys, correlational studies and epidemiological research. As noted earlier, it is important to define the specific terms, including the variables, that are to be included in a study and express them precisely in the research question, aims or objectives.

FEASIBILITY

As stated earlier, and as can be seen in Figure 9.2, it is essential at this early stage of the research process to consider the feasibility of the proposed study at the same time as identifying the research question. Any proposed study needs to be timely, and whether it is a good time to undertake such a study will become evident from your reading around a proposed research topic. It must be self-evident that the research question being considered has not already been answered and that it is still relevant. At the same time, it must also be clear that there is value in trying to answer the question through the proposed study, that the study will be cost-effective, that it is significant and that resources are available to conduct the study. One key resource is the availability of participants for a proposed study. There is no point posing valuable and significant research questions if access to participants is near impossible. In preparing the research question, it is also important to involve others, particularly service users, patients and carers. You may think your research question is important and should be answered by undertaking a research study but your patients may have different priorities that need to be considered. Similarly, when a research topic does not readily fit in with an institution's research priorities there may be problems in getting permission to conduct the research. Furthermore, when you need to seek funding for a research project it is worth considering whether the research topic will match any potential funders' research priorities.

Whether a proposed research study is feasible is also determined by ethical considerations. Chapter 8 provides an overview of the ethical principles that need to be considered when conducting research. However, it is essential that any proposed research starts from the premise of being based on sound ethical principles. Any ethics committee (NHS, social services or university) will expect a clearly set out main research question and any other **secondary research** questions. All proposals and protocols prepared for potential funders will also require explicit research questions. The research question is thus crucial.

THE LINK BETWEEN THE RESEARCH QUESTION AND METHOD USED

Research questions should drive the chosen methodology for a research study. In the earlier example, there is an indication of what type of methodology might be used to answer the question. A hypothesis would lead to thinking of an experiment such as a randomised controlled trial comparing different types of mobilisation (bed rest or walking for 30 minutes). A question such as 'How do patients move following lower-limb burns and how does this influence wound healing?' might lead to an observation type of study that also has some wound measurement component. A research question such as 'Why are some patients better able to mobilise than others?' would prompt a study involving interviews with different groups of patients, whereas a research question such as 'What is the lived experience of mobilising after lower-limb burns?' suggests a phenomenological study (see Chapter 15 for an explanation of this type of research).

In other chapters in this book, there are debates about how the research may be driven by the particular beliefs of the researcher and how it may lead to the asking of particular research questions that will be answered by a particular approach to the research. For example, a researcher with a scientific background might pose a research question that leads to the prediction of a specific outcome (a hypothesis) and an experimental study. Conversely, a researcher influenced by interpretivism/naturalism might pose a research question and suggest a methodology where the researcher and the researched are not objectively separated, such as in action research.

This chapter has focused on developing the research question at the beginning of the research process and then designing an appropriate study to answer the question or meet the aims of the study. Although the background, experience and expertise of the researcher are clearly important, it is the research question that should drive the research. In a profession such as nursing, that has broad interests and is influenced by a wide range of paradigms, it is inevitable that an eclectic approach to research will be embraced. However, it is crucial that a research design should be chosen to answer the research question, not the research question adapted to fit the study design.

Reflective exercise

Can you develop a research question that would answer a current issue/problem in your clinical practice? Remember not to try to solve everything in one question; if need be, focus on one aspect of the problem/issue.

CHAPTER SUMMARY

- A clearly defined problem or gap in current knowledge is an important prerequisite for any research and this is framed in the form of a research question.
- Developing a research question is the first stage in the research process.

- The research question:

  o identifies a gap in knowledge or a problem
  o focuses attention on directly relevant and significant issues that need to be researched
  o guides and focuses the research study
  o leads to an appropriate research design.

- The research question can be used for literature searching and undertaking systematic reviews and provides guidance for clinical audit.
- The research question enables ethics review bodies and funding organisations to identify whether a study is justifiable and worth doing.
- Sources for research questions include clinical experience, professional issues, theoretical frameworks and policy imperatives.
- A research aim is a description of the intention or broad purpose of the research.
- Research objectives explain how the research question will be answered.
- A hypothesis is a statement of the expected relationship between or among the things being studied; it goes further than a research question and predicts an outcome.
- A variable is an 'object' that is being investigated in a research study and is considered to be capable of varying.
- A good research question is one that is clearly expressed and focused on a researchable problem.
- The research question is the driver for the choice of research methodology and design.

Journals with good examples of research questions, aims, objectives and hypotheses

- *Clinical Effectiveness in Nursing*
- *Health and Social Care in the Community*
- *International Journal of Nursing Studies*
- *Journal of Advanced Nursing*
- *Nurse Education in Practice*
- *Nurse Education Today*
- *Nurse Researcher*
- *Nursing Research*

WEBSITES

Department of Health: www.dh.gov.uk – has details about research funded by the Department of Health and any invitations to tender for new projects under their R&D pages.

Medical Research Council: www.mrc.ac.uk – includes opportunities for projects funded by the Medical Research Council.

National Institute for Health and Care Excellence: www.nice.org.uk – for details of published clinical guidelines and those in progress, and how to develop guidelines.

National Institute for Health Research Central Commissioning Facility: www.nihr.ac.uk/about/central-commissioning-facility.htm – gives guidance on the aims and scope for applications to the Research for Patient Benefit programme.

RDInfo: www.rdinfo.org.uk – for guidance on how to start a research project, including a flow chart that guides the reader through turning an idea into a research question.

Service Delivery and Organisation Programme: www.sdo.nihr.ac.uk – has details of research about the NHS Service Delivery and Organisation research programme. Also available is a checklist for researchers who are preparing proposals, with a section on research questions and research objectives.

To access further resources related to this chapter, visit the companion website at https://study.sagepub.com/mouleaveyard3e

REFERENCES

Allen, J., Gibbons, K., Beckmann, M., Tracy, M., Stapleton, H. and Kildea, S. (2015) 'Does model of maternity care make a difference to birth outcomes for young women? A retrospective study', *International Journal of Nursing Studies*, 52: 1332–42.

Bahorski, J.S., Hauber, R.P., Hanks, C., Johnson, M., Mundy, K., Ranner, D., Stoutamire, B. and Gordon, G. (2015) 'Mitigating procedural pain during venipuncture in a pediatric population: A randomised controlled trial', *International Journal of Nursing Studies*, 52 (10): 1553–64.

Harding, R., Beesley, H., Holcombe, C., Fisher, J. and Salmon, P. (2015) 'Are patient–nurse relationships in breast cancer linked to adult attachment styles?', *Journal of Advanced Nursing*, 71 (10): 2305–14.

Jiang, Y., Ye, Z.P., You, C., Hu, X., Liu, Y., Hao, L. and Lin, S. (2015) 'Systematic review of decreased intracranial pressure with optimal head elevation in post-craniotomy patients: A meta-analysis', *Journal of Advanced Nursing*, 71 (10): 2237–46.

McKeon, J. and McKeon, P. (2015) 'PICO: A hot topic in evidence based practice', *International Journal of Athletics Therapy and Training*, 20 (1): 1–3.

Melendez-Torres, G.J., Grant, S. and Bonell, C. (2015) 'A systematic review and critical appraisal of qualitative metasynthetic practice in public health to develop a taxonomy of operations of reciprocal translation', *Research Synthesis Methods*. DOI 10.1002/jrsm.1161.

O'Rourke, H., Fraser, K., Duggleby, W. (2015) 'Does the quality of life construct as illustrated in quantitative measurement tools reflect the perspective of people with dementia', *Journal of Advanced Nursing*, 71 (8): 1812–24.

Ordas, B., Fernandez, D., Ordonez, C., Marques-Sanchez, P., Alvarez, M.J., Martinez, S. and Pinto, A. (2015) 'Changes in use, knowledge and beliefs and attitudes relating to tobacco among nursing and physiotherapy students: A 10 year analysis', *Journal of Advanced Nursing*, 11 (10): 2326–37.

Straus, S.E., Galsziou, P., Richardson, W. and Haynes, R.B. (2010) *Evidence-based Medicine: How to Practice and Teach EBM*, 4th edn. New York: Churchill Livingstone.

10
WRITING A RESEARCH PROPOSAL

Learning outcomes

The chapter will enable you to:

- Understand the steps involved in preparing a research proposal
- Appreciate the role of a research proposal as a mechanism for applying for research funding
- Discuss the probable content of a research proposal
- Understand the function and details of full economic costing

Nurse researchers are often required to submit a **research proposal** for a variety of audiences and student nurses can be asked to provide a research proposal as a basis for their dissertation. These can include proposals for local research monies or development opportunities, those sent in response to external funding calls, to meet ethical approval requirements or as part of academic assessment requirements. Frequently, proposals are required when seeking staff development funding support for academic study, such as for Master's and doctoral-level study. Though many of the elements discussed in this chapter may have some relevance for potential doctoral students, they are specifically directed at students writing a dissertation proposal and those responding to a competitive tendering process in order to secure research monies to complete a specific piece of research.

In developing a research proposal the nurse needs to consider how best to prepare the application and make decisions about its content. University-based researchers responding to calls from external bodies will also need to consider using **full economic costing** packages to generate predicted project costs.

In this chapter, we outline the steps involved in preparing to submit a research proposal for a dissertation and for funding. We review the likely structure such a proposal would follow, identifying key information that might be provided to support an application. We also discusses the use of 'full economic costing' to cost research undertaken by universities.

PREPARING A DISSERTATION OR PROJECT PROPOSAL

As part of undergraduate or postgraduate studies students are often required to prepare a research project plan or dissertation proposal, often preceding the execution of the project. In preparing a project plan you will need to meet any assessment criteria and address assignment guidelines. In particular you might be asked to think about the following:

- What problem will you look at?
- Are there specific questions to answer?
- What does the literature tell you about the current related research and understanding of the issue?
- Will you involve the public in your study?
- How will you answer your question? What type of research approach/design will you use?
- Are there any ethical and research governance issues to address?
- How will you collect and analyse data?
- How will you disseminate your findings?
- What will your plan of work be and timetable for completion?
- Are there any cost issues associated with the study?

The problem

It is possible that, through your experiences of care delivery as either an undergraduate student or as a member of staff, you will have identified problems or issues that you might want to explore as part of a research project. It is important to discuss these ideas with staff in practice and academia to see whether it might be feasible to explore these further. It is important to be realistic in what you want to look at and identify an issue that it is reasonable to consider in the time and cost envelope available. You will also need to know that other researchers have not already addressed the problem through completing an initial review of the related literature (see Chapter 6).

Research question(s)

You will find specific information on how to develop research questions in chapter 9 and should be prepared to develop questions to answer your problem. The question(s) need to be concise and are a description of exactly what you intend to answer and obtain information about. The development of questions can be difficult and you may need to develop them over time as part of an iterate process, informing the development through a literature review and discussions with others.

Literature review

At the proposal stage you may not have time to complete a detailed and complete critical review of the literature but should have undertaken an initial search and critical review in order to support the need for the study. Chapters 4–6 can assist you in the search and review processes, whilst Chapter 20 provides information on how to undertake a systematic review of the literature. At the proposal stage, showing evidence of identifying search parameters and terms, the results of an initial search and critical review of a proportion of the literature using a recognised framework such as that in Chapter 5 will probably be required. The review should confirm that the problem you are considering is an issue and that further project work is required to identify possible answers. The review should also help inform the development of the research question(s), which outline the specific areas the project will seek to address through data collection.

Involvement of the public

Often student projects do not include members of the public; however, they can be included as advisers to projects. Members of the public are often linked to research units and centres in universities and can offer advice on research design, recruitment, data collection tools and dissemination. Depending on the focus of your study it might be helpful to discuss the potential to involve the public and also explore any cost implications of inclusion.

Research design and data collection

The research design includes the plan of the research and the structure of what you are planning to do. It will need to include your approach to the research and how you intend to collect and analyse data that will help you answer your research question(s) and potentially generate outcomes from the research that benefit patients and/or healthcare delivery and staff. There are a number of chapters in the book that will help you think about research design, data collection and analysis (see Chapters 11, 14–19 and 21–27). These include chapters on the most commonly used approaches and data collection tools.

It is worth noting here that many studies in healthcare are evaluation or outcome-based studies (see Chapter 16). These are increasingly important as they are used to assess the effectiveness, quality and impact of care delivery. You could use an evaluation study to investigate how well an intervention or practice is working and can determine good practice and the need for change. Evaluations ideally consider three stages in the process of introducing change; using or collecting data that captures the before, during and after phases. You should remember that this is the ideal and frequently you may only be able to collect data in the second stage, the during/implementation phase. Data might also be collected for other purposes during the implementation phase and if available to use can help in the data collection process. Evaluations can also be complex and consider the cost-effectiveness of treatments or practices, and can be used to inform the commissioning of services (DH, 2012).

Dissemination

You may be required to present a dissemination strategy for your project. This could include presenting your work within a university or clinical setting, at a conference or at a public engagement event – one where members of the public will be present. There are different ways of presenting your work such as a poster presentation, leaflet, digital presentation, academic paper, journal club or research meeting (see Chapter 28). It is important to think about the audience and also whether any costs might be involved.

Timeframe and costs

Assessment submission dates and budgets will need to guide your timeframe for completion and the process you engage with. Ideally you should develop a Gantt chart (see later in the chapter) for your proposed work that identifies all activities involved in the study and when they should take place. This will guide your project when it starts. In addition, any costs associated with the project should be presented alongside how you intend to cover them. This may involve you thinking about applying for external or small internal pots of money that might be available.

PREPARING AN APPLICATION FOR FUNDING

Identifying funding opportunities

Information about research bidding opportunities can be presented through a number of forums and mechanisms. Often, advanced intelligence is received through specific networks operating within a specialist field. Funding calls can be advertised in the press or emailed to specific mailing lists. Most organisations funding research advertise new research opportunities on their websites. In the UK these include the Association of Medical Research Charities (www.amrc.org.uk), National Institute for Health Research (www.nihr.ac.uk), Economic and Social Research Council (www.esrc.ac.uk), the Wellcome Trust (www.wellcome.ac.uk), along with a number of other funders. Universities will often employ staff to collect a list of funding opportunities to circulate to key research staff, and a similar system operates within the NHS – the world's largest publicly funded health service – through the R&D units. Organisations, such as the Higher Education Academy (HEA) – who help institutions discipline groups and all staff to provide the best possible learning experience for their students – provide information highlighting research opportunities to members.

Not all research-funding opportunities are advertised as part of specific funding rounds. A number of charities and other healthcare organisations have identified monies available to support research related to their specialism. Researchers can submit more general proposals that relate to the aims of the funding body, one example being the Resuscitation Council (UK) (www.resus.org.uk), funder of a variety of research projects in the field of resuscitation through small grants. The National Institute for Health Research also offer open calls in some of their funding streams, allowing researcher-led submissions at particular points of the year.

At present, nursing research doesn't have a specific funding body and though there are a number of funding opportunities the competition is often high. Those proposals most likely to succeed in meeting the aims and objectives of the call are succinct and focused, have relevance and demonstrate an ability to complete the research. Writing proposals is a skill and one that requires development over time. A number of strategies can be employed to maximise success, such as the use of research design services and specialist input and advice in methodology, statistical testing and health economic. Despite investment of time, energy and expert input, not all bids are successful and for some funders the success rate might be as low as 20 per cent. Learning from rejection is important, so any opportunities for feedback should be sought and used to consider review and either inform resubmission or submission to another funder.

> ## Reflective exercise
>
> Have a look at a call for research proposals. You could search the National Institute for Health Research (www.nihr.ac.uk) website, which often has current research calls. Look at the submission template – what kinds of information do the researchers need to provide? Remember, these are complicated bids which often take several months to develop and require expert teams that can include academics, clinicians, health economists, statisticians and have public involvement.

Background work

When a call is received it is important to consider how the research relates to an existing research record and how a current profile can support the proposal. A proposal is more likely to be successful if the researcher can demonstrate a clear area of expertise in the field and present a profile of previous research and publications that relate to the call. At this stage, it is worth considering who may form the research team. Depending on the scope of the bid, strategic decisions may need to be taken regarding the composition of any bidding team. Most healthcare research projects will involve more than one person, attracting a team who bring different strengths to the proposal. Collaboration is often a requirement of those funding research. For example, healthcare research may benefit from a team composed of a number of different healthcare professionals, reflecting an interprofessional approach. Collaboration between healthcare providers and university staff is often desirable, bringing the expertise of clinical specialists, statisticians, methodologists and health economists together. Research can benefit from service user involvement, national or international links; the presence of industry and European funding requires the inclusion of different European-based partners.

It is also important to clarify the aims and objectives of the call, visiting websites or accessing other background information. It may be possible to speak to the funders to ascertain further detail. Some funders, such as the Joint Information Systems Committee (JISC) who fund e-learning based research, run Town Planning meetings and invite possible bidders to attend sessions that provide further bid information and opportunities to ask questions. Funders may also offer an opportunity to attend a forum or event where members may work together to develop a grant application.

The bid should also be discussed internally with R&D departments or within local research communities. It is also important to alert the institution of a possible bid opportunity so that appropriate departments and staff can offer help with reading through proposals, funding advice and can ensure any internal processing systems are followed.

Planning the writing

Often, the time to respond to a call is limited, though this will vary according to the funder and the details of the bid. A number of funders request expressions of interest that can be a couple of pages in length. Full bids can take some time to develop, though often the available response time is less than a month. It will be important to look at what material is readily available to support the bid. For example, can a previous academic paper or literature review be updated for use? The guidance for proposal submissions varies across funders and any submission not meeting these is likely to be discarded. It will therefore be crucial to follow the guidance and either allot members of the team to undertake the development of parts of the bid or agree some sort of writing programme.

Content of the proposal

The content and presentation requirements are likely to be outlined by the funder. This may be very prescriptive and should be followed as failure to meet the requirements set out in the call can lead to it being discarded without consideration. Often funders provide headings that need to be used and identify a word limit. There is usually the requirement to submit supporting CVs and often a need to demonstrate support from employers and any partner organisations involved in the bid. The Economic and Social Research Council, the UK's leading research and training agency in economic and social research, provides one suggested template with accompanying guidance notes on how to write a good application (www.esrc.ac.uk/funding/). The proposal example below (Figure 10.1) was written in response to a call from a local healthcare provider. Looking at the structure of this, it includes the project title, details of the project team, background, aims and objectives, methods, timetable for completion, and budget costs. The CV of the lead investigator was also required.

Figure 10.1 Research proposal

Title: Evaluate a Service Improvement Initiative: Early Supported Discharge Team for Stroke Patients

Research Team: The research team will be drawn from the [name omitted].

Background

The Early Supported Discharge (ESD) Team was established in July 2008, funded from the closure of 10 beds at [name omitted]. The initial team of 10 included occupational therapy (OT), physiotherapy, speech and language therapy and dietitian input at Band 7, along with a Band 6 physiotherapist, OT and a Band 6 nurse. In addition, there were Band 4 and 3 OT technicians and Band 3 physiotherapy support. The inception of the team coincided with a peer-based Clinical Review of Stroke Services designed to identify compliance with the National Stroke Strategy (2007) in each of the south-west health communities. It reported in October of 2008, suggesting those patients being discharged from in-patient rehabilitation units, whose discharge is dependent on accessing further rehabilitation and who meet the criteria for early supported discharge, should be able to access ESD teams.

The aim of the service was to meet national and local stroke priorities and provide a seamless, high quality, evidence-based ESD service for patients affected by stroke. It also aimed to deliver a cost-effective service for the Trust. An interim report produced by the ESD team in 2009 [reference omitted] provided a positive evaluation of the service. It reported reduced length of stay by an average 13.5 days, saving 1094 bed days and increasing patient satisfaction, with 86% of patients being satisfied/highly satisfied with the ESD service. This evaluation was focussed on measuring achievement of the aims of the service, and there was a desire to capture the learning from this service improvement development that might have national relevance for care developments in ESD for stroke patients and staff. This was particularly relevant as this type of development is in its infancy with only a limited number of current examples in the United Kingdom (UK), such as the Walsall initiative [reference omitted].

This proposal sets out the aims and methods to be used to gather further evaluation data by an external evaluation team. This will enable an external review of the effectiveness of this service improvement development that might have national relevance for care developments in early supported discharge for stroke patients.

Aims

To examine the process of new service implementation and make recommendations for future initiatives

Objectives

- To map the process of implementing a new service initiative in the community
- To explore the views of key stakeholders in the development of new patient care pathway from acute to community setting
- To explore the composition and roles of the members of the interdisciplinary team
- To evaluate the team member experiences of the initiative

Methods

A participatory approach is proposed to engage the ESD team members in aspects of developing the research design

The research will comprise two phases:

Phase One – will capture the experiences and learning of the inter-disciplinary ESD team members about this development of the service. Data will be collected from members of the inter-disciplinary ESD team members through individual semi-structured interviews. The interview questions will be designed and collated by the research team, with input from the ESD team.

Phase Two – will explore external key stakeholder perspectives on the ESD team development. Individual semi-structured interviews will be conducted with four stakeholders. The interview questions will be designed and collated by the research team, with input from the ESD team.

Data Analysis

The interviews from both phases of the evaluation will be transcribed, read through and coded individually by the research team. The codes will be discussed, agreed and the emergence of themes will be discussed.

Ethical approval for both phases will be obtained from the Faculty Ethics Committee at [name omitted] and the project will be registered with the Trust Research and Development unit. Informed consent will be obtained from all participants. They will be given an information sheet about the research and all sign a consent form.

Issues of anonymity will be discussed with the team and stakeholders at the outset. It must be acknowledged that it might not be possible to anonymise data in such a way as to fully protect the identity of individual members. The evaluation team will pay particular attention to presenting data in a way that would not be attributable to individuals but this cannot be fully guaranteed. As part of this process, key themes will be returned to the participants for comment and all participants will be offered the opportunity to check drafts of the final report.

Time line

We envisage a 12-month project commencing in May and ending in April.

May–June		Ethical approval Developing interview schedules 1st Advisory board meeting
June–September	Phase 1	Data collection and analysis Identify sample for phase 2
October–February	Phase 2	Data collection and analysis 2nd Advisory board meeting
March/April		Final report Final advisory board meeting Prepare conference abstracts and publications

There will be an advisory board in place with representation from [name omitted] and the key stakeholders from the community, SHA, ESD team and service users.

Costs

Project manager and lead

(Lead the project, attend advisory board meetings, lead on ethical approval, process, data collection and analysis, final report writing)

- £13,000

Research fellow

(support with data collection, transcription, ethical approval, final report)

- £3,500

(Continued)

Figure 10.1   (Continued)

Statistician

(support with data analysis from ESD data capture)

- £2,100

Administrative support

(organisation of interviews, transcription support)

- £1,500

Travel for data collection approx. £200

Cost of consumables and final report £50

Cost for three advisory board meetings £300

Conference/publication costs £1,000

Total = £21,650

References

Department of Health, 2007 National Stroke Strategy, London, The Stationery Office.

In developing a proposal, it should be remembered that its function is to provide clear justification of the need for the study and detail how the study will be completed in order to achieve the aims and objectives and address the research questions or problems. The proposal is therefore likely to include the following:

- research problem and background
- aims and objectives
- research methods
- data collection
- data analysis
- ethical approval issues
- project team and management
- outputs
- dissemination
- budget (see full economic costing)
- curriculum vitae.

Increasingly, the funder of health and social care research will also expect service user involvement in the research, and including reference to this in the proposal is helpful. It may, for example, include having service users named as research partners and involved in designing the research, in its implementation. Service users and carers may also be engaged as members of an advisory or steering group for the project. The decision to involve service users needs to be taken early on, especially if they are to form part of the research team. There are also implications for the research budget, which may need to include user costs (DH, 2006).

Research background, aims and objectives

This section of the proposal should be made really clear to the funder. It needs to present the existing research in the field and give justification for the research. In nursing research, it should be possible to argue the potential benefits of the research to nursing care and patient experience. The background should be used to demonstrate the bidder's expertise, referencing publications and highlighting experience in the field. An opportunity to refer to work of potential scrutinisers should be taken and it is important to demonstrate a wide and current knowledge base. A word limit may be imposed on this section and therefore any inclusions must have relevance. It may also be possible to make a statement here about the credibility of the research team and their ability to complete the research. Clarity will also be aided if the research aims and objectives are set out in achievable terms. Funders will always be concerned that the expected outcomes are achievable within the timeframe and budget set out.

Often, the call will include the aims and objectives the funders want to achieve which can aid the researcher. For example, in Figure 10.1 the aim of the funders was clearly laid out to include evaluating the process of new service implementation in order to make recommendations for future initiatives. The aim appears in the proposal and is reflected through the proposal objectives. It may also be helpful to review the general philosophy, aims and objectives of the funding body and to reflect these within the proposal. It is important to reiterate the need to write achievable aims and objectives and to ensure that the remainder of the proposal demonstrates how these will be met.

Proposed investigation

The proposal needs to make clear what kind of research design is going to be used and outline the stages of the research. This detail needs to be presented in the opening lines with a rationale for the adoption of particular approaches if required. Details on a number of research designs and methods are presented in Chapters 11, 14–19, 21–25 and can be used to support proposal writing. The amount of detailed description required on the methods, sample, data collection and analysis would depend on the funder. There should be sufficient information presented to make clear how the sample will be selected and composed, how data will be collected, from where and by whom and clear statements about the processes of data analysis should be provided. The funders need to understand what sampling approach will be used (see Chapter 12), and what sample size will be used, and be confident that the sample can be accessed within the timeframe. It would add strength to the proposal if the bidders can demonstrate previous use of the suggested methodologies and convey an understanding of the strengths and weaknesses of the approaches suggested.

The bid may suggest the need for pilot work to test out data collection approaches or tools. It may also identify the involvement of a statistician to support the analysis of numerical data and refer to a power calculation to support sample size generation. It should be clear to the funders that the design, sample, methods of data collection and analysis are consistent with the aims and objectives of the study. For example, in Figure 10.1 the objectives include mapping the new service implementation and exploring the experiences and composition of the Early Supported Discharge (ESD) team and external stakeholder views on the process. To achieve these objectives, the researchers interviewed the teams asking questions about roles and the process of team development and implementation. In addition, stakeholder views on the process of team inception and implementation were explored through interviews.

Ethical issues

Much research conducted within healthcare will require ethical approval to meet research governance requirements (see Chapters 7 and 8). Some funders require evidence of ethical approval prior to proposal review, such as the Resuscitation Council (UK). The proposal will need to outline the ethical approval processes that will be put in place and identify these in the project timeline. Nursing research is likely to meet the requirements for researching ethically in the UK set out by the Research Governance Framework for Health and Social Care (DH, 2010). Researchers will seek ethical approval from the National Research Ethics Service (NRES) (www.nres.nhs.uk; see Chapter 7). This will address how issues such as the provision of participant information and informed consent will be managed. Additionally, the proposal can outline processes in place to manage and store research data in line with the Data Protection Act, which makes new provision for the regulation of the processing of information relating to individuals (The Stationery Office, 1998).

PROJECT MANAGEMENT

Most funders want to be confident that the planned work is likely to be completed in the funding timeframe, often one or two years. To help funders make this judgement a timeline of work, or Gantt chart, should be included. Figure 10.1 suggests a work schedule for a 12-month project. This provides a plan of work and highlights the key activities. Depending on the funder, a more detailed plan of work may be required. The funder may also want to see evidence that the schedule will be monitored by a steering group or advisory body and can request feedback on progress in a formal interim report. It is advisable to write an initial plan of work that is realistic. A project lasting one year should expect to spend three to four months gaining ethical approval, accessing a sample and preparing for data collection; a further three or four months should be spent collecting and analysing the data, with the final months used for collating and presenting the results.

The funders will also need to be confident that the research team have the skills and expertise to complete the research. The curriculum vitae (CV) of the project manager will be reviewed and possibly those of the project team members. Where a more novice researcher is leading a proposal, it will be important to demonstrate that research support and mentorship is in place. This may come from the mentorship of a more experienced researcher or through a steering group.

Dissemination

Outputs from research are becoming increasingly important to funders in health and social care. Not only is the generation of a report, conference papers and publications expected, but also other forms of dissemination can be supported. These might include hosting a website related to the project, holding events that will disseminate the results to relevant professional groups, and providing reports in various formats that might be more applicable to users and other consumers of research. The report can also be produced digitally and the executive summary can be made available as a podcast. The project may have other outputs such as toolkits, teaching materials or new developments. The dissemination of these will need some consideration, and the distribution or marketing may be governed by a contractual agreement made with the funder at the outset of the project. The issue of intellectual property rights will need consideration, as it is important to know who owns the copyright of any products. Often these are owned by the institution(s) employing the research team, though agreements can be put in place that reward the individual employees. In research projects where such issues are likely to arise legal advice should be sought.

Curriculum vitae

The proposal will need to include the CV of the lead investigator at least and possibly require a two-page submission from each member of the team. These can be gathered at the early stages of developing the proposal. A template may be offered that should be used by all involved. Alternatively, if no template is suggested, the following headings may be used:

- name and contact details
- current employer and position
- employment history
- educational qualifications
- research experience
- relevant publications
- conference presentations.

The CV must include those aspects of research activity and experience that are relevant to the bid. It should support the application and demonstrate research capability.

Full economic costing

Full economic costing (fEC) relates to the costing and charging of research under-taken by universities in the UK. It is a research costing methodology introduced by the government in 2005 following the Transparency Review that was originally insti-gated in 1998. The review was undertaken to demonstrate the full costs of research and other publicly funded activities in higher education. The review was completed to improve accountability for the use of public money and suggested that government departments and other purchasers of contracted research undertaken by universities must expect to pay nearer the costs of their research. The costs relate to three areas, as shown in Table 10.1.

Table 10.1   Examples of research costs

Directly incurred costs	Costs directly related to the project, including research assistant pay, travel, subsistence, equipment, external consultants, consumables, printing and stationery, IT hardware and software
Directly allocated costs	The principal investigator and co-investigator costs, estates and other directly allocated costs such as major facilities, centrally sourced technicians
Indirect costs	Contribution to centrally shared costs

The use of fEC is mandatory and most universities have access to web-based sites that enable calculation of the total cost of research based on the input of directly incurred and directly allocated costs. Any nurses undertaking research within universi-ties or as part of a university-based project team will need to use fEC, though it should be noted that not all charities fully fund fEC and may not pay for all directly allocated or indirect costs. Research councils usually pay 80 per cent of the fEC.

There are a number of things to consider when developing a research proposal. It is always advisable to work closely with the tender documents provided by the funder, in particular looking at the aims and objectives. Expert support can be helpful in develop-ing the proposal which should be presented in the format requested. There are other considerations that need to be made, including the composition of a bidding team, which should include all the skills required and relevant expertise. The bid should include relevant background literature and methodology, make reference to patient and public involvement, and ethical approvals required, and provide information on the project timeline and costing. The funder will also need to know about project manage-ment and how staff will work as a team to deliver the project. Table 10.2 provides a list of key Do's and Don'ts.

Table 10.2   Key Do's and Don'ts of research proposal development

Do	Don'ts
Look at the aims and objectives of the call closely	Submit a proposal without addressing the aims and objectives of the call and funder

Do	Don'ts
Undertake background work, e.g. literature review, think about expertise and current or previous related work	Bid in areas where previous expertise and experience is crucial if you and the bidding team have none
Consider the best team to respond and have partners in place if appropriate	Bid if partnerships are needed and these are not in place or are tenuous
Follow the guidelines for submission closely and make sure any internal reviewers and support staff, e.g. research office have access to these	Ignore the guidelines for submission
Follow any submission templates to structure the report	Ignore the submission template
Provide all of the information requested, e.g. CVs	Leave out essential information requested by the funder
Get expert support, if available, from colleagues with previous experience of the funder and from staff with expertise in costing and bidding	Undertake proposal development alone without taking advice from those with more experience
Include reference to ethical approvals as required and have these in place if needed	Ignore the need for ethical approval if required and forget to obtain approval prior to submission if needed
Make it clear in the bid who will project manage and oversee the project to completion	Submit a proposal without making clear who is the project manager taking responsibility for completion
Include a clear dissemination strategy appropriate to the bid and funder	Omit a dissemination strategy

CHAPTER SUMMARY

- Nurse researchers are often required to submit a research proposal for a variety of audiences.
- When writing the proposal it is worth reviewing existing and available expertise and potential team membership.
- Whether the proposal relates to individual work as part of academic study or to larger grant applications, it will need to address a number of areas and include statements about the research problem and background, aims and objectives, research methods, ethical approval, project team and management, service user engagement, outputs and dissemination.
- If submitting a proposal to an external funding body, a clear Gantt chart of proposed work and timeframe would be required along with detailed costing of the project.

SUGGESTED FURTHER READING

Becker, L. (2014) *Writing Successful Reports and Dissertations.* Los Angeles: Sage. This text offers guidance on how to write reports and dissertations.

Denicolo, P. and Becker, L. (2012) *Developing Research Proposals*. London: Sage. This text offers guidance on how to develop and write research proposals for dissertations and funded research.

Kenner, C. and Walden, M. (2009) *Grant Writing Handbook for Nurses*, 2nd edn. London: Jones and Barlett. This text specialises in how to write a proposal to secure a research grant.

WEBSITES

Association of Medical Research Charities: www.amrc.org.uk – provides information on a range of medical research charities that offer grant funding.

Department of Health: www.dh.gov.uk – provides information on research and healthcare policy.

Economic and Social Research Council: www.esrc.ac.uk – UK's largest funding body for research related to social and economic issues. Offers grants in these areas.

Higher Education Academy: www.heacademy.ac.uk – provides services to higher education including teaching development grants, scholarships and some research monies.

Medical Research Council: www.mrc.ac.uk – aims to improve human health through medical research. Offer grants, fellowships and studentships.

National Institute for Health Research: www.nihr.ac.uk – commissions and funds NHS, social care and public health research. Also offers fellowships.

National Research Ethics Service: www.nres.nhs.uk – provides information on the requirements for ethical and R&D approvals.

Royal College of Nursing Research Society: www.rcn.org.uk – promotes excellence in care through research. Hosts an annual international research conference, provides three awards and supports with ethics and **patient and public involvement in research**.

Wellcome Trust: www.wellcome.ac.uk – promotes excellence in research for health including grants in areas such as public engagement and health and ethics.

 To access further resources related to this chapter, visit the companion website at https://study. sagepub.com/mouleaveyard3e

REFERENCES

Department of Health (2006) *Reward and Recognition: The Principles and Practice of Service User Payment and Reimbursement in Health and Social Care*, 2nd edn. Available at: www.dh.gov.uk (accessed 30 July 2015).

Department of Health (2010) *Research Governance Framework for Health and Social Care*, 2nd edn. Available at: www.dh.gov.uk (accessed 16 July 2015).

Department of Health (2012) *Health and Social Care Act*. Available at: http://services.parliament. uk/bills/2010-12/healthandsocialcare/documents.html (accessed 30 July 2015).

The Stationery Office (1998) *The Data Protection Act 1998*. Available at: www.legislation.gov.uk (accessed 30 July 2015).

PART 3
DOING RESEARCH

11
RESEARCH APPROACHES AND DESIGN

Learning outcomes

This chapter will enable you to:

- understand what is meant by the research design
- identify the components of a research design
- consider designs available within qualitative and quantitative approaches

The development of the research design is an important part of the research process. The design is the plan of how the research aims, objectives, hypothesis and question(s) will be answered. The literature review can inform the development of the design. The researcher may be able to replicate a previous design or take elements of it into a new study. There are a number of designs available to the researcher. Research questions may also require the researcher to work with a design that incorporates different research approaches. The research design will include the approach that can be described as quantitative, qualitative or a combination of both, such as case study research, which can include a range of data collection methods.

The design is a map of the way in which the researcher will engage with the research subject(s) in order to achieve the outcomes needed to address the research aims and objectives. Therefore, the selection of a design will depend on a number of factors such as the research question that needs addressing, the skills and expertise of the researcher, the resources available for the project, and will need to take account of data access and ethical approvals.

In this chapter, we explore the research designs used by the nurse researcher to address those research questions, aims and objectives set out in research and we review the elements which compose research design.

CHOOSING A RESEARCH DESIGN

In selecting the **research design**, the nurse researcher needs to focus clearly on the research question(s) and purpose of the study. The purpose of the research design is to ensure that the evidence collected allows the researcher to try and answer the research question(s). The design is therefore the plan of the research that will provide the evidence needed to answer the research question. It is likely to include the following:

1. The research questions to be addressed
2. The research approach – qualitative, quantitative or both
3. The selection of sites and participants or source of data
4. Ethical considerations for the study
5. A timeline for the research
6. The resources available for the research
7. Methods of data collection
8. Methods of data analysis.

The list above presents the processes to be completed in the research and should also draw on the skills and expertise of the researcher. Whilst researchers may have greater skills in qualitative or quantitative research approaches, the differences between these are increasingly blurred and the skills required to undertake both can be reflected across the team members. For example, it can be irrelevant to try to compartmentalise particular designs or methods into either qualitative or quantitative research. It is important to remember that some surveys will draw on qualitative evidence, whilst historical research may use quantitative data (Yin, 2014).

Different research designs and methods can be used within the research approach adopted. The selection of design will be affected by a number of practical factors. The research team will need to think about the time available for the research and the resources and costs of particular data collection methods. For example, if the researcher has a limited budget and timeframe for research, then a longitudinal study that includes observational techniques will not be practical.

There is also a need to ensure that the research complies with ethical requirements for a study in healthcare (see Chapters 7 and 8). A design that might cause unnecessary harm to the patients involved is unlikely to be approved.

The choice of research design is also dependent on access to participants, research subjects or research data. There is little point designing a study to capture data from thousands of respondents if there are limited numbers available. Equally, there can be difficulties in designing studies involving particular vulnerable groups if they are difficult to access.

There isn't a perfect research design, and frequently decisions about aspects such as sampling and data collection methods will be guided by the practicalities of research endeavour, as discussed above. Our own research experiences have demonstrated that often decisions about data collection methods are taken based on availability of resources or participants. For example, individual face-to-face interviews may be preferable, yet telephone-based interviews may be conducted, as access to busy nursing staff spread across a range of clinical practice environments can be problematic. However, the researchers need to be confident that the methods of data collection used will not compromise the quality of the information accessed, as ultimately the research needs to be robust and collect data that will address the research questions. The focus of the research design has to be about whether it is appropriate to gain the evidence needed to answer the research question. There are issues of validity and reliability that need considering in the selection of a design. The design and methods of data collection used must be able to obtain the evidence needed in a robust way to address the research problem. For example, if we wanted to look at patients' views and experiences of service delivery, there would be little point developing an **experimental design** that is more focused on testing cause-and-effect relationships. We would need to think about a design that allows the research team to investigate patient views and experiences, taking a more qualitative approach and exploring experiences and views through data collection methods that could include interviews, focus groups and recording of diaries or journals.

Prior to considering different research designs, it is important to highlight the main aspects of different **qualitative** and **quantitative research approaches**, which as mentioned are frequently combined.

RESEARCH APPROACHES

Qualitative and quantitative research approaches have in the past been presented as competing and divergent positions, but more recently there is recognition of the need to use a range of approaches to address the questions of nursing research. The contrasting elements of qualitative and quantitative research are described in Table 11.1. Qualitative research, in the crudest sense, is research that aims to generate data that comprises words and pictures. Qualitative research is most commonly part of an interpretivist approach and can be viewed as constructivist (Guba and Lincoln, 1994). Interpretivists in the broad sense simply believe that the social world needs to be interpreted to be understood. Qualitative researchers often tend to be focused on language, perceptions and experiences in order to understand and explain behaviour. In nursing research, an interpretivist position would be used to describe and understand people's experiences of care, trying to understand the individual and their interactions with others. It acknowledges that there is no single truth or one understanding, but celebrates individual differences. For example, someone admitted to hospital may be anxious and upset, though the same person may not experience subsequent hospital admissions in the same way. Individuals can react to the same experience in different ways, and each of us can react to the same experiences in different ways.

Qualitative research may be used to look at issues such as the patient experience or the views of healthcare staff. To gain these insights the researcher needs to interact with the study participants. The researcher engages with the participant in a meaningful way to gain a holistic picture of life experiences and uses observation and interviews as the main methods of data collection to facilitate an interactive and subjective approach (Bryman, 2012). The results are not normally open to generalisation and wide application but describe the local context and can be open to transferability to other contexts.

Quantitative research often generates research data that can be analysed numerically using statistical techniques. Quantitative research tends to be driven by a positivist or scientific approach or by, more latterly, a post-positivist approach. Positivism emerged in the Enlightenment and was in part a reaction against the idea that knowledge was handed down by God and could only be interpreted theologically. Broadly, positivist approaches stress the importance of testing and measurement and believe scientific truths exist even in the social world. Positivists have tended to believe that through the controlled testing of variables, cause-and-effect relationships can be determined and the truth established. Positivists argue that the scientific method can also be used to study social phenomena, and that universal laws exist that can explain human behaviour in an objective way. They would suggest that there is one truth and objectivity.

Post-positivist beliefs, developed in the mid-twentieth century, recognise that social phenomena cannot be understood through uncovering universal laws, and that it is problematic to predict a cause-and-effect relationship that is true for all. For example, a universal law would suggest that our person admitted to hospital experiencing anxiety and upset would always feel this on every admission and everyone else would feel the same way. Post-positivist research seeks to look at relationships or correlations between variables being measured (see Chapter 26). The post-positivists maintain some of the processes of empiricism, answering hypothesis or research questions through a scientific approach. Numerical data is obtained through formal methods of data collection, which are objective and free from bias (Burns et al., 2014).

Whilst acknowledging the different philosophical positions, it should be remembered that other factors influence the design selection, such as available funding, research skills, timeframe available, ethical approval and access to the research sample. Additionally, the researcher will need to give foremost consideration to the research

Table 11.1 Contrasting elements of qualitative and quantitative approaches

	Qualitative	Quantitative
Philosophical origin	Interpretivist	Positivist
Researcher relationship with subject	Close	Distant
Researcher position in the research	Often insider	Outsider
Research strategy	Unstructured	Structured
Relationship with theory	Develops, interprets	Tests
Data collection	Observation, interviewing	Instruments
Type of data	Rich, individual	Hard, reliable
Data analysis	Interpretation	Statistical
Findings	Unique, transferable	Generalisable

problem and questions that need to be addressed. The research design selected needs to obtain the evidence required to address the research problem.

Induction and deduction

The production of knowledge through scientific method is often categorised as being through two approaches to generating knowledge, called 'induction' and 'deduction'. In practice, many research approaches cannot be categorised as purely inductive or purely deductive, but are rather a mixture of the two. However, the two terms are useful tools in helping us to understand different approaches to producing knowledge through the research process.

Induction or **inductive reasoning** is a process of starting with the observations and details of an experience, our observations of something, that are used to develop a general understanding of phenomena. Specific observations and descriptions are made and used to develop a theory or hypothesis of a more general situation that can be tested or investigated further. For example, whilst on the ward our observations of patients may show a tendency for better sleep patterns if relaxation therapies are used before the ward lights are switched off for the night. These observations could be developed into a theory or a hypothesis. The hypothesis is a statement of predicted relationship (see Chapter 9), which if based on the initial observations would suggest that 'the use of relaxation therapies before night time will lead to patients having better patterns of night time sleep'. Typically, induction is seen as part of qualitative and quantitative research where the aim is to develop concepts and themes from the interpretation of observations and interviews.

Deduction or **deductive reasoning** starts with the development of a general theory about something, which is then tested, through undertaking further observations or by developing tests. Drawing on the example above, testing would look to measure whether there is a relationship between the use of relaxation therapies and the quality of patients' sleep. Researchers aim to deduce how the theory works and identify causal relationships through controlled testing or experimentation. Data obtained will be used to either verify the theory or discount it. Deduction is seen as being part of quantitative research as it looks to test theories or hypotheses for correlations and relationships. For example, the researchers would want to test the relationship between the use of relaxation therapies and patients' sleep.

QUALITATIVE APPROACHES

Qualitative approaches focus on understanding social settings; often in nursing this will be the ward or community environment. They facilitate exploration of relationships and human experience within the research setting and enable face-to-face, personal contact in data collection. Three qualitative approaches – **phenomenology**, **ethnography** and **grounded theory** – which are most frequently used in nursing research have their traditions in anthropology, sociology and psychology (Polit and Beck, 2014).

The researcher may be required to engage over a period of time with the research setting in order to collect data using methods where the researcher can become the research instrument. The researcher can work with a range of data collection methods. These can include observations, interviews, group discussions and the analysis of contextual data, diaries, letters and other documents. These methods allow the researcher to gain insight into the social context of the research, to gain in-depth data from the participants, and to enable them to 'tell their story' and provide rich data about personal experiences, feelings and thoughts. The data are usually recorded on to audio, video or digital recording for verbatim transcription and analysis (see Chapter 27). A process of thematic analysis is used to identify key meanings and interpretations from the data. This involves a process of breaking the data into key units of meaning through a coding process, re-ordering data and drawing interpretations that are often verified by the participants (see Chapter 27). The process is described as data reduction, display, conclusion drawing and verification (Miles et al., 2013).

The researcher may maintain a reflective diary or field notes recording the research events. These reflections are used in a similar way to our employment of reflective practice in nursing. The researcher uses the records to consider their role and influence in the research and in interpreting the data. A necessary emphasis is placed on this as the researcher is often immersed in the research setting and study and will need to take opportunities for reflexivity in which actions and analysis are critically reviewed. Diary recordings and field notes can form part of the data analysis, which is usually prolonged and leads to the construction of narratives and validated interpretations of participant experiences.

The three approaches of phenomenology, ethnography and grounded theory are discussed in greater detail in Chapter 15, with a brief description provided here.

Phenomenology

Phenomenological approaches are grounded in philosophy and psychology and aim to explore the lived experience of humans within the context of that experience (Smith et al., 2009). A nurse researcher would employ such an approach if the research sought to find out how patients or staff experienced a particular phenomenon, to discover the meaning of the phenomenon. This approach can be selected if the nurse researcher wants to explore the experience of those caring for elderly relatives and consider their perception of the world as a carer and experiences of being a carer in today's society.

In phenomenological research a number of methods of data collection can be used; interviews that are in-depth and focus on the experience that is being explored are most common. Data can also be collected through diaries, autobiographies, written accounts, journals and conversations. The research example 11.1 collected data through semi-structured interviews. These methods all allow the researcher to collect data about people's experiences that should provide an in-depth reflective account for analysis.

Research example 11.1

Phenomenology

Lee et al. (2012) used a hermeneutic–phenomenological approach to analyse qualitative interviews conducted in Malaysia with 40 healthcare professionals. The semi-structured interview guides were used to explore the professionals' views on the barriers to starting insulin therapy in people with Type 2 diabetes, the incidence of which has doubled in the last 10 years. The results identified that three main areas affected initiation. Firstly, patients often preferred complementary therapies and mistrusted insulin. Secondly, professionals held long-standing negative attitudes to the prescription of insulin, some of which were a legacy from previous poor guidelines for administration. Finally system issues such as communication and language challenges affected initiation.

Ethnography

Coming from the tradition of anthropology, ethnography means a 'portrait of people' and involves writing about people and culture. Ethnographic approaches tend to be about using observational data collection methods, often over a long period. Ethnographers aim to gain an understanding of the culture and social norms of a particular group, such as nurses, by studying behaviours through fieldwork (Hammersley and Atkinson, 2007). Through ethnography the nurse researcher would attempt to learn from members of a particular cultural group and understand their world as it is lived and perceived (Polit and Beck, 2014). An example is given in Research example 11.2. This approach can be used to answer questions about patients' experiences of a long-term treatment plan or student nurses' experiences of a pre-registration programme of study.

Research example 11.2

Ethnography

Thomson (2011) used ethnography to examine relationships and roles within health and social care, occupying an 'insider' research role. The study focused on exploring the everyday lives of healthcare professionals. Thomson was a senior lecturer with experience of physiotherapy practice whilst collecting data. The approaches to data collection included observations and interviews. In addition, Thomson used a reflexive approach, recording field notes and using these to reflect on her position within the study. Thomson's experience of healthcare practice enabled familiarity with the context, language used and roles. Thomson reflected on the effectiveness of the approach used over a prolonged time period, which facilitated an in-depth exploration of the practice of healthcare professionals.

Grounded theory

Developed in the 1960s by sociologists Glaser and Strauss (2008), grounded theory aims to develop hypotheses and theories from the data collected through observations and interviews with humans in their own environments. Grounded theory usually starts with specific observations and analysis of the data collected to generate a theory, therefore usually working in an inductive way, but can develop to use deductive reasoning.

The researchers initially develop themes and hypotheses from observations using an inductive approach. These hypotheses can be subjected to further observations to try to verify relationships and correlations, using a deductive approach. Induction, however, plays the greatest role in grounded theory. The researchers use the emergent themes from the analysis of observations or interviews to undertake theoretical sampling. The use of theoretical sampling is shown in research by Abid-Hajbaghery (2007), reported in Research example 11.3. Analysis of initial data from registered nurses identified issues related to management. Abid-Hajbaghery explored these further by interviewing key managers. Grounded theory also attempts to compare similar findings in the data through a constant comparison method to try to gain a wider perspective of the issues arising in the study.

Research example 11.3

Grounded theory

Abid-Hajbaghery (2007) aimed to clarify the concept of evidence-based nursing and explore the factors influencing its use by Iranian nurses.

Grounded theory (see Chapter 15) was used as it allows the identification, description and explanation of interactional processes that occur between and amongst individuals and groups in a particular social context (Strauss and Corbin, 2015).

Twenty-one registered nurses formed an initial purposive sample, selected because of their length of experience and full-time employment, followed by theoretical sampling. Initial interviews with staff nurses were coded to reveal management issues that were then explored with key staff. Observations were also conducted in clinical settings.

Data collection and analysis were simultaneous, and interview and observational data were reviewed concurrently to allow for constant comparisons.

Two main categories emerged from the data: 1) Nurses' perceptions of evidence-based nursing, and 2) factors affecting evidence-based nursing.

QUANTITATIVE RESEARCH

Quantitative research seeks to generate numerical data that can be analysed using statistics. It emerged from a positivist position, which has developed more latterly into a post-positivist approach. Put crudely, positivism seeks to generate understanding from phenomena that are observable and generates scientific knowledge from verified facts (Bryman, 2012). Its approach seeks to be formal, objective, rigorous, controlled, and a systematic process is followed to generate knowledge. Post-positivists recognise that social phenomena cannot be understood through uncovering universal laws, and that it is problematic to predict a cause-and-effect relationship that is true for all. Post-positivists look at relationships or correlations between variables being measured (see Chapter 26) and maintain some of the processes of empiricism, answering hypotheses or research questions through a scientific approach.

Quantitative approaches are often used to describe new phenomena, such as whether a newly discovered drug treatment is better than existing prescriptions, or they can be used to test the effectiveness of alternative therapies on cardiac care patients.

The origins of quantitative research lie in the work of Fisher (1971), who developed the ideas of the hypothesis (a statement of predicted outcome tested by the researcher), research design and statistical analysis. Today nurse researchers use these methods to measure cause-and-effect relationships (see Chapter 14). The 'true experiment' has since been developed to include the quasi-experiment (Shadish et al., 2002), used to test a cause-and-effect relationship where conditions are less controlled. **Quasi-experiments** are used in social science and healthcare research where it is often impossible to control and limit the effect of a number of variables, or to randomly allocate patients to groups (see Chapter 14). An experiment may be used to test the relationship between a particular treatment and its effect or outcome responses.

Correlation studies can be a precursor to experimental or quasi-experimental research, aiding the development of a hypothesis (Burns et al., 2014). Correlation research aims to identify the strength of a relationship between two variables, gauged through statistical testing that identifies results between a perfect positive (+1) to perfect negative (−1). Correlation may be used to measure the relationship between information provision and well-being.

Descriptive research is also used to generate nursing knowledge for practice. These approaches aim to describe phenomena, provide a description of what exists and present frequency measures that can be used to develop hypotheses for testing. These approaches can consider questions such as: What are the completion rates on particular nursing programmes? How many hours a day do nurses spend in completing electronic patient records? What are patient's attitudes to physiotherapy services in rehabilitation?

Quantitative designs

Nurse researchers employing quantitative research will be addressing hypotheses that look to measure cause-and-effect relationships, seeking to measure the correlation relationship between two different phenomena or wanting to describe phenomena about which little is understood. Data collection will be structured with information being gathered from a representative sample (see Chapter 12); often the researcher may be detached from the process. Statistical analysis of collected data is aimed to accept or reject any predicted cause-and-effect relationship or describe a new phenomenon and generate a new hypothesis.

Though a number of different types of research design exist, those mainly used within nursing research include:

- Experimental
- Quasi-experimental
- Survey.

These designs are discussed in detail in Chapter 14, with brief explanations provided here. Further designs include evaluative studies (see Chapter 16), case studies, action research (see Chapters 18 and 19) and Delphi technique (see Chapter 17).

EXPERIMENTAL RESEARCH

A hypothesis will usually guide an experimental design that sets out to test a cause-and-effect relationship. The nurse researcher will include elements of control, randomisation and manipulation. Simply, the researcher will identify a specific research population, and randomly allocate these to an experimental or treatment group and a control group. The researcher will introduce and manipulate particular variables with the treatment group and measure the effect on particular pre-defined outcome measures. The outcome measures will be taken from the control group, who did not receive the intervention, and the data will be subjected to statistical comparison. A Research example is given below.

Research example 11.4

Randomised Controlled Trial

Silva et al. (2010) used a randomised controlled trial to see whether behaviour change interventions were effective in promoting physical exercise and weight control behaviours in women. In total a sample of 239 was accessed, who met a series of inclusion criteria. These were: aged between 25 and 50 years, not pregnant, free from major illness and have a recorded body mass index of between 25 and 40 kg/m². The use of inclusion criteria allowed the researchers to control a number of variables, which could affect the research outcomes, such as very large differences in weight. The women were randomised into either the control or experimental group. The control group received general health improvement guidance whereas the experimental group received the intervention based on self-determination theory that promoted autonomous forms of exercise and intrinsic motivation. The researchers recorded weight and exercise levels over a 12-month period for both groups and compared the data to look for any statistically significant difference in measurement between the groups. Those women on the self-determination programme had achieved the greatest weight loss and higher levels of physical activity suggesting the programme they had received was more effective than the health improvement guidance delivered to the control group.

QUASI-EXPERIMENTAL RESEARCH

This approach mirrors that of the experimental design in many respects, with the use of a hypothesis to establish a cause-and-effect relationship. Often the design is employed when factors make one or more elements of control, manipulation or randomisation difficult to achieve.

Research example 11.5

Quasi-experimental

Holmila et al. (2010) used a quasi-experimental approach to introduce an intervention to control teenage drinking. The study did not assign intervention sites randomly and therefore randomisation of the sample was not achieved. The intervention sites were chosen purposively and the controls were matched according to a number of local characteristics. This meant the study was a quasi-experimental design. Whilst there was a control group this was matched to the experimental sites and random allocation was not achieved. Manipulation was achieved as the experimental sites received an additional intervention and outcomes from both sites were measured and compared.

SURVEYS

Surveys can be used to gather data, through self-reporting, about an identified and specific population. This data is collected through postal, telephone, or online question-naires, **structured interviews** or even observations (Burns et al., 2014). Thus, the survey can be used to collect data as part of quasi-experimental (Abramson and Abramson, 2008) descriptive and correlation studies. Research example 11.6 provides an example.

Research example 11.6

Online survey

Bruns et al. (2012) used an online survey to access physicians at three different sites across Brazil. In total, 41,847 physicians were invited to respond by email. The survey tool included 21 questions related to the measurements undertaken of the fetal heart as part of routine scanning in pregnancy. The final response rate was 467 and whilst lower than might have been expected, respondents were secured from across Brazil and provided sufficient data for meaningful analysis.

Reflective exercise

Most of us have completed a survey; these can be market research surveys com-pleted when you are shopping or telephone surveys asking about service received. Next time you complete a survey think about what the survey is trying to find out. Do you think the questions asked will help the researchers find out what they are most interested in? How long is the survey? How is it administered? Could the survey be improved in any way?

TRIANGULATION IN RESEARCH

Triangulation in research draws on multiple methods, combining both qualitative and quantitative approaches in one research study to address the research questions, aims and objectives (Denzin, 2009). Nurse researchers may choose to triangulate research approaches in order to address complex nursing problems and combine study of relationships and human experience with measuring causality or correlation. For example, a combined approach may be used to explore questions about patients' ability and experiences of coping with living with a chronic condition, such as cardiac fail-ure. It is suggested that operating with a triangulation of methods will require team expertise in each area and a commitment to maintain the philosophical underpinning of both approaches (Burns et al., 2014). A mixed methods approach is frequently used and is increasingly popular. For example, a study aiming to look at a new intervention and measure economic benefits may include a survey conducted with a large number of patients, which includes health economic measures. The survey will have to collect initial baseline data prior to the new intervention and then will be repeated after a period of time to measure any changes. The survey tool can also act to support recruitment for individual interviews, by inclusion of a final question that asks participants to volunteer for a second stage of data collection. The design might also include interviews with wider stakeholders such as staff delivering the intervention.

Chapter 21 highlights the different levels of possible triangulation and discusses the perceived benefits and issues associated with combining research approaches. It is suggested that through triangulation in data collection some of the concerns related to weaknesses of particular approaches can be lessened (Denzin, 2009). However, not all support this view and there remain concerns that weaknesses may be exaggerated and that the difficulties of attempting to combine differing philosophical positions within one approach affect the trustworthiness of any claims. It is also suggested that the readers of research employing triangulation should be aware of the need to understand and review the strengths and weakness of a combined study considering issues of trustworthiness and rigour (see Chapter 13) in reviewing how a triangulated approach is used to answer specific research question(s).

CHAPTER SUMMARY

- The selection of the overall research approach must be appropriate to the study.
- The research design includes the approach, methods of data collection and analysis that will be used to address the research questions, aims and objectives.
- There isn't a perfect research design, and frequently decisions about aspects such as sampling and data collection methods will be guided by the practicalities of the research endeavour.
- The main qualitative designs include phenomenology, ethnography and grounded theory.
- The main designs used in quantitative research include experimental, quasi-experimental and survey.

SUGGESTED FURTHER READING

Andrew, S. and Halcomb, E. (eds) (2009) *Mixed Methods Research for Nursing and the Health Sciences*. Oxford: John Wiley and Sons Ltd. This text introduces missed methods designs and offers advice on their conduct, providing a range of exemplar examples.

Cresswell, J. and Piano Clarke, V. (2011) *Research Design: Qualitative, Quantitative and Mixed Methods Approaches*, 3rd edn. Los Angeles: Sage. A comprehensive guide to mixed methods approaches. The book discusses a range of designs in detail.

Punch, K. (2011) *Introduction to Social Research: Quantitative and Qualitative Approaches*, 3rd edn. London: Sage. This book provides a detailed description of both quantitative and qualitative design and mixed methods. It includes coverage of ethics and using the Internet in research.

WEBSITES

Research methods tutorials: www.socialresearchmethods.net/ – this site offers resources for applied social research and evaluation.

National Centre for Research Methods: www.ncrm.ac.uk – offers training and information on research methods.

To access further resources related to this chapter, visit the companion website at https://study.sagepub.com/mouleaveyard3e

REFERENCES

Abid-Hajbaghery, M. (2007) 'Factors facilitating and inhibiting evidence-based nursing in Iran', *Journal of Advanced Nursing*, 58 (6): 566–75.

Abramson, J. and Abramson, Z. (2008) *Survey Methods in Community Medicine*, 6th edn. Oxford: John Wiley and Sons Ltd.

Bruns, R., Junior, E., Nardozza, M., Martins, W. and Moron, A. (2012) 'Measurement and planes assessed during second-trimester scans in Brazil: An online survey', *The Journal of Maternal-Fetal and Neonatal Medicine*, 25 (11): 2242–7.

Bryman, A. (2012) *Social Research Methods*, 4th edn. Oxford: Oxford University Press.

Burns, N., Grove, S. and Gray, J. (2014) *The Practice of Nursing Research: Appraisal, Synthesis and Generation of Evidence*, 7th edn. St Louis, MO: Saunders Elsevier.

Denzin, N. (2009) *The Research Act: A Theoretical Introduction to Sociological Methods.* NJ: Transactional Publishers.

Fisher, R. (1971) *The Designs of Experiments.* New York: Hafner Publishers.

Glaser, B. and Strauss, A. (2008) *The Discovery of Grounded Theory: Strategies for Qualitative Research.* Chicago, IL: Aldine Transactions.

Guba, E. and Lincoln, Y. (1994) 'Competing paradigms in qualitative research', in N. Denzin and Y. Lincoln (eds), *Handbook of Qualitative Research.* Thousand Oaks, CA: Sage. pp. 105–17.

Hammersley, M. and Atkinson, P. (2007) *Ethnography: Principles in Practice*, 3rd edn. NY: Taylor and Francis.

Holmila, M., Larlsson, T. and Warpenius, K. (2010) 'Controlling teenager's drinking: Effects of a community based prevention project', *Journal of Substance Use*, 15 (3): 201–14.

Lee, Y-K., Lee, P-Y. and Ng, J. (2012) 'A qualitative study on healthcare professionals' perceived barriers to insulin initiation in a multi-ethnic population', *BMC Family Practice*, 13 (1): 28–38.

Miles, M., Huberman, A. and Saldana, J. (2013) *Qualitative Data Analysis: A Methods Sourcebook*, 3rd edn. Thousand Oaks, CA: Sage.

Polit, D. and Beck, C. (2014) *Essentials of Nursing Research: Appraising Evidence for Nursing Practice*, 8th edn. Philadelphia, PA: Lippincott Williams & Wilkins.

Shadish, W., Cook, T. and Campbell, D. (2002) *Experimental and Quasi-experimental Designs for Generalised Causal Inference*, 2nd revised edn. NY: Houghton Mifflin Houghton.

Silva, M., Viera, P., Countinho, S., Minderico, C., Mathis, M., Sardinha, L. and Teixeria, P. (2010) 'Using a self-determination theory to promote physical activity and weight control: A randomised controlled trial in women', *Journal of Behavioural Medicine*, 33: 110–22.

Smith, J., Flowers, P. and Larkin, M. (2009) *Interpretative Phenomenological Analysis: Theory, Method and Research.* London: Sage.

Strauss, A. and Corbin, J. (2015) *Basics of Qualitative Research: Techniques and Procedures for Developing Grounded Theory*, 4th edn. Thousand Oaks, CA: Sage.

Thomson, D. (2011) 'Ethnography: A suitable approach for providing an inside perspective on the everyday lives of health professionals', *International Journal of Therapy and Rehabilitation*, 18 (1): 10–17.

Yin, R. (2014) *Case Study Research: Design and Methods*, 5th edn. Thousand Oaks, CA: Sage.

12
SAMPLING TECHNIQUES

Learning outcomes

This chapter will enable you to:

- Understand definitions of a research population and sample
- Appreciate the need for different approaches to identifying sample size within quantitative and qualitative research
- Appreciate the different sampling techniques used in qualitative and quantitative research
- Discuss the strengths and weaknesses of different sampling strategies available
- Appreciate the ethical issues involved in sample access

Nurse researchers will invariably need to employ sampling techniques in their research to make the project manageable. The time and expense involved in research projects prohibits data collection on the scale seen in the national census, involving the entire population. Therefore, researchers will want to ensure that the sample size and composition are appropriate to the study to strengthen the research outcomes and conclusion drawing. The process of sample selection is a crucial stage in the research process, with poor sampling techniques having the potential to compromise the research findings. A number of sampling strategies exist for use in both qualitative and quantitative or mixed-methods research, none being an exact science as each has individual strengths and weaknesses. In this chapter, we consider the ways in which nurse researchers select populations and samples. The discussion reviews a number of recognised sampling techniques that fall within probability and non-probability-sampling strategies, identifying the strengths and weaknesses of the different approaches available.

DEFINING THE POPULATION AND SAMPLE

The researcher will be interested in collecting information or data from a particular **population** whose composition meets specific criteria. For example, nurse researchers might be asking research questions about undergraduate nursing students or service users suffering from particular mental health problems. These groups form the target population. Depending on the area of research interest, the population might be large, such as all nurses employed within the United Kingdom (UK), or defined more narrowly as practising children's nurses within the UK. Populations need not always include human subjects, and could incorporate documents, events or objects.

Nurse researchers will often set specific parameters before selecting the sample, limiting the study population through the use of inclusion or eligibility criteria. These are criteria that the population members either must have (inclusion) or should not have (exclusion). The criteria for inclusion or exclusion might relate to age, gender, professional qualifications or diagnosis. Those studies using quantitative methods will hope to sample from an accessible population in order to generalise the research findings to the wider target population. For example, the target population may include all patients recovering from a myocardial infarction in the UK, yet the researchers will work with an accessible population composed of those patients who meet the eligibility criteria.

A **sample** is a subset of the population, selected through sampling techniques. Polit and Beck (2014) suggest that the entities making up a sample are known as elements. Frequently nursing research will see individual patients or nurses as elements within a sample, though elements may be documents or biological specimens. Nurse researchers employ sampling strategies to enable them to work with a sample, as it is unrealistic and uneconomic to collect data from an entire population. As researchers are working with a sample it is important, particularly in quantitative research, that the sample selected is representative of the target population, being as similar as possible to the population to which the results will be generalised (LoBiondo-Wood and Haber, 2014). If there are major differences between the target and accessible population, these should be acknowledged by the researcher as a limitation of the study, as this can impact on the generalisability and transferability of the research outcomes. For example, differences between the target and accessible population would exist if a study was aiming to recruit children's nurses who were members of an ethnic minority group, but was unable to achieve these criteria when recruiting from an accessible sample. Though there is no guaranteed method of achieving a representative sample, the use of **sampling frames** and plans can assist the process.

SAMPLING FRAMES

A sampling frame is developed to include all of the possible members of the population who might be eligible for inclusion in the final sample. It will be composed of a list of all of the patients, nurses, cases or events in the accessible population, established through the use of eligibility criteria. Those included in the sampling frame will therefore reflect as closely as possible the characteristics of the target population. The nurse researcher employs the sampling frame to identify the sample group. Many sampling frames are already in existence that can be used by researchers. Those wanting to study nurses and midwives could draw on the Nursing and Midwifery Council register, and universities hold lists of students enrolled on nursing courses that can be accessed. It should be noted, however, that the researcher might experience difficulties if the sampling frame is incomplete or inaccurate. In some cases it may not be possible to generate such a frame-work. Nurse researchers exploring questions with drug and alcohol users would not have access to a sampling frame and might find it difficult to construct one. Inaccuracies in a sampling frame may lead to errors in the generated sample. These systematic errors occur as the sampling frame is lacking particular elements of the population, a problem that cannot be remedied unless the frame is corrected.

It is also important to note that sampling frames have limited relevance to qualitative research, which does not seek to generalise the findings of research to a wider population. The types of sampling approaches used in these cases are discussed later in the chapter.

SAMPLE SIZE CALCULATION IN QUANTITATIVE RESEARCH

Nurse researchers undertaking quantitative research will want to determine the size of the sample required so that the study can be powered to ensure any statistical differences between groups in intervention and comparison studies can be shown. A statistician often completes the calculation of the required sample size, a power calculation, in the design stage. For example, research by Moule et al. (2006) aimed to compare the results of two groups of nursing students, those who had completed nursing skill simulation training and a second group of non-completers. A power calculation suggested that the research should include a minimum of 62 participants in both the simulation and the control groups in order to demonstrate significant results at an 80 per cent confidence level. This meant that the significance level was set at 20 per cent and any significant results achieved would mean the researchers could be 80 per cent confident that the results were related to a real difference between the simulation and control groups. However, there was a 20 per cent chance that a real difference would not be detected. Usually the greater the power, such as increasing to a 95 per cent confidence level, the larger the sample size required.

The statistician will consider the outcomes being measured, tools of measurement and the expected differences between the groups in order to complete a power calculation. Those studies unable to achieve a sample size great enough to achieve the power required are seen as flawed. In some cases a pilot study may be completed and the results used to power a larger study.

SAMPLE SIZE IN QUALITATIVE RESEARCH

We have seen that a specific **sample size calculation** is needed to support quantitative research where the final sample size is intrinsic to the data analysis. In contrast, qualitative researchers have no specific rules of sample size to work with. Smaller sample sizes of 6 to 10 might be used to describe the experience of a population; however, when the researcher wants to look at variation across the group members, then the sample size should be larger (Polit and Beck, 2014). Ultimately, the size of the sample should be based on the need to obtain sufficient information to address the research questions.

Often, qualitative researchers will aim to achieve data saturation. This is achieved when the researcher fails to identify any new data from the participants, and at this stage sampling should cease.

PROBABILITY SAMPLING

Probability sampling is characterised by the use of random selection to obtain sample members. The use of random selection occurs when the elements of a population, be that individuals, events or objects, have an equal chance of being included in the final sample. This approach to sampling allows the researcher to state the probability of an element of the population appearing in the sample. It reduces sampling errors and bias and increases sample representativeness, thus giving increased confidence in the sample. It is the preferable approach when a representative sample is required and is therefore often employed in quasi-experimental and experimental designs. However, bias can be present within random samples, resultant from random errors and systematic errors. Random errors are those occurring randomly within the final sample. For example, a randomly selected sample may have an over-representation of a particular ethnic group. Increasing the sample size used can reduce the chances of this type of sampling error. Systematic errors occur as a result of inaccuracies in the sampling frame and cannot be corrected through increasing the sample size. Correction would require changes to the sampling frame that remove inaccuracies. There are four commonly used probability-sampling approaches: **simple random sampling**, **systematic random sampling**, **stratified random sampling** and **cluster** or **multi-stage sampling**.

Simple random sampling

A simple random sampling approach to identifying a sample is rigorous, but often time-consuming. The principles of simple random selection as described here are duplicated across the different random sampling approaches. There are a number of approaches that can be used to achieve randomisation, with the website www.randomisation.com providing an electronic resource for researchers. The nurse researcher will draw on the sampling frame to select a sample as a subset of the population. For example, if the researcher wanted to access patients recovering from resuscitation events, the sampling frame would include all patients meeting the eligibility criteria within an acute hospital. The sampling frame might include a wider sample group of perhaps all those nurses working as Cancer Nurse Specialists across the UK. The simplest way of identifying a sample is from the frame generated electronically. A list of random numbers from, say, 0 to 99 or greater can be used to select pre-numbered elements from the sampling frame. Statistical packages such as Statistical Packages for Social Scientists (SPSS) can generate random numbers to enable sample selection.

There are various advantages to this sampling approach. It removes the potential biases of the researcher from the selection process; any differences seen in the characteristics of the sample and population have occurred by chance, and as the sample size increases the probability of selecting a non-representation sample decreases. However, some disadvantages are also noted. Those reviewing research using this sampling approach must recognise the limitations of the sampling strategy that can emerge if the researchers have been unable to list the target population. Research example 12.1 gives an example of simple random sampling strategies.

Research example 12.1

Example of simple random sampling

Simple random sampling was used in research based in Nigeria. The research undertaken by Onwujekwe et al. (2009) explored whether community-based health insurance was an equitable strategy for funding healthcare provision. Community-based health insurance is a form of voluntary health insurance that is increasingly being implemented in Africa. The insurance system is designed by and for the people and is expected to improve the health system for the community. Systematic random sampling was applied within 10 local government areas engaged in the scheme. All households in the areas were assigned numbers that were then used to select a simple random sample. In total 455 households were selected from the numbered list in one area and 516 in the second area.

Systematic random sampling

This approach to sampling is best employed when a 'database' is available that can be used to organise the sample to allow systematic selection. For example, if researchers wanted to systematically sample qualified nurses in the UK, they could ask the Nursing and Midwifery Council for access to the current database of qualified nurses. The sampling must start at a random point in the population, not necessarily with the first identified member. The researcher must know the total population size and the number of the sample required to allow calculation of the sampling gap (Burns et al., 2014). For example, if the population is 1,000 and 100 participants are required for the research, then every 10th member of the population will be sampled as 1,000/100 = 10. The initial sample selection would occur between numbers 1 and 10, with the tenth person included thereafter. If number 8 were initially selected, then the sample would include numbers 18, 28, 38 and so on. See Research example 12.2 for a further example. Whilst this approach should eliminate bias, it should be remembered that the approach relies on the original list being accurate and free from any bias in its generation.

Research example 12.2

Example of systematic random sampling

Uzodike et al. (2015) used systematic sampling in South Africa to access adult patients attending a primary healthcare antiretroviral therapy clinic. The population had attended the clinic between June 2011 and June 2012. In this period, 1,633 patients received treatment at the clinic. A sample of 488 charts, a total of 30 per cent of this population, was selected for the study. Systematic random sampling was used to select every third file in the clinic until the sample size was achieved.

Stratified random sampling

Nurse researchers might use a stratified random sampling technique when certain characteristics of the population are needed to address the research questions. It may be the case, for example, that particular age groups are required, grades of nursing staff, gender, ethnic groups or staff with particular levels of experience (see Research example 12.3). A study might want to access 200 surgical patients at different treatment stages arranged into four strata. It might include those patients currently receiving treatment and those six weeks, six months and one year following surgery. The participants are randomly selected to represent the four strata identified. Greater commonality in the sample is expected within each of the strata than across the four different strata.

The researcher can undertake proportionate sampling, ensuring that all the strata have the same total number of participants. If selecting a proportionate sample for the example above, each of the four strata would have 50 participants. Alternatively, there may be justification for selecting for a disproportionate sample. Research canvassing the views of nurses might want a sample stratified into males and females. A proportionate sample would see equal numbers of males and females included; however, this does not represent the total population of nursing, which employs more females than males. It might therefore be appropriate to select a disproportionate sample with a greater number of females than males in the strata. An alternative approach is to maintain strata of equal proportions and attach weighting to the findings of the strata to equalise the effect of the different strata sizes.

It is suggested that stratified sampling can challenge the researcher (LoBiondo-Wood and Haber, 2014). First, the sampling approach requires access to an initial list composed in a way that allows sampling in the strata required. Second, it can be difficult to ensure that the different sample proportions are achieved and, finally, the process can be time-consuming.

Research example 12.3

Example of stratified random sampling

Stratified random sampling was used by Vuorenmaa et al. (2013) as part of research with parents in Finland. The sampling approach was used to select participants for a study that evaluated the validity and reliability of a scale used with parents, the Finnish Family Empowerment Scale. To access a stratified random sample, the Population Register Centre information system was used. This held information on parents with children aged between 0 and 9 years. The children were stratified into a number of age groups; 0-1 years, 2-5 years, 6, 7, 8 and 9 year olds. Parents were selected from the six groupings. These were used to ensure that participating parents would be using different types of health and education services such as child health clinics, day school, pre-school and primary school services.

Cluster sampling

Cluster sampling is a term used interchangeably with multi-stage sampling. It is often employed when simple random sampling is too expensive and complex to organise and when the individual elements of a population are unknown. Cluster or multi-stage sampling involves a staged approach to sample selection that uses an initial sampling frame. Sample selection usually narrows from large to small clusters, such as selecting one health region from the initial sampling frame, then selecting one hospital from that region and finally selecting to one or two wards within the hospital. From these wards individual patients or staff can be recruited.

This approach can enable the nurse researcher to access samples at a small cost using a random sampling approach. Weaknesses in the approach can exist if the samples are closely associated and similar, as they originate in the same locality (Bowling, 2014). This may mean that a larger sample size is required to increase precision (Burns et al., 2014).

NON-PROBABILITY SAMPLING

Non-random methods are used to select elements for inclusion in **non-probability sampling**. This means the researcher is unable to state the chances of elements of the population appearing in the final sample. Often, non-probability sampling is employed by qualitative researchers who use different techniques from those seen in quantitative research to access their samples. Most qualitative researchers are not concerned with measuring specific attributes of a sample in order to generalise the findings to a wider population. Instead, the focus of qualitative research is to gain understanding, experience and meaning from the most appropriate sample. The main methods of sampling used include **convenience** or **accidental**, **quota** and **purposive sampling**. Samples can also be described as being generated through **network** or **snowball** techniques. It should be noted that though most commonly seen in qualitative research, these sampling approaches might be used in quantitative research if the researcher is unable to access data necessary to support random sampling techniques.

Convenience (accidental) sampling

Gathering information from those cases or people locally available is known as using a convenience or accidental sample. A market researcher who canvasses in the local supermarket or street corner will gather opinion and views from an accidental sample of shoppers and pedestrians who happen to be in the location at the time. This approach excludes all other members of the population who shop elsewhere. Nurse researchers often draw on the local community of staff and patients to form a sample of convenience (see Research example 12.4). Conducting interviews with staff employed in the local hospital trust, student nurses at the local university or patients within a particular Accident and Emergency department would constitute the use of a convenience sample.

Often, the sample is composed of those who volunteer or self-select, which can lead to concerns that those recruited have given their time because they have a particular view to present. A researcher accessing a convenient sample of healthcare staff to ask about the use of computers in the workplace may find that those volunteering are either keen to use computers or have a real dislike of information technology use in the work-place. The risk of introducing bias in this sampling approach is far greater, therefore, than in any other sampling technique (LoBiondo-Wood and Haber, 2014).

Research example 12.4

Example of convenience sampling

Kovačič and Kovačič (2011) undertook a pilot study to gather information on the immediate and short-term effects of relaxation therapy on the self-esteem of patients with breast cancer. A convenient sample of 32 patients was recruited from an accessible population of women from the local hospital in Slovenia. The sample was a convenient sample because it was drawn from a local population of women, easily accessed by the researchers. The researchers did have some inclusion criteria set for the sample – all had to be female and have had breast cancer surgery; in addition all were between the ages of 19 and 44. The women were randomised into the experimental group (n = 16) and the control group (n = 16). Both groups received the standard physiotherapy treatment for one week and the experimental group was given additional relaxation training and a relaxation tape to practise at home. The effect of the relaxation treatment was measured through the use of an outcome measure, a questionnaire measuring self-esteem, used at 1 and 4 weeks and also prior to radiation treatment. The findings showed statistically significant differences in self-esteem scores between the groups, with the experimental group achieving higher self-esteem.

Quota sampling

In order to use quota sampling, the researcher must have some knowledge of the composition of the population of interest in order to identify specific strata in the population. The researcher ensures the strata are included in the sample. For example, if researching diabetic treatments, then the inclusion of patients with diabetes from different age ranges may be important. Sample numbers would be selected to represent the proportions of patients in different age bands receiving treatment. If there are 1,000 patients receiving diabetic treatment and the final sample size is 100 or 10 per cent, then the proportion of each age group who should be included in the sample needs calculating. If 20 per cent, or 200 of the original 1,000 treated for diabetes are aged under ten years, then 20 per cent of the 200 will be selected, requiring the researcher to select 20 participants from the age group 0–10. See Research Example 12.5 for a further example.

The criteria for selection could include gender, ethnicity, socio-economic status, employment, educational level or diagnosis. The sampling technique should reduce the chances of over- or under-representation, but bias can still exist. This can occur if those included in the sample are not typical members of the population.

Research example 12.5

Example of quota sampling

Robb et al. (2010) aimed to assess awareness of three National Cancer Screening Programmers for breast, cervical and bowel cancer in the UK. The populations they were interested in included ethnic minority groups, in particular the six largest minority groups in the UK (Indian, Pakistan, Bangladeshi, Caribbean, African and Chinese). The team used a quota sampling approach to ensure they were able to include members of the different populations in the research. The sample included 1,500 adults from the six ethnic minority groups who completed a questionnaire on awareness of the screening programmes and took part in face-to-face interviews. In this research the quota levels for the six ethnic minority groups was high; in some research quota numbers will be much smaller. In this example the criteria for selection was related to ethnicity and quota sampling was used to try to reduce over- or under-representation of the six different groups.

Purposive sampling

Often used in qualitative research, purposive sampling aims to sample a group of people or events with a specific set of experiences or characteristics. The technique can also be referred to as 'judgement sampling', as the researcher is making a judgement about the composition of the sample, selecting participants who they believe have either experienced a particular episode or have a set of knowledge that relates to addressing the research question (see Research example 12.6). Patton (2015) identifies several strategies that can be employed in purposive sampling, including extreme or deviant case sampling (extreme and unusual cases), typical case sampling (average or typical cases) and criterion sampling (cases where pre-determined criteria exist).

A purposive sample has an over-representation of a particular group and is not representative of an entire population being studied. For example, if the research question is aiming to review emerging new roles in nursing, the researcher may select a purposive sample of modern matrons who are believed to undertake a relatively new role in a particular way. The selection is based on the researcher's judgement and selection of those modern matrons practising in a variety of different ways.

It is suggested that purposive sampling can also be used to pilot questionnaires or develop hypotheses for further study (Bowling, 2014). Purposive sampling has also been employed within experimental designs to access patients receiving a particular treatment. Obviously the results from such a study could not be generalised, as the sampling approach is non-randomised, though research outcomes could inform treatment development.

Research example 12.6

Example of purposive sampling

Chang et al. (2011) employed purposive sampling in research that aimed to explore the care needs of older patients in intensive care units.

The criteria for purposive selection identified by the researcher included patients:

- aged 65 or older
- who had never been admitted to intensive care before
- with no cognitive and mental impairment
- willing and able to participate.

In total, 35 patients were included in the sample, based in one of three district hospitals. The researchers wanted to explore the expectations of care delivery whilst in intensive care and the areas of care that should be improved or strengthened. In order to address these questions the researchers needed to sample purposively and collect data from older patients who had experienced intensive care delivery in recent weeks. The sampling criteria were also limited to those patients experiencing intensive care for the first time. This ensured patients spoke of recent experiences as an older person, rather than perhaps considering past experiences.

Network (snowball) sampling

Network or snowball sampling is the approach used when nurse researchers are aiming to select hidden samples. The researcher will need to draw on networks to identify the sample, often involving a third party in sample access. For example, researchers aiming to recruit the homeless, victims of abuse or other hidden populations may access some participants through hostels or self-help groups, using convenience-sampling methods. They then rely on the initial sample to draw on their networks to recruit further partici-pants. Burns et al. (2014) warn that such sampling techniques, whilst recruiting subjects with the knowledge and expertise to provide information for the study, have inherent biases because selection is not independent, as members of the sample are known to one another. Therefore, whilst the researcher bias can be reduced, there is the high potential for sample bias being introduced. However, the approach is often the only one available to researchers sampling populations who are less accessible.

CHAPTER SUMMARY

- An appropriate sample size and composition is crucial to strengthening the research outcomes and conclusion drawing.
- Nurse researchers will often set specific parameters, limiting the study population through the use of inclusion or eligibility criteria.
- A sample is a subset of the population, selected through sampling techniques.
- A number of sampling strategies exist for use in both qualitative, quantitative or mixed-methods research that fall within probability and non-probability-sampling techniques.
- A sampling frame and specific sample size calculation can be used to support probability sampling for quantitative research.
- Probability sampling is characterised by the use of random selection to obtain sample members.
- There are four commonly used probability-sampling approaches: simple random sam-pling, systematic random sampling, stratified random sampling and cluster sampling.
- Non-random methods are used to select elements for inclusion in non-probability sampling as qualitative researchers are concerned with gaining understanding, experience and meaning from the most appropriate sample.

- The main methods of sampling used include convenience or accidental, quota and purposive sampling. Samples can also be described as being generated through network or snowball techniques.

SUGGESTED FURTHER READING

Field, L., Pruchno, R., Bewley, J., Lemay, E.P., Jr. and Levinsky, N. (2006) 'Using probability vs. nonprobability sampling to identify hard-to-access participants for health-related research: Costs and contrasts', *Journal of Aging and Health*, 18 (4): 565–83. This article offers a comparison of the recruitment costs and participant characteristics associated with the use of both probability and non-probability sampling.

Suresh, K. and Chandrashekara, S. (2012) 'Sample size estimation and power analysis for clinical research studies', *Journal of Human Reproductive Sciences*, 5 (1): 7–13. The paper presents the essentials in calculating power and sample size.

WEBSITES

Site that provides online randomisation: www.randomization.com.

Site on clinical trials by the National Cancer Institute that includes a discussion on randomisation: http://www.cancer.gov/clinicaltrials/understanding/what-is-randomization.

To access further resources related to this chapter, visit the companion website at https://study.sagepub.com/mouleaveyard3e

REFERENCES

Bowling, A. (2014) *Research Methods in Health: Investigating Health and Health Services*, 4th edn. Berkshire: Open University Press.

Burns, N., Grove, S. and Gray, J. (2014) *The Practice of Nursing Research: Appraisal, Synthesis, and Generation of Evidence*, 7th edn. St Louis, MO: Saunders Elsevier.

Chang, C-W., Chen, Y-M. and Ching-Ching, S. (2011) 'Care needs of older patients in the intensive care units', *Journal of Clinical Nursing*, 21: 825–32.

Kovačič, T. and Kovačič, M. (2011) 'Impact of relaxation training according to Yoga in Daily Life®System on self-esteem after breast cancer surgery', *Journal of Alternative and Complementary Medicine*, 17 (12): 1157–64.

LoBiondo-Wood, G. and Haber, J. (2014) *Nursing Research: Methods and Critical Appraisal for Evidence-based Practice*, 8th edn. St Louis, MO: Mosby Elsevier.

Moule, P., Wilford, A., Sales, R., Haycock, L. and Lockyer, L. (2006) 'Can the use of simulation support pre-registration nursing students in familiarising themselves with clinical skills before consolidating them in practice?', Faculty of Health and Social Care, University of the West of England, Bristol. Available at: http://hsc.uwe.ac.uk/net/research/ Data/Sites/1/GalleryImages/ Research/NMC%20Final%20Report%20UWE.pdf (accessed 28 July 2015).

Onwujekwe, O., Onoka, C., Uzochukwu, B., Okoli, C., Obokeze, E. and Eze, S. (2009) 'Is community-based health insurance an equitable strategy for paying for healthcare? Experiences from southeast Nigeria', *Health Policy*, 92 (1): 96–102.

Patton, M. (2015) *Qualitative Evaluation and Research Methods*, 4th edn. Thousand Oaks, CA: Sage.

Polit, D. and Beck, C. (2014) *Essentials of Nursing Research: Appraising Evidence for Nursing Practice*, 8th edn. Philadelphia, PA: Lippincott Williams & Wilkins.

Potter, Y. and Justham, D. (2012) 'Washing and changing uniforms: Is guidance being adhered to?', *British Journal of Nursing*, 21 (11): 649–53.

Robb, K., Wardle, J., Stubbings, S., Ramirez, A., Austoker, J., Macleod, U., Hiom, S. and Waller, J. (2010) 'Ethnic disparities in knowledge of cancer screening programmes in the UK', *Journal of Medical Screening*, 17 (30): 125–31.

Uzodike, N., Ross, A. and Harbor, O. (2015) 'Adherence by a primary healthcare clinic in KwaZulu-Natal to the national HIV guidelines', *South African Family Practice*, 57 (3): 198–202.

Vuorenmaa, M., Halme, N., Astedt-Kurl, P., Kaunonen, M. and Perala, M. (2013) 'The validity and reliability of the Finnish Family Empowerment Scale (FES): A survey of parents with small children', *Child: Care, Health and Development*, 40 (4): 597–606.

13
RIGOUR AND TRUSTWORTHINESS IN RESEARCH

Learning outcomes

This chapter will enable you to:

- Understand the terms 'reliability' and 'validity' in quantitative research
- Describe how reliability and validity can be assessed in quantitative research
- Understand how rigour and trustworthiness can be established in qualitative research
- Explain the four dimensions of trustworthiness

Nursing research has its traditions in qualitative and quantitative methods, though is increasingly employing mixed method designs, combining both approaches in addressing research questions. A number of chapters in this book discuss the research approaches and methods that can be used (see Chapters 11, 14–19 and 21) and refer to the need for rigour, trustworthiness, validity and reliability in their application. In this chapter we explain what these concepts mean and how they can be evaluated within nursing research.

RIGOUR, VALIDITY AND RELIABILITY IN QUANTITATIVE RESEARCH

Nurse researchers working with quantitative methods have sought to ensure **validity** and **reliability** in their methods of data collection to maintain the **rigour** of the study. Validity and reliability are related to the data collection methods and tools employed in the research and to the extent that the researcher has been able to limit any bias in data collection processes. Having a valid and reliable data collection tool affords **credibility** to the instrument and subsequent research findings.

Validity

Validity is a measure of whether a data collection tool accurately measures what it is supposed to. In nursing practice we use validated measurement tools to record data on a daily basis. Such examples include the use of recording devices to measure a patient's blood pressure and pulse. Three types of validity measures are available to the researcher; **content validity** (being the most basic), **criterion-related validity** and **construct validity**.

Content validity

Content validity is concerned with the ability of the measure; say the questions in a questionnaire, to collect data about the phenomena under study. If we are interested in how much knowledge someone has on resuscitation, a pre-test can be developed to cover all aspects of the knowledge required. There is no one way of determining the content validity of this pre-test. One approach would be to get an expert review. Experts in the field might be asked to look at the questions and comment on whether they represent the range of questions that might be asked in relation to resuscitation. They might also comment on any questions included that are irrelevant. Another way of validating the content of a questionnaire is through the calculation of a content validity index (CVI). To do this a panel of experts would review the questionnaire and rate the relevance of the questions to the subject. For example, a basic life support pre-test may include questions on maintaining safety, assessment for circulation and breathing, and the delivery of chest compressions. The panel would decide which of these questions were 'very important', 'important', or 'not important'. The index is calculated to reflect the level of agreement seen across the panel member ratings. If all of the members felt a question was 'not important' it might be removed. An example is given in Research example 13.1.

Research example 13.1

Example of the generation of content validity

Gillespie et al. (2012) employed expert review panels as part of a process of determining the content validity of the *Perceived Perioperative Competence Scale-Revised* (PPCS-R). The development of the tool involved a series of expert panel reviews to identify the speciality standards that define competent practice in the perioperative environment. Initially, eight conceptual domains of competence were identified and included, technical and procedural knowledge, practical knowledge and aesthetic knowledge, also communication, teamwork, co-ordination and clinical leadership. An original 120-item questionnaire developed from literature and pilot work was reduced to a 98-item scale through two rounds of assessment using the content validity index mentioned above. This tool was tested with 345 nurses in Australia. As a result a 94-item tool was further developed and tested with a sample of 1,138 Operating Room nurses. Finally a 40-item tool was achieved. The application of the scales confirmed an initial hypothesis that nurses with more clinical experience and perioperative qualifications had higher levels of perceived competence.

The term 'face validity' can also be used. This implies that the measure appears to measure what it is intended to, 'on the face of it'. This judgement follows a review of the questionnaire, but not necessarily by a subject expert. The questionnaire could be given to one person, such as a colleague, to review. Alternatively, a number of participants might be asked to review the questionnaire and identify issues such as questions that don't make sense or those that might be difficult to interpret and answer.

Criterion-related validity

A second type of validity measure is criterion-related validity. In using this, the nurse researcher will attempt to measure the validity of the data collection tool by comparing its findings with those collected from another method. The results obtained by the measure to be validated might be compared with those obtained through another validated questionnaire. If the scores are closely correlated, then the tool can be described as having criterion-related validity. Two types of criterion-related validity exist: concurrent and predictive.

Concurrent validity describes the ability of two measures administered at the same time (concurrently) to achieve correlated outcomes. A survey measuring patients' nutrition whilst in hospital can have concurrent validity if the results identifying those patients who are undernourished correlate with nurses' observations of patients' dietary requests and feeding habits.

Predictive validity describes the ability of the measure to determine the possible difference between the current and future measures of the same criteria. For example, a tool that measures the attitudes of nurses to computer use in the workplace now, will have predictive validity if the findings are consistent with future behaviour and attitudes towards computer use. So if the tool finds that nurses have a negative attitude to computers, then it will have had predictive validity if nurses in the future react to computers in a negative way.

Construct validity

Polit and Beck (2014) suggest that establishing construct validity is more challenging than content or criterion-related validity as it involves making a judgement relating to what the instrument is measuring. In other words, how much is a questionnaire able to measure the criterion or constructs it is intending to measure, such as health, anxiety or empathy? These constructs are complex and therefore challenging to measure. The researcher would draw on the relevant literature to try to identify the different facets of the construct and use these to develop the questions in the questionnaire. For example, health might include facets of being free from disease, mentally and physically able, and in a state of well-being. The questions would need to identify the presence or absence of these facets to measure how healthy someone is.

Different techniques exist that allow researchers to measure construct validity. The use of 'known-groups technique' is one example (Polit and Beck, 2014). In this technique two groups known to differ in the attributes to be measured on the construct are asked to complete the questionnaire. For example, asking two groups of patients with different levels of experience to complete the questionnaire can validate a measure of anxiety on hospitalisation for surgery. One group would include those being admitted for a surgical procedure for the first time; the second group would be composed of patients who have had more than one previous operation. The two group scores would be compared to see if there was any difference in the group responses. We would expect that the patients being admitted for surgery for the first time would be more anxious than those with previous experience. If no difference was seen, then we might be concerned about the validity of the questionnaire.

Reliability

Reliability is the consistency with which a tool measures what it is intended to. Within nursing practice a number of tools have to be not only valid in what they measure, but also reliable. Therefore the instruments used to record blood pressure, pulse and temperature not only have to take accurate measures of these vital signs, but also need to do so every time they are used. The nurse researcher is interested in three measures of reliability that include the stability of a measure, its internal consistency and equivalence.

Stability

Test–retest procedures enable researchers to establish whether a measure is stable, in other words, whether it obtains the same measurements when used on the same person at different times. Ward et al. (2009) applied the same attitude measure to a range of healthcare practitioners on two separate occasions. The scale measured attitudes towards information technology. In order for the tool to be deemed stable, the results when compared should be similar, or if different the change should be accounted for. If, for example, the staff involved in the study had completed computer training and become more involved in computer use in between the two measurements, that might account for a change in attitude, probably in a positive direction.

Internal consistency

The split-half technique is employed in measuring internal consistency. It is used with questionnaires that have a total score and measure a specific criterion. The questions are split into two groups and scored, then compared to see if they are similar. If this is the case, the questionnaire is said to have high internal consistency, as all questions are measuring the same criterion.

Equivalence

A test of equivalence is more usually applied in observational research when a number of researchers are collecting data using a schedule (see Chapter 26). Inter-rater reliability can be measured when two or more trained observers use the tool to record independent observations of the same event.

A reliability coefficient is calculated to show the strength of relationship between the observer recordings. This is illustrated in Research example 13.2.

Research example 13.2

The use of inter-rater reliability measures

Fang-Meei et al. (2012) evaluated an interview version of a tool used to screen suicide risk in hospitalised patients. A two-hour training course was provided for 54 general nurses caring for hospitalised patients. The tool was used by the nurses to screen the risk of suicide in 205 patients diagnosed with either chronic obstructive pulmonary disease or lung cancer. The nurses compared their assessments with those of their trainers within a 24-hour period. The patients completed a repulsion of life scale and symptom distress, following the nurses' assessment. The inter-rater reliability between the nurses and their trainers was strong at .85. The nurses' screening of suicide risk also correlated significantly with repulsion to life and symptom distress rated by the patients. Given the significant results it was suggested that the training might be introduced more widely to improve nurses' assessment of suicide risk.

RIGOUR AND TRUSTWORTHINESS IN QUALITATIVE RESEARCH

In considering the maintenance of rigour within qualitative research, we can see that the validity and reliability measures employed in quantitative research are not transferable. Data collection in qualitative research can involve the research participants as part of co-enquiry methods (see Chapter 15) and the researcher is often involved with participants rather than remaining detached. Data is collected using a number of methods that are neither standardised nor necessarily structured. Qualitative researchers in nursing are hoping to present the 'truth' and describe the insider or 'emic' view and therefore need to use alternative approaches to support rigour in their research. For a number of years the research community has been challenged to find a way to meet these demands.

Lincoln and Guba (1985) have developed criteria for establishing the rigour and **trustworthiness** of qualitative research. The criteria aim to allow the researcher to demonstrate how the interpretations presented in the data, and conclusions drawn, reflect participants' experiences. Four key components are included: **credibility**, **dependability**, **confirmability** and **transferability**.

Credibility

The data presented in any qualitative research report or publication has to be seen to be credible, just as quantitative data needs to be seen as valid. Those reading the research must believe that the data presented is a 'true' representation of the participants' view, experience or belief. Readers must have confidence that the interpretations remain faithful to the insider view. A number of steps can be taken that support claims for credibility. These can include the use of triangulation in data collection and prolonged engagement in the field. Researchers can also employ expert review processes and member checking, asking the participants to review the analysis and interpretation.

Triangulation can be used to enhance credibility, as discussed in Chapter 21. This might involve obtaining more than one data source in a study about a particular phenomenon, using more than one researcher to collect data or drawing on multiple methods of data collection. For example, the research may be designed to study one phenomenon using data collected through both observations and interviews. See Research example 13.3.

Research example 13.3

The use of triangulation in data collection

Bunkenborg et al. (2013) explored nursing practice in an in-hospital situation in Denmark, focusing on monitoring practices. The research was driven by the recognition that sub-optimal care in a general hospital setting can lead to patient deterioration which results in intensive care admission, cardiac arrest or sudden death. A qualitative design was used that triangulated methods of data collection including **structured observations** and individual interviews. In total 13 nurses were recruited to the study. They were observed for seven hours over ten observation periods. The researcher was known to the participants and collected data on how the nurses gathered patient information, prepared for ward rounds and communicated information with their medical and nursing colleagues. Semi-structured interviews were undertaken following the observations, which explored their experiences of bedside hospital practices of observation, assessment, monitoring and communication. The findings suggested clinical monitoring practice varied between nurses according to their different levels of professionalism.

Investing more time in the field and prolonging the length of engagement with participants will aid the development of trust with the researcher and enhance credibility. Immersion in the culture will facilitate the development of understandings that can be more readily corroborated over a prolonged period of observation.

Researchers can approach expert reviewers, such as fellow researchers, as objective peers to establish credibility. They can review the processes of sampling, data collection and analysis, and explore recordings of audio- or videotape or field notes. What Maxwell (1992) refers to as 'descriptive' and 'interpretative' validity can only be provided by the participants themselves, through a process of member checking. Descriptive validity refers to verifying the factual accuracy of the account. Interpretative validity refers to the emic account, to confirm what the participants meant in what they said or did. This involves returning the data and interpretations to the participants for their reactions and to confirm the credibility of the qualitative data.

A further measure of credibility relates to the researchers themselves and their ability to act as research instruments, as collectors and interpreters of the data. The reader of qualitative research might want to satisfy themselves of the credibility of the researcher, their qualifications and research experience.

Dependability

Qualitative data cannot be seen as credible unless its dependability is known; its ability to stand the test of time. Establishing dependability can be seen as a parallel process to that of confirming reliability in quantitative data. Lincoln and Guba (1985) suggest that an audit trail of the research can assist in establishing the dependability and confirmability of the research. As audit trails are so closely linked to confirmability, a fuller discussion is provided below.

Confirmability

Confirmability is a measure of the objectivity of the data. To confirm the objectivity, the researcher presents an audit trail of the methods, presentation of data and analytical processes presented as a decision trail, which are subjected to external audit by a reviewer introduced towards the end of the study. The findings are then subjected to an audit to establish the trustworthiness of the data. However, difficulties arise when it is impossible to completely follow a decision trail. In addition, data analysis is affected by researcher immersion in the field and data that bring uniqueness to the interpretation. It is suggested that an independent auditor could not replicate the uniqueness of a study and may well form different conclusions when following an audit trial (Sandelowski, 1998).

Transferability

Researchers need to demonstrate the extent to which the research findings can be transferred from one context to another by providing a 'thick description' of the data, as well as identifying sampling and design details. Thick description is the thorough description of the research setting and research processes to enable the reader to establish how transferable the results are. This component is therefore similar to that of generalisability seen in quantitative research, though it should be remembered that in qualitative research there is interest in transferring rather than generalising the results.

Often it is beyond the scope of most publications to provide an in-depth discussion of the maintenance of rigour and trustworthiness in nursing research, though papers in the *Journal of Advanced Nursing* are asked to address this.

Reflective exercise

When you are reading a research paper for an assignment think about the following:

1. Does the paper have a specific section that makes explicit how rigour and trustworthiness was achieved?
2. If you are reviewing quantitative research think about how rigour, validity and reliability were achieved?
3. If you are reviewing qualitative research think about how rigour and trustworthiness were achieved?
4. If it isn't clear how rigour and trustworthiness were achieved, then how does this affect the quality of the findings?

CHAPTER SUMMARY

- Maintaining rigour and trustworthiness is important to the quality of the overall study.
- Validity and reliability in methods of data collection are important to maintaining the rigour of quantitative studies.
- Validity is a measure of whether a data collection tool accurately measures what it is supposed to.
- Three types of validity measures are available to the researcher, with content validity being the most basic, others including criterion-related and construct validity.
- Reliability is the consistency with which a tool measures what it is intended to.
- The nurse researcher is interested in three measures of reliability that include the stability of a measure, its internal consistency and equivalence.
- Criteria have been developed to establish the rigour and trustworthiness of qualitative research to include the four key components of credibility, dependability, confirmability and transferability.

SUGGESTED FURTHER READING

LoBiondo-Wood, G. and Haber, J. (2014) *Nursing Research: Methods and Critical Appraisal for Evidence-based Practice*, 8th edn. St Louis, MO: Mosby Elsevier. Chapter 15. This chapter discusses the purposes of reliability and validity and gives detail on how to critique the reliability and validity of measurement tools.

Morse, J. (2015) 'Critical analysis of strategies for determining rigor in qualitative inquiry', *Qualitative Health Research*, 25 (9): 1212–22.

Polit, D. and Beck, C. (2014) *Essentials of Nursing Research: Appraising Evidence for Nursing Practice*, 8th edn. Philadelphia, PA: Lippincott Williams & Wilkins. Chapter 16. This chapter provides information on reliability, validity and trustworthiness in qualitative research.

Rolfe, G. (2006) 'Validity, trustworthiness and rigour: Quality and the idea of qualitative research', *Journal of Advanced Nursing*, 53 (3): 304–10. An article offering a review and discussion of the issues of validity, trustworthiness and rigour as part of delivering quality in qualitative research.

WEBSITES

To access further resources related to this chapter, visit the companion website at https://study.sagepub.com/mouleaveyard3e

REFERENCES

Bunkenborg, G., Samuelson, K., Akeson, J. and Poulsen, I. (2013) 'Impact of professionalism in nursing on in-hospital bedside monitoring practice', *Journal of Advanced Nursing*, 69 (7): 1466–77.

Fang-Meei, T., Sinkuo, C., Mei-ben, C., Jyu-Li, H., Shirling, L. and Sing-Ling, T. (2012) 'Evaluating the suicide risk-screening scale used by general nurses on patients with chronic obstructive pulmonary disease and lung cancer: A questionnaire survey', *Journal of Clinical Nursing*, 21 (4): 398–407.

Gillespie, B., Polit, D., Hamlin, L. and Chaboyer, W. (2012) 'Developing a model of competence in the operating theatre: Psychometric validation of the perceived perioperative competence scale-revised', *International Journal of Nursing Studies*, 49 (1): 90–101.

Lincoln, Y. and Guba, Y. (1985) *Naturalistic Inquiry*. Newbury Park, CA: Sage.

Maxwell, J. (1992) 'Understanding and validity in qualitative research', *Harvard Educational Review*, 60: 415–42.

Polit, D. and Beck, C. (2014) *Essentials of Nursing Research: Appraising Evidence for Nursing Practice*, 8th edn. Philadelphia, PA: Lippincott Williams & Wilkins.

Sandelowski, M. (1998) 'The call to experts in qualitative research', *Research in Nursing and Health*, 21: 467–71.

Ward, R., Glowgoska, M., Pollard, K. and Moule, P. (2009) 'Developing and testing attitude scales around IT', *Nurse Researcher*, 17 (1): 68–78.

14

EXPERIMENTAL DESIGNS

Learning outcomes

This chapter will enable you to:

- Understand the characteristics of experimental and quasi-experimental designs
- Appreciate the design of randomised controlled trials
- Explain the strengths and weaknesses of experimental designs
- Show an awareness of the ethical considerations of experimental research

There is a long tradition of using experimental research to support the development of nursing knowledge and practice. Experimental designs are employed to test the effectiveness of treatments and interventions, such as whether one drug treatment is more effective than a comparable product. Many people would argue that experiments are the only way to find out if a treatment or intervention truly works. Hence, they are very important in health care. In this chapter, we discuss this key research design and consider the main experimental approaches used to generate outcomes to support healthcare practice. Additionally, we highlight the application of the design in research practice and identify ethical considerations of use.

WHAT IS AN EXPERIMENTAL DESIGN?

Experiments can conjure up an image of people in white coats within laboratories working with test tubes. These images fail to show the true extent of experimental research. Such research can take place in a number of settings, and **experimental designs** can be used to test either a research hypothesis or question (see Chapter 9). Commonly, the research hypothesis is written as a statement that sets out the relationship between the independent (treatment or intervention) and dependent (outcome) variables and predicts an outcome. The hypothesis can be expressed as a 'null' hypothesis

(H_o), suggesting there is no expected relationship. The hypothesis stated is never truly proven or not, but accepted or rejected through the research.

For example, experimental research could test the following hypothesis:

Relaxation therapy will slow the effects of cachexia in cancer patients (H_1)

This could be expressed as a null hypothesis:

Relaxation therapy is not effective in reducing the effects of cachexia in cancer patients (H_0)

In the above example, the independent variable and intervention is the use of relaxation therapy, with the dependent variable being the effects on cachexia. The study population is patients with cancer. In order to address the research hypothesis using an experimental design, certain characteristics will need to be in place. These include manipulation, control and randomisation.

Manipulation

The researcher will manipulate the independent variable, in this case the relaxation therapy, and then observe the effect on the dependent variable, the cachexia (condition of the late stages of cancer). The manipulation can involve delivering the intervention to one group of cancer patients (the experimental group) whilst withholding it from another set of patients (the control group). A pre-test–post-test design may be used to measure the effect of treatment, as discussed below. A pre-test–post-test design allows the researcher to record what changes were caused by the relaxation therapy, and compare these with data from the members of the control group.

Control group

The control group consists of research participants who are often selected because they possess similar characteristics to members of the experimental group. Data are collected from the control group and compared with findings from the experimental group. This allows the researchers to look at the effect of the independent variable on the experimental group. Thus, the level of cachexia will be measured in the cancer patients not receiving relaxation therapy and compared with those in the experimental group who were administered the treatment. This gives the researcher information about how effective the relaxation therapy (independent variable) is.

Randomisation

Researchers will use computer programmes to randomise study participants from the population into either the experimental or the control group. All participants should have an equal chance of inclusion in either group and will be comparable. This will limit systematic bias that could affect the cachexia (dependent variable). In our example, if the patients in the control and experimental groups are very different, say in age or grade of cancer, this could lead to differences in the measurement of cachexia (dependent variable) that need not necessarily be linked to the use of relaxation therapy, but to original differences between patients in the two groups.

Pre-test–post-test design

The pre-test–post-test design, sometimes known as the before-and-after design, is commonly used to measure change in experimental research. It includes randomisation of participants into either the experimental or control groups. Using our example, the researcher will collect baseline data from the cancer patients prior to (pre-test) the intervention or relaxation therapy. Examples of baseline data may be recording of vital signs, hormonal levels or stress levels. The same measures are taken after the intervention as a post-test. Then the pre-test and post-test measures are compared. This gives a measure of the effect of the independent variable (relaxation) on the dependent variable (cachexia) for each patient and the whole group.

There are a number of other possible approaches that can be taken. These include factorial design (two or more variables are simultaneously manipulated) and cross-over design (exposing participants to more than one treatment at different points of the research) (Polit and Beck, 2014).

Limitations of experimental research

Though experiments offer the best approach to test a hypothesis and measure a cause–effect relationship, there are some limitations to their use in healthcare research. These limitations often relate to the need to manipulate variables, which may mean either the experimental or control group can be disadvantaged, something the ethical approval processes will scrutinise (see Chapters 7 and 8). The ethical standpoint taken will reflect the current evidence base, therefore if there was significant evidence to suggest that manipulation of relaxation therapy was potentially harmful, then testing of (H_1) or (H_0) above would be unlikely to secure ethical approval.

The Hawthorn effect (see Chapter 24) is the researcher impact on behaviour and performance (Roethlisberger and Dickson, 1939). This effect could have an impact on the research participants and subsequently on the dependent variable measures.

Internal and external validity

To establish the true relationship between the two variables being tested and nothing else, the researcher tries to limit the effect of any other variables that can be internal or external to the study. Internally, these can be biases or confounders. Biases may result at any stage of the study in the sample selection, data collection, analysis and interpretation of the results. The random allocation of matched participants aims to reduce sample bias. This, along with large sample sizes, also helps reduce confounding variables that may affect the dependent variable. In the example given above, a confounding variable may work in the same or a different way from the independent variable (the relaxation therapy), affecting the outcomes and dependent variable (the cachexia).

In order for the research findings to be generalisable to a wider population, external validity must be confirmed. This would enable the researcher to be confident in making recommendations for wider practice based on the research findings. To maximise external validity, the research participants must be selected and allocated randomly to either the experimental or the control group. The participants are not likely to be the same as the target population, but should be representative of them. For example, if the researcher is trying to look at patients' attitudes to rehabilitation therapy in cardiac care, then they may set inclusion and exclusion criteria to ensure that the initial population consists of cardiac patients, and to ensure that the results can be generalised back to a cardiac population.

RANDOMISED CONTROLLED TRIALS

To evaluate how effective interventions are, the **randomised controlled trial (RCT)** is seen as the 'gold standard' research design, used by medicine for some time. Randomised controlled trial findings are often used to inform the development of National Institute for Health and Care Excellence (NICE) guidelines, which are current recommendations published to enable healthcare professionals to improve outcomes for patients by ensuring their practice is up to date. Additionally, drug trials are often classified into the four stages shown in Table 14.1.

Within nursing there is the potential to employ RCTs to measure the effectiveness of practice delivery, comparing existing practices or evaluating new practices against those in existence, in order to provide an evidence base for practice. Whilst RCTs could support the development of a scientific base for nursing, it should also be acknowledged that the suggested criteria which must be met for a clinical trial in nursing (Burns et al. 2014), require the use of large patient samples, randomised into comparison groups to test a hypothesis. Research questions in nursing will not always be open to hypothesis development and testing.

The RCT requires randomisation of the patients to the control and intervention groups, and often participants are 'blinded'. This is where participants, care-givers and those making outcome assessments in the trial research team do not know which intervention is being received. This helps to reduce bias because those directly involved are not aware of those receiving the new treatment or intervention. The control and intervention groups are from the same population, the only difference in treatment being that the intervention being tested is delivered to the intervention group only. In Research example 14.1 the intervention group received a behaviour change intervention and the control group did not.

Research example 14.1

A randomised controlled trial (RCT)

Silva et al. (2010) used a randomised controlled trial design to see whether behaviour change interventions were effective in promoting physical exercise and weight control in women. Using a sample of 239 women who met a series of inclusion criteria, the sample was randomised into one of two groups. The experimental group received the intervention based on self-determination theory that promoted autonomous forms of exercise and intrinsic movement. In comparison the control group received a more standard treatment. Both weight and exercise taken were measured at various points over a 12-month period for both groups. The women in the experimental group showed increased weight loss and higher levels of physical exercise when compared to the women in the control group. This suggested the self-determination theory-based programme had a beneficial effect. We can see in this study that the three elements of randomisation, control and intervention group were present. The outcome measures were collected for both groups and enabled the researchers to conclude that the self-determination theory-based programme could be introduced with benefit for the women.

Table 14.1   Classification of clinical trials

Phases	Definition
Phase I	Initial screening of the drug to see if it is safe, perhaps using healthy human volunteers.
Phase II	Small study to develop a protocol or design to test the drug; often carried out with a small group of patients.
Phase III	Final testing using the protocol with a large set of patients to allow comparisons to be drawn.
Phase IV	Post-regulatory approval studies that include monitoring of the drug in use for adverse effects; long-term effects on morbidity and mortality.

Given the importance of RCTs to the development of evidence-based practice, guidelines have been produced for authors to follow when presenting their findings. The CONSORT reporting of clinical trials (www.consort-statement.org/) is expected by a number of key nursing journals. These guidelines include headings and suggested content to support rigorous presentation. A range of critical review frameworks such as CASP (www.casp-uk.net) (see Chapters 5 and 6) can be used to help those reading RCT papers to appraise the strengths of the trial, its validity and reliability.

CROSS-OVER TRIALS

A cross-over trial is a longitudinal study in which participants receive both treatments (Senn, 2002). For example, if a trial is comparing treatment A and treatment B, then the participants will receive both A and B treatments as part of the study. The participants will receive both the intervention or experimental treatment and the standard treatment or placebo. These trials are often used in healthcare and can be part of experimental and observational studies.

There are two main benefits to this design. Firstly, the design reduces any patient variability because the comparison of treatment is made on the same patient. Secondly, the design requires fewer participants reducing the resource needed and recruitment demands (Senn, 2002; Jones and Kenward, 2014). However, the design also has some potential limitations. The 'order' of receiving the treatment can impact on the outcomes; thus receiving treatment A or B first can affect the outcome. The first treatment can also lead to unintended effects on second treatment 'carry over' and affect the outcome. To try and limit this effect the researchers can leave a period of time between the two treatments or interventions, known as the 'wash out' (Bose and Dey, 2009).

Research example 14.2

Cross-over trial

Jo et al. (2015) employed a cross-over study to compare the effectiveness of 2-minute switched cardio-pulmonary resuscitation (CPR) and rescuer-limited CPR in an in-hospital setting in Korea. Rescuer-limited CPR was defined as that where the rescuer determined the length of resuscitation time rather than this being a 2-minute timeframe as recommended by international guidelines. In total, 90 medical students took part and were randomised into two groups of 23 and 22 pairs. One group completed the 2-minute switched CPR followed by two hours rest and then completed rescuer-limited CPR. The second group completed the reverse procedure with rescuer-limited CPR taking place first. The researchers found that the rescuer-limited CPR achieved a greater number of effective chest compressions and of a more consistent quality that the 2-minute switched CPR. This design reduced the impact of rescuer variability and the two-hour resting time or 'wash out' between the two CPR delivery approaches limited any unintended effects on outcome.

QUASI-EXPERIMENTS

Having considered the characteristics necessary to conduct an experiment or RCT, it should be apparent that not all nursing research questions could be open to testing through such a rigorous true experimental design. When at least one of the three components of a true experiment (manipulation, control group, randomisation) is missing from a study, this is known as a **quasi-experimental design**. The study identified below doesn't make clear a process of randomising the study participants. They do have an intervention or experimental group and a control group, but these are not matched and equivalent. This means there may have been differences between members of the two groups, which could have an impact on the research outcomes. The two groups have a different experience – one the new intervention education delivered by the breastfeeding buddies, whilst the control group receive the existing education delivery, which is nurse-led. Both groups complete the same questionnaires and interviews to collect data about their learning and intention to breastfeed, and these results are used to compare whether the new intervention has been effective.

Research example 14.3

Quasi-experimental research

Rempel and Moore (2012) undertook a non-equivalent control group quasi-experimental study to evaluate a prenatal breastfeeding class, involving two groups. The experimental/intervention group included participants of a peer-led session led by breastfeeding buddies. Breastfeeding mothers, who had received training, provided information and demonstrated breastfeeding techniques. The second (control) group attended an established hospital-based breastfeeding nurse-led session. The researchers wanted to compare a range of outcomes to see if the intervention of the buddy-led session was as effective as the nurse-led session. Women attendees were asked to complete a questionnaire immediately prior to the sessions, and telephone interviews were conducted after one week and one and six months post partum. The findings suggested that the volunteer peer-developed and peer-led prenatal breastfeeding session was effective in providing breastfeeding education. Breastfeeding outcomes among mothers who attended this peer-led session were similar to those of mothers who attended an established nurse-led session

Sometimes there may be ethical or practical constraints that prevent an experimental or RCT design being used (Grove and Mohnkern, 2009). For example, if nurses wanted to look at the effectiveness of a new way of managing patient medication through self-administration, it would be difficult to research this within one setting, as having two systems running might cause confusion for patients and staff. It might be possible to organise the changes across two wards, introducing the new system within one whilst maintaining current practice in the other. In this example, a new intervention is being introduced and compared with existing practice. There isn't true randomisation into control and experimental groups, but similar groups are being compared. This design doesn't allow the researcher to control for all of the extraneous variables, thus the cause-and-effect relationship measured isn't as certain, but strong. Thus, the researchers cannot be certain that any benefits to patient care seen in the intervention group are directly attributed to the change in medication administration. The stepped-wedge cluster-randomised trial is one example of a design where data from the same groups are compared that is increasingly seen in use in healthcare.

STEPPED-WEDGE CLUSTER-RANDOMISED TRIALS

The stepped-wedge cluster-randomised trial is particularly used in the evaluation of services. Cluster groups (for example, wards or community areas) are randomised at regular intervals, known as steps, and moved from the control group to the intervention group under evaluation. All the clusters involved provide both control and intervention data (Hemming et al., 2015). The design usually involves the selection of the clusters, a control period for each cluster when pre-intervention data can be collected, and then time to prepare for the intervention. The intervention is then applied to each cluster on a rolling basis for a defined period of time, when data is again collected. The number of clusters involved and the time spent within the intervention period is determined by sample size calculations.

The design could be used, for example, if a new information technology (IT) system is being introduced and evaluated. The clusters could include ten wards, and each ward will complete a control period when baseline data can be collected, then a preparation period, followed by the implementation of the IT system. Wards one to ten will be rolled through this pattern spending equal amounts of time in each stage, but at different times in the study, as shown in Research example 14.4 below.

Whilst this approach supports the evaluation of practice change there are some limitations in its use. The time taken to apply the design to a number of clusters can be considerably longer than an RCT, power calculations undertaken can be more complex, and there can be recruitment and retention issues. Finally, the implementation of the design needs careful planning as any further changes in practice delivery that might impact on the evaluation have to be avoided during the implementation period (Dreischulte et al., 2013).

Research example 14.4

Stepped-wedge cluster-randomised study

Hill et al. (2015) used a stepped-wedge cluster-randomised study in Australia to examine the effectiveness of individualised falls prevention education for patients and staff. In total, eight rehabilitation units were involved that were randomly allocated over a 50-week period. After a ten-week control period, two units commenced the educational intervention. Subsequent units were allocated into the intervention at ten-week intervals until all were included. The researchers found that individualised patient and staff education led to a reduction in falls in wards where the elderly patients were receiving rehabilitation. We can see that this study used the rehabilitation wards as clusters and each received a control period and preparation for the intervention, followed by a period of intervention study on a rotational basis.

There are a number of quasi-experimental designs available, such as the 'pre-test and post-test' sometimes known as the 'before-and-after'. Comparison group design with pre-test and post-test are the most prevalent (Grove and Mohnkern, 2009). In this design the participants are not randomly selected; the experimental group receives the intervention and the comparison group either receives no treatment or the treatment that is normally used (see Table 14.2).

Table 14.2   Comparison design

Group type		Design stages	
Experimental group	pre-test	treatment	post-test
Comparison group	pre-test	no treatment	post-test

If it is not possible to conduct a pre-test, such as when measuring the impact of a rehabilitation programme where there is no pre-test data, then a post-test measurement design is used that measures post-test data only. Such designs are limited by the lack of a comparison pre-test, which can threaten the studies' validity (Grove and Mohnkern, 2009).

Table 14.3　Do's and don'ts of experimental design

Do's	Don'ts
Do use to measure cause–effect.	Don't use when not trying to establish cause and effect.
In a pre-test and post-test design, do measure the outcome before and after intervention to allow for comparison and measure effect.	In a pre-test and post-test design, comparisons cannot be made if pre-test and post-test data are not available.
Do include elements of randomisation, control and manipulation in an RCT.	Don't undertake an RCT without elements of randomisation, control and manipulation.
Do use a quasi-experimental design if unable to include all three components of an RCT.	Don't use a quasi-experimental design if all three components of an RCT are used.
Do seek ethical approval for experimental research.	Don't undertake experimental research without having gained ethical approval.

Reflective exercise

Think about your practice. Have you been involved in any research with patients or the public, which has used a quasi-experimental design? Or have you ever been the subject of quasi-experimental research? What would you expect to see happening in research that used this design? What would the potential ethical issues be?

ETHICAL ISSUES ASSOCIATED WITH EXPERIMENTAL AND QUASI-EXPERIMENTAL DESIGNS

Experimental and quasi-experimental designs are used to measure the effectiveness of a treatment or procedure, comparing this with existing practice in order to develop evidence-based care. Such research results in patients receiving treatments that have not been tried or tested, and therefore there are possible disadvantages to being a member of either an experimental or a control group. It may be the case that patients will want to be part of the experimental group, in the hope that a new possible treatment may be more effective than those currently in use. This can lead to difficulties recruiting patients to the control group. To try to overcome these potential problems, researchers can obtain patient consent to take part in the research prior to allocation to either the control or the experimental group. However, as informed consent includes an option for patients to withdraw from the study at any time without prejudice, retention in the control group population may become an issue as the study progresses. Experimental designs should be subjected to Ethical Committee Approval (see Chapters 7 and 8). The ethics committee members will want to ensure that the research will 'do the patient no harm' and that the benefits of the research are likely to outweigh any potential risks to the participants. Table 14.3 gives a list of do's and don'ts.

CHAPTER SUMMARY

- Experimental research can take place in a number of settings, and such designs are used to test either a research hypothesis or a question. An experimental design includes characteristics of manipulation, control and randomisation.
- Experimental designs offer the best approach to test a hypothesis and measure a cause–effect relationship, though there are some limitations to their use in health-care research.
- Randomised controlled trials are the 'gold standard' research design for use in evaluating the effectiveness of interventions.
- Usually at least one of the three components of a true experiment is missing from the quasi-experimental design (manipulation, control group, randomisation).

SUGGESTED FURTHER READING

Shadish, W., Cook, T. and Campbell, D. (2001) *Experimental and Quasi-experimental Designs for Generalized Causal Inference*. Boston: Houghton Miffin Company. This text gives detailed information on experimental and quasi-experimental designs. It explores some details in depth, like causation.

Jones, B. and Kenward, G. (2014) *Design and Analysis of Cross-over Trials*, 3rd edn. London: Chapman Hall. This text presents short case studies of issues relating to sample size estimation and other issues of cross-over trials.

WEBSITES

CASP critical review framework: www.phru.nhs.uk/casp/casp.htm – this website presents a framework which can be used to guide the critical appraisal of research papers. It includes frameworks for both qualitative and quantitative research designs.

Centre for Reviews and Dissemination: www.york.ac.uk/inst/crd – part of the National Institute for Health Research, which provides a database of the effectiveness of health and social care interventions and systematic reviews.

CONSORT (reporting on clinical trials): www.consort-statement.org/ – the CONSORT guidelines are presented which are used to structure the presentation of clinical trial papers in a number of healthcare journals.

To access further resources related to this chapter, visit the companion website at https://study. sagepub.com/mouleaveyard3e

REFERENCES

Bose, M. and Dey, A. (2009) *Optimal Cross-over Designs*. Singapore: World Scientific.

Burns, N., Grove, S. and Gray, J. (2014) *The Practice of Nursing Research: Appraisal, Synthesis, and Generation of Evidence*, 7th edn. St Louis, MO: Saunders Elsevier.

Dreischulte, T. Grant, A. Donnan, P. and Guthrie, B. (2013) 'Pros and cons of the stepped wedge design in cluster randomised trials of quality improvement interventions: two current examples', *Trials*, 14 (Suppl 1): 087. Available at: www.trialsjournal.biomedicalcentral.com/articles/10.1186/1745-6215-14-31-087 (accessed 13 May 2016).

Grove, N. and Mohnkern, S. (2009) *Study Guide for Understanding Nursing Research: Building an Evidence-based Practice*, 6th edn. St Louis, MO: Saunders.

Hemming, K., Haines, T., Chilton, P., Gilling, A. and Lilford, R. (2015) 'Stepped wedge cluster randomised trial: Rationale, design, analysis and reporting', *BMJ*, 350: h391. Available at: www.bmj.com/context/350/bmj.h391 (accessed 29 September 2015).

Hill, A-M., McPhail, S., Waldron, N., Etherton-Beer, C. and Ingram, K. (2015) 'Fall rates in hospital rehabilitation units after individualised patient and staff education programmes: A pragmatic, stepped-wedge, cluster-randomised controlled trial', *The Lancet*, 385 (9987): 2592–9.

Jo, C-H., Cho, G-C., Ahn, J-H., Park, Y-S. and Lee, C-H. (2015) 'Rescuer-limited cardio-pulmonary resuscitation as an alternative to 2-min switched CPR in the setting of an in hospital cardiac arrest: A randomised cross-over study', *Emergency Medical Journal*, 32 (7): 539–43.

Jones, B. and Kenward, G. (2014) *Design and Analysis of Cross-over Trials*, 3rd edn. London: Chapman Hall.

Polit, D. and Beck, C. (2014) *Essentials of Nursing Research: Appraising Evidence for Nursing Practice*, 8th edn. Philadelphia, PA: Lippincott Williams & Wilkins.

Rempel, L. and Moore, K. (2012) 'Peer-led prenatal breast-feeding education: A viable alternative to nurse-led education', *Midwifery*, 28 (1): 73–9.

Roethlisberger, F. and Dickson, W. (1939) *Management and the Worker*. Cambridge, MA: Harvard University Press.

Senn, S. (2002) *Cross-over Trials in Clinical Research*, 2nd edn. Chichester: Wiley.

Silva, M., Viera, P., Countinho, S., Minderico, C., Matois, M., Sardinha, L. and Teixeria, P. (2010) 'Using self-determination theory to promote physical activity and weight control: A randomized controlled trial in women', *Journal of Behavioural Medicine*, 33: 110–22.

15

QUALITATIVE RESEARCH APPROACHES

Learning outcomes

This chapter will enable you to:

- understand the three main qualitative research approaches
- identify the differences between the approaches

Nurse researchers tend to use qualitative research approaches to look at questions around life experiences, beliefs, motivations, actions and perceptions of patients and staff. Rather than aiming to test a hypothesis, as is often the case in quantitative research, qualitative approaches look to support the interpretation and understanding of human experience. They allow the researcher to focus on interpreting social settings, such as the ward or community environment.

Qualitative approaches facilitate the exploration of relationships and human experience within the research setting. Three main approaches are used: phenomenology, ethnography and grounded theory. Whilst all are qualitative research approaches, they differ in many respects, including in overall aim, data collection methods and analysis.

To enable understanding of individual experience and perception, the researcher works closely with participants during the research; this can be through the process of data collection. Researchers use interactive methods of data collection, and often the participants are involved in verifying the interpretation of meaning drawn from analysis of the data. The findings can be presented as a set of descriptions, themes, theories and frameworks or models for practice.

In this chapter, we discuss phenomenology, ethnography and grounded theory as the main qualitative approaches. We start by revisiting the characteristics of qualitative research (see Chapter 11) and the role it plays in developing nursing knowledge. For issues associated with maintaining rigour in qualitative research, see Chapter 13.

QUALITATIVE APPROACHES

There are a number of key characteristics shared by qualitative research approaches:

- Qualitative research is most commonly part of inductive reasoning, starting with a set of observations of a situation and moving to the generation of ideas and in some cases theory.
- The setting for the research is usually 'natural' and the researcher is immersed within it.
- The focus of the research is generally the views, experiences and perceptions of the participants.
- The researcher aims to take a holistic view, seeing the whole picture.
- Data collection and analysis may interrelate and be flexible and reflexive.

Inductive reasoning

Typically, induction or inductive reasoning is seen as part of qualitative research, where the aim is to develop concepts and themes from the interpretation of observations and interviews. Inductive reasoning is a process of starting with the details of an experience or our observations of something, and using these to develop a general understanding of phenomena. Specific observations and descriptions are made and used to develop a hypothesis and theory of a more general situation that can be tested. The researcher enters the research arena ready to learn and aims to gather a range of material, which is interrogated and open to scrutiny in order to draw understandings. The researcher will be trying to gain a clearer picture of the problems and issues through the analysis of data gathered through observations and discussions. This inductive approach to research is therefore helpful in exploring those areas of practice and care where there is currently limited understanding or where the current explanations are limited and fail to reflect individual experiences. Say, for example, a new practice role has been developed and implemented within cancer care. Using an inductive approach would allow the researcher to explore the patient, manager and new practitioner perspectives and experiences of the role that might further inform its use and development. Through observations, the researcher would be trying to identify what the issues and problems might be and what is happening as a result of implementing the role. The researcher would analyse the data collected and reflect on the meaning of this, whilst also thinking about their own preconceptions in relation to the research.

A variety of data collection methods such as observation, interviews and analysis of written data, is used to generate ideas, concepts and possibly theory. Often, researchers work with participants, who verify or check interpretations. Researchers are keen to ensure impartiality in analysis and present interpretations that reflect the participant perspective.

Natural setting

Qualitative nurse researchers are interested in collecting data in the natural or real-world setting. The researcher is aiming to follow the participants into their 'natural environment', which in healthcare could be a range of clinical or community care settings or a home environment. In studying the real world, the researcher will not set up an intervention study or experiment, but will undertake a natural experiment. The researchers are observing behaviour as it occurs naturally and will make no attempt to intervene or make a change in the environment. The researcher will enter a real-life environment to study particular phenomena. This could include observing the impact of the implementation of a new policy in practice or the introduction of a new staffing role. Denzin and Lincoln (2011) suggest that study in the natural setting allows researchers to make sense of and interpret phenomena. The natural experiment enables the researcher to study practice that cannot be manipulated in an experimental study, for example there may be ethical issues preventing an experimental study of those receiving treatment for mental health issues; however, it may be possible to gather data from this group by entering a 'natural' healthcare setting. One disadvantage of researching in the natural setting, however, is the potential for researchers to draw different interpretations from the same observed behaviour. Depending on the qualitative approach, data collection may require the researcher to be present in the research setting for prolonged periods, for example to collect observational data of nurses working within a particular care environment. They can collect data using a range of techniques, including a record of occurring events, notes and audio or video recordings. The researcher is unlikely to observe everything but will select samples, either deciding to record observations at particular points in time over perhaps a week or undertaking situational sampling, and observing different situations or settings for a specific period of time.

Reflective exercise

Think about setting up an observational study in the setting you are currently working in. What would some of the challenges be? Could observations be undertaken in the setting? How could data be collected? What preparation would be needed for the staff, the setting and the patients? Are there any ethical issues that would prevent observations taking place?

Participant perspective

Qualitative researchers believe that participants or research subjects are able to provide data on their experience of the social world that others can interpret and make sense of. The relationship between the researcher and participant is important to the achievement of the research. LoBiondo-Wood and Haber (2014) suggest that the research may influence the participants, but that the researcher is also affected and should be open to the participants, to avoid attaching their own meaning to the experience. The researcher needs to remain open to the ideas of the participants gained through listening and observing.

Holistic view

The nurse researcher is interested in the entire and whole human experience. The researcher will want to explore the complete experience, considering the context and interrelated factors affecting the participant. For example, when considering the user experience of someone with a mental health condition, it could emerge that a number of situations are important components of the experience. The workplace, home situation, family relations, friends, healthcare staff and treatments can all impact on the overall experience. Through listening to the individual's complete story, these interrelated aspects will emerge.

Interrelated processes

A number of data collection methods are available that can be used flexibly. The researcher can collect data through interviewing, conducting focus group discussions, observing practice delivery and interactions or analysing video or digital recording, written diaries and text. Whilst there may be an initial suggested number of participants or observation episodes, the final sample total will be determined as the research progresses. The researcher has the scope to either increase or reduce the number of interactions involved depending on the quality of the data obtained during the data collection process, and provided any changes sit within the ethical approval obtained. For example, Huang et al. (2008) wanted to understand the coping experiences of carers living with a schizophrenic family member. Purposive sampling and in-depth, face-to-face interviews were used to collect data. The research team was unclear initially what the total sample size would be. As data collection and analysis progressed, they felt they had reached data saturation, and didn't need to collect any further data when the sample size comprised 10 carers (5 men and 5 women).

The process of data collection is flexible and can be guided by the participants. Open questioning, starting the interview with an overall question, allows the researcher to react to the interview situation and explore particular aspects or issues in more depth. The researcher will want to gain insight into the experiences and perceptions of the participant so will use data collection techniques to effectively achieve this. This process requires some skill and training and may require some innovation and creativity in approach, using the interaction to gain deeper insight into the main issues.

PHENOMENOLOGY

Phenomenological approaches emerged from philosophy, with the origins being traced to Immanuel Kant in the eighteenth century (Moran, 2000), though popular views site the origins with the work of German philosopher Husserl in the twentieth century, who developed a philosophy that sought to describe human experience as legitimate without the need for external analysis (Sokolowski, 2000). The adoption of this work followed, particularly by Heidegger. Phenomenologists believe it is possible to understand human behaviour by describing and interpreting human experience within the context of that experience. They believe that meaning and truth can be drawn from people's lived experiences. In other words, through accessing and interpreting the experience of a patient with cancer, we can draw meaning and understanding of what it is like to live with cancer.

There are some important ideas underpinning **phenomenology**. First, phenomenological research seeks to gather life experiences, describe them and reflect on them. Everyday experiences were described as 'life world' by Husserl, though they are more usually known as 'lived experiences'. These 'lived experiences' provide powerful data that can give insights useful beyond the immediate case of research, described by Husserl as 'essences'. Common themes can be seen within the data that relate to the context and time of collection. These are presented in the data to show how themes identified in people's stories are linked and related. For example, Sweeney et al. (2007) explored the experiences of people living with a supra-pubic catheter. Data was collected through in-depth interviews with six adults living in the community who had a supra-pubic catheter for long-term urinary bladder drainage. Interpretation of the data occurred via thematic analysis of the participants' stories. They presented two distinct but interrelated themes: adjustment to life with a catheter and feelings of being unprepared or supported as they learned to live with a supra-pubic catheter. These two common themes were used to present the 'essences' of the six people living with a supra-pubic catheter.

The second concept seen in phenomenology is that of 'bracketing'. Husserl suggested researchers needed to remove their preconceptions from the field of data collection through 'phenomenological reduction'. This was meant to enable the researcher to enter the field with an open mind and be able to study phenomena without the burden of preconception. Often, researchers will write down or record their preconceptions in some way and acknowledge them in order to be disciplined in data collection and to ensure they are aware of their own views and open to listening to the experiences of others.

As nursing works with a patient-centred approach to care delivery and attempts to keep the patient at the forefront, phenomenology can provide an important evidence base for practice. A number of researchers, such as Sweeney et al. (2007), have used phenomenology to try to understand the experiences of patients and provide descriptions and reflections that can help nurses gain insight into the patient's 'lived experience'. Having some understanding of 'what it is like' can support the development of empathy and patient-centred care.

Phenomenological research in nursing is usually described as having two main branches: descriptive and interpretive.

Descriptive phenomenology

The approach was conceived initially by Husserl (1962) and is also associated with Giorgi (1997). Descriptive phenomenology seeks to see researchers enter the field with an open mind, leaving preconceptions behind. Researchers should seek to complete descriptions that encompass a full range of everyday life experiences, which are gathered by participants through what is heard, seen, felt, remembered, acted on and decided (Polit and Beck, 2014). Given the need to be open-minded, one of the main aspects of this approach is the concept of 'bracketing'. The researcher identifies any preconceived ideas and beliefs about the phenomenon under study, recognises and withholds these from the research. The researcher will record a reflexive journal or diary of the research to help maintain 'bracketing', recording their thinking and views. Despite this, there can be difficulties in trying to 'remove' beliefs and preconceived thoughts from a research process.

The researchers are interested in identifying the 'essences', those themes that best describe the lived experience, what is common but also where the differences might be. For example, in looking at the lived experience of clients with learning disabilities and a period of hospitalisation, we may find that there are common experiences of preparation for admission and poor discharge planning, though there may be differences in these experiences based on whether the admission was planned or an emergency.

Interpretive phenomenology

Research example 15.1

Interpretive phenomenology

Griffiths et al. (2011) used interpretive phenomenology to gain an understanding of children's perspectives of having cancer. The children were interviewed at two points in time, at six monthly intervals, following a successful application for ethics approval. The children were aged between 8 and 16 years and were patients of a pediatric oncology unit. A total of nine families were included in the study. At the time of the study, the children were at different stages of treatment for a wide range of cancers. The interviews were semi-structured and asked a range of questions including: What are the hardest parts of your life? What are the hardest parts about being sick? The interviews were recorded and transcribed, and analysis began with reading the complete transcripts. Initial themes were noted and then further reading enabled identification of meaning units, which were attributed with a code. Each code reflected the meaning unit, one example being the impact of diagnosis. This process of analysis was repeated for each transcript individually. Each transcript was then imported into a software analysis package and recoded, and the codes were grouped into clusters of codes to represent a theme. Sub-themes were also identified and cross-referencing between the transcripts and themes took place involving the research team. Finally, five themes were identified: the experience of illness, the upside of being sick, refocusing on what is important, acquiring a new perspective, and the experience of returning to well-being.

Heidegger, as a student of Husserl, developed interpretive phenomenology. He felt that understanding the lived experience was more important than merely describing it; he termed **hermeneutics** the understanding of human experience. Interpretive phenomenologists do not 'bracket' themselves. Hermeneutic phenomenologists aim to be open to any new perspectives, but they may draw on preconceptions to enable them to appreciate what is new and different. Polit and Beck (2014) suggest the goal of the approach is to discover understanding, wisdom and possibilities from the study of another world. In the example above, the researchers use a semi-structured interview guide of open questions in order to explore the experiences of the children and allow them to talk fully about their lives with cancer.

Hermeneutic phenomenologists are more likely to develop 'fusions of horizons' than 'essences'. The presentation is less concerned with providing a specific conclusion presented by descriptive phenomenologists, but offers a story or picture that allows the reader to draw interpretations and meaning for their own use.

Phenomenologists work with purposive samples (see Chapter 12), including participants who have the relevant 'lived experiences' to talk about in the study. For example, the study above sought to ensure that the participants included in the study had experiences of living with cancer. Not all studies will draw on current experiences, as in our research above, but can access stories retrospectively. Data collection is generally through in-depth interviews (see Chapter 23), as in our example, which can allow the interview to be guided by the participants. Experiences can also be accessed through diaries and autobiographies. Data are analysed to identify interrelated themes and insights through processes of qualitative data analysis, as described above (also see Chapter 27). As in our example, data are analysed to ensure that meanings are extracted, which requires reading the whole text several times and a process of coding which facilitates the identification of themes and sub-themes.

There are a number of different approaches used to support analysis; Van Manen (2010) presents a less systematic method, though approaches to analysis, such as that proposed by Giorgi and Giorgi (2003), can be used. This systematic approach, as described by Griffiths et al. (2011), involves reading the text, dividing it into meaning units, identifying meaning units in transferable and general ways, presenting common themes and experiences, and illustrating these using quotations from the text to support their findings (see Giorgi and Giorgi, 2003). Sweeney et al. (2007) report a process of data analysis that includes being immersed in the data throughout the process of data collection and undertaking analysis by reading and re-reading the data:

> Immersion occurred at interview, during the transcription of the text, listening to the audiotapes, and during the reading and re-reading of the data. Through thematic analysis of the textual data, interpretations were reconstructed to reveal common meanings and understanding of 'what it is like to live with a supra-pubic catheter'. (2007: 420)

ETHNOGRAPHY

Hammersley and Atkinson (2007) suggest there is some disagreement about the term **ethnography**, with diversity in definition and process. They go on to suggest that anthropological traditions (the study of humankind) of the approach are reflected in ethnography, which is seen as involving the ethnographer participating, in either overt or covert ways, as part of people's lives for an extended period. During this time, the researcher listens, watches and asks questions in an attempt to uncover the issues that are the focus of the research.

Ethnography means a 'portrait of people' and involves writing about people and culture, providing descriptions of a group, such as intensive care nurses, and the culture they work in, the routines, rituals and customs of the intensive care unit and the roles of the people within it. An ethnographic approach is used to describe and interpret how the behaviour of people is influenced by the culture they live in. It is characterised by the researcher entering the 'natural' field to gather in-depth data. The researcher is described as 'going native', a phrase developed by the early studies of ethnographers such as Margaret Mead, who lived among the tribes of Papua New Guinea in the 1930s in order to understand them (Haralambos and Holborn, 2013). As well as being characterised by the researcher entering the field and being immersed in the culture, the approach aims to gather the (emic) 'insider' perspective, so that a 'thick' and detailed analytical description can be provided of the people and culture. Ethnography would be seen as part of an inductive approach, where specific observations and details of an experience are used to develop a general understanding of phenomena.

In presenting an ethnographic study, the nurse researcher will produce a rich and holistic description of the cultural setting. Interpretations of the culture are drawn, describing behaviour patterns seen. This is illustrated in Research example 15.2.

Research example 15.2

An ethnographic study

Fry (2012) used ethnography to study how beliefs impacted on contemporary emergency department triage practices in Australia. She was working full time whilst undertaking the study and though not involved in the delivery of emergency care at the time, she had experience as an emergency clinician. A purposive sample of ten Triage nurses at Clinical Nurse Specialist level was selected to take part in the study. Ethical approval was in place prior to data collection. The 12-month study was undertaken in four emergency departments. The data collection involved non-participant observation and participant interviews. Observations were scheduled to occur at the weekends and bank holidays and included memo taking. In total, 200 hours of observations were recorded. As a non-participant observer, Fry chose a passive observer role.

Ethnographers use the term **emic perspective** to mean gaining the insider view, as in our research example above, gathering data from those inside the culture, those who understand the rules, ways of working and are part of the culture. The researcher going into the setting to gather data who is not an insider would have an **etic perspective**, entering the culture from the outside. The ethnographer, through their 'etic' position, presents the 'emic' perspective in a story that describes the culture and the positioning of the people within it.

The sample used is often purposive, as we see in the research by Fry (2012) above (see Chapter 12). Fry selected specific settings and populations to study how beliefs impacted on contemporary emergency department triage practices in Australia. In other research, this might include selecting settings such as maternity care, intensive care, student nurses studying mental health or patients' rehabilitation in recovering from spinal injury. The selection is systematic (Hammersley and Atkinson, 2007) to ensure that participants have the necessary experience and immersion in the culture to provide the 'emic' perspective.

As with other research approaches, the ethnographer needs to operate under ethical principles (see Chapters 7 and 8) and gain ethical approval for the study, as described in the example above. It is less likely that ethical approval would be given for participant observation methods that included a covert observation role, where the researcher role is hidden. The researcher will be expected to operate with informed consent in place, allowing participants the scope to consent to take part in the research, with an option to withdraw from the study at any time without prejudice.

As in the approach taken by Fry above, data are predominantly collected through participant observation (see Chapter 24). Ethnographers will observe practice, interactions and behaviours, listen to conversations and ask questions. Fry adopted a passive role in the research, observing the practice of the nurse consultants as they worked. Researchers may also gather data from documentation and through interviews. Ethnographers will maintain a fieldwork diary, recording their initial thoughts and interpretations of the culture. Ethnographic researchers may well operate from a position of reciprocity in the research, where the intimacy of the relationship between the researcher and the participants is acknowledged and the researcher 'gives something back' to the participants. The development of reciprocity is advocated by Hammersley and Atkinson (2007), who believed the ethnographer should avoid merely exploiting the participant.

Data are analysed using the processes described in Chapter 27, which enable the researcher to interact with the data to develop key themes. The key stages include organisation of data such as a fieldwork diary, observational records and other data, reading and re-reading, reviewing observations, coding the data, reducing the codes to larger categories, looking for patterns across the categories and organising the data into themes and sub-themes. The process may also include a process of verification of the analysis with the participants.

Fieldwork allows the researcher to produce a detailed account of the group culture and working, described as **thick description**. The thick description is an analysis of the group culture, a view of its patterns of working, member relationships, meanings and functions.

GROUNDED THEORY

Grounded theory was developed in the 1960s by sociologists Glaser and Strauss (1967). It is a method that usually starts with specific observations and an analysis of data collected to generate ideas or a theory, therefore usually working in an inductive way, but can develop to use deductive reasoning. Its whole purpose is to generate theories or hypotheses (see Chapter 9), and it is often used to study new research areas. The theory emerges from systematically collected and analysed research data. Once the hypotheses or theories are developed, they can be tested through deductive research, an approach that tests a hypothesis through mainly quantitative designs, and the results will either support the predicted hypothesis or not.

Research example 15.3

The use of grounded theory

Khadivzadeh et al. (2015) used a grounded theory approach when studying fertile couples' experiences of having their first child in Iran. In-depth interviews were used to collect data from 45 participants. The researchers used Strauss and Corbin's (2008) constant comparative method, with three levels employed; open, axial and selective coding. After the initial face-to-face interview, participants completed a questionnaire providing data on family fertility history. Data analysis began during the interviews and continued throughout transcription. Open coding was used to identify subcategories from which categories were developed as analysis progressed. Interviews continued until data saturation was achieved. The transcription and coded data were checked by peers and participants, as part of 'member checking'. This supported the trustworthiness of the study (see Chapter 13).

Grounded theory has its foundations in the 'symbolic interactionism' developed by Margaret Mead in the 1920s and 1930s, which focuses on explaining social processes, such as the way people make sense of social interactions and interpret them. It has the potential to support our understanding of human behaviour and how people interact. It is therefore important in supporting the study of nursing and healthcare, where the understanding of human interaction and behaviours are important for improving care delivery and practice. The example above uses grounded theory in this way, to study the experiences of first-time parents in Iran. Grounded theory may also be used to develop nursing practice. For example, the design could be employed to develop an approach to managing the care of first-time parents in the hospital that supports them. Through data collection and analysis, a theory can be developed about what happens when first-time parents are confronted with prenatal care and delivery and about how the parents manage the experience.

Grounded theory is very much 'grounded' in the field. For example, the research problem is often identified in the field, as was the issue reported above. The types of research questions that might be explored include: What is happening in the research setting? What interactions occur in the setting? What are people's experiences and what do they mean? How is work organised? What is needed to improve things? Thinking of our Research example 15.3, the questions may have included: What factors affected your decision to start a family? How confident did you feel about starting a family? What was your first childbearing experience like? The processes of sampling, data collection and analysis occur simultaneously. Nurse researchers will identify a sample, collect some data, analyse the data and identify categories, then describe the emerging issues before re-entering the process of sample, collection and analysis. Data collection employs in-depth interviews in the main, as seen above, though observations and documentary analysis may also be used. It is suggested that up to 50 participants might be involved in in-depth interviewing (Polit and Beck, 2014).

A process of theoretical sampling is used, where the emerging issues guide the sample selection. The initial sample will be composed of key individuals in the research setting who will be able to talk about the research issue – perhaps in our example this would be the ward manager. Data are analysed, and as concepts and issues emerge the researcher will select further samples, either individuals or events, that they believe will provide further insight and contributions to developing the initial findings. So, for example, analysis of data may suggest that the researchers need to interview key staff involved in patient admissions. This can raise some challenges for the researcher as initial ethical approval processes may not account for the scope of the sample used and there may be a requirement to have ongoing dialogue with the ethics committee.

The researchers employ 'constant comparison' to identify the main problem and develop and refine the emerging categories, as seen in the example above. The categories identified from the new data collected are compared constantly with the initial identified categories. Researchers look for commonalities and differences in the data and use this process to collapse the number of categories. Data collection becomes more focused as time progresses and the researchers concentrate on the key emerging theoretical issues in data collection. The process of data analysis includes: constant comparison, data coding, reduction of codes and development of categories, developing links between the categories and developing a core category used to develop a theory. In our example above, Khadivzadeh et al. (2015) used axial coding to identify subcategories from which categories were developed as analysis progressed. Research exploring first-time parents' experiences of child birth generated the following code: 'Caring for my family integrity', which included categories of, 'gaining confidence, evaluating situational conditions to make a decision, managing child bearing across the life course and parental role attainment' (p. 62). Over the years, different versions of grounded theory have emerged, with both Glaser and Strauss developing their thinking, along with other researchers. Glaser maintains his original view that the theory should emerge through constant comparison and should be grounded in the data; however, more recently he has suggested that in the later stages of analysis, external theories can be brought into the research analysis and theory development. He still suggests that grounded theory doesn't require the application of models and strategic approaches (see Gibbs, 2010). This position is at odds with the new thinking of his previous partner, Strauss. Strauss has also gone on to publish with Corbin, presenting an approach to grounded theory that challenges some of the earlier thinking presented in the 1960s (see Strauss and Corbin, 2008). Strauss and Corbin offer a more structured approach to grounded theory, providing a model with instruction on how to develop categories, a position opposed by Glaser. New theorists have also developed new versions of grounded theory. Gibbs (2010) suggests Charmaz takes a constructivist position. This proposes that the researcher constructs their interpretation of the world, so they have a particular way of seeing things in the world. It is suggested that this construction is used to interpret the data and that the categories and theories developed are constructed by the researcher. This brings a different dimension to grounded theory, where it is suggested that the interpretation of data and the development of the theory are influenced by the researcher perspective.

CHAPTER SUMMARY

- The three main qualitative research approaches are: phenomenology, ethnography and grounded theory.
- Qualitative research can be described as 'inductive reasoning'.
- Inductive reasoning starts with a set of specific observations of a situation and moves to the generation of a general theory or hypothesis.
- The qualitative research setting is 'natural' and the researcher is immersed within it.
- The researcher gains the views, experiences and perceptions of the participants.
- The researcher aims to take a holistic view, seeing the whole picture.
- Data collection and analysis may interrelate and be flexible and reflexive.
- Phenomenology aims to explore the life experience of individuals and explain what it means.
- Ethnography is used to describe and interpret how the behaviour of people is influenced by the culture they live in.
- Grounded theory starts with a set of observations of a situation and moves to the generation of ideas and theory. Its whole purpose is to generate hypotheses or a theory. Different versions have developed over time.

SUGGESTED FURTHER READING

Hammersley, M. and Atkinson, P. (2007) *Ethnography: Principles in Practice*, 3rd edn. London: Routledge. This is a text which provides detailed information on ethnography and refers to the theory and application.

Seale, C., Gobo, G., Gubrium, J. and Silverman, D. (eds) (2007) *Qualitative Research Practice*. London: Sage. This text concentrates on presenting the methods used and the use of them in the field.

Strauss, A. and Corbin, J. (2008) *Basics of Qualitative Research: Grounded Theory Procedures and Techniques*, 3rd edn. London: Sage. Concentrating on the grounded theory approach, this text considers the theory and practical application of it.

WEBSITES

Qualitative Health Research: http://qhr.sagepub.com – a peer-reviewed monthly journal that includes international and interdisciplinary qualitative health research.

Qualitative Inquiry: http://qix.sagepub.com – a peer-reviewed journal presenting an interdisciplinary forum for qualitative methodology in healthcare and human sciences.

 To access further resources related to this chapter, visit the companion website at https://study.sagepub.com/mouleaveyard3e.

REFERENCES

Denzin, N. and Lincoln, Y. (2011) 'Introduction: The discipline and practice of qualitative research', in N. Denzin and Y. Lincoln (eds), *Handbook of Qualitative Research*, 4th edn. Thousand Oaks, CA: Sage. Chapter 1, pp. 1–20.

Fry, M. (2012) 'An ethnography: Understanding emergency practice belief systems', *International Emergency Nursing*, 20 (3): 120–5.

Gibbs, G. (2010) 'Grounded theorists and some critiques of grounded theory', University of Huddersfield. Available at: www.youtube.com/watch?v=hik-NKtI_vY&feature=mfu_inorder&list=UL (accessed 3 November 2015).

Giorgi, A. (1997) 'The theory, practice and evaluation of the phenomenological method as a qualitative research procedure', *Journal of Phenomenological Psychology*, 28: 235–60.

Giorgi, A. and Giorgi, B. (2003) 'The descriptive phenomenological psychology method', in P. Camic, J. Rhodes and L. Yardley (eds), *Qualitative Research in Psychology: Expanding Perspectives in Methodology and Design*. Washington, DC: American Psychology Association. pp. 243–74.

Glaser, B. and Strauss, A. (1967) *The Discovery of Grounded Theory*. Chicago, IL: Aldine.

Griffiths, M., Schweitzer, R. and Yates, P. (2011) 'Childhood experiences of cancer: An interpretative phenomenological analysis approach', *Journal of Pediatric Oncology Nursing*, 28 (2): 83–92.

Hammersley, M. and Atkinson, P. (2007) *Ethnography: Principles in Practice*, 3rd edn. London: Routledge.

Haralambos, M. and Holborn, M. (2013) *Sociology, Themes and Perspectives*, 8th edn. London: Collins.

Huang, X., Sun, F., Yen, W. and Fu, C. (2008) 'The coping experiences of carers who live with someone who has schizophrenia', *Journal of Clinical Nursing*, 17 (6): 817–26.

Husserl, E. (1962) *Ideas: General Introduction to Pure Phenomenology*. New York: Macmillan.

Khadivzadeh, T., Roudsari, R-L., Bahrami, M., Taghipor, A. and Shavazi, J-A. (2015) '"Caring for my family integrity": Fertile couples' first childbearing experience in the urban society of Mashhad, Iran', *Human Fertility*, 18 (1): 60–9.

LoBiondo-Wood, G. and Haber, J. (eds) (2014) *Nursing Research: Methods and Critical Appraisal for Evidence-based Practice*, 8th edn. St Louis, MO: Elsevier Mosby.

Moran, D. (2000) *Introduction to Phenomenology*. London: Routledge.

Polit, D. and Beck, C. (2014) *Essentials of Nursing Research: Appraising Evidence for Nursing Practice*, 8th edn. Philadelphia, PA: Lippincott Williams & Wilkins.

Sokolowski, R. (2000) *Introduction to Phenomenology*. Cambridge: Cambridge University Press.

Strauss, A. and Corbin, J. (2008) *Basics of Qualitative Research: Grounded Theory, Procedures and Techniques*, 3rd edn. London: Sage.

Sweeney, A., Harrington, A. and Button, D. (2007) 'Supra-pubic catheters: A shared understanding, from the other side looking in', *Journal of Wound, Ostomy and Continence Nursing*, 34 (4): 418–24.

Van Manen, M. (2010) *Researching Lived Experience: Human Science for an Action-sensitive Pedagogy*, 2nd edn. New York: State University of New York Press.

16
EVALUATION AND OUTCOMES-BASED RESEARCH

Learning outcomes

This chapter will enable you to:

- understand evaluation research and its role in healthcare and healthcare services
- identify the way different research designs can be utilised in evaluation research
- describe some of the outcome measures that are used in evaluation research
- appreciate the practicalities associated with the conduct of evaluation research in healthcare and healthcare services

Evaluation research is a systematic assessment which is used to provide useful feedback about a particular programme or project (Patton, 2015). Evaluation is consequently of prime importance within the health service as we have a continued emphasis on promoting an evidence-based approach to the delivery of care. For this aim, the National Institute for Health and Care Excellence (NICE) and the National Service Frameworks were established to promote a base for good quality and cost-effective clinical interventions and to demonstrate effectiveness not only of healthcare innovations but also of existing procedures and interventions as a way of confirming that available resources are used in the most effective and efficient way. Evaluations of healthcare interventions and services are also undertaken outside this framework. This chapter explains what evaluation research is, why we do it and how to do it. Evaluation research in healthcare is frequently based on a collection of data about the structure, inputs, process, output and outcomes of a service, and these will provide the main guide for the chapter, alongside discussion of the practicalities associated with undertaking evaluation research projects.

EVALUATION: WHAT IS IT AND WHY DO IT?

Evaluation research is a form of applied research. Applied research is designed to investigate a current practical problem. Similarly, evaluation research will normally be undertaken when you want to find out how well an activity, policy or practice is working, and/or what its impact is. Evaluation research and audit are often linked together in health services. However, it is important to remember that audit records that a change has or has not occurred, whereas evaluation is concerned with determining the reasons why, as well as what, change(s) have occurred.

In everyday use, evaluation refers to the making of judgements about the worth or value of something. This can be a subjective assessment, such as determining the literary merit of a new book. Evaluation can also refer to a more formalised or systematic process undertaken by researchers or professional evaluators. Such a formal type of evaluation is effectively a 'disciplined enquiry' in which scientific procedures are used to collect and analyse information or data about an intervention, such as a policy, practice or service (Lincoln and Guba, 1986).

Evaluation is a form of research and makes use of the tools and techniques of basic research, applying them to research questions about need, efficiency, effectiveness, appropriateness and acceptability. Many of the research methods that have been discussed in this book can be used for evaluation, for example, experimental methods, surveys and questionnaires and qualitative designs. The literature review method can also be used as a tool for evaluation. Realist reviews (Wong et al., 2010), are specifically designed for evaluation purposes.

As with all research, evaluation research is associated with demands/requirements to ensure that healthcare delivery is of a consistently high quality, is evidence-based, effective and efficient. It has been suggested (Gray, 2008) that decision making by healthcare practitioners, managers and policy makers (regardless of the way decisions are made or the level at which they are taken) is usually informed by three sets of factors:

1. Values held by the individuals making the decisions
2. Available resources
3. Evidence derived from research about what denotes good and effective practice.

A reliance on evidence to underpin the decision-making process has become more noticeable with increasing pressure on resources and a need to 'justify' the 'worth' of any intervention. This is closely related to the concept of evidence-based practice which is discussed in detail in Chapter 29. These pressures are reinforced by an increasing awareness of what medicine can do on the part of potential users of healthcare services and of their rights to care. In the UK, the role of NICE in determining best practice, the development of National Service Frameworks (NSFs) (DH, 1997), clinical governance (DH, 1999) and a general call for the practice of evidence-based care (DH, 1996) have all served to create a demand for evaluations of existing healthcare practices and services. This reliance on evidence-based practice is linked to an expectation that any new intervention and new ways of working are formally evaluated to ensure that they are actually delivering the care expected and meeting patients' needs in terms of quantity and quality, quite apart from their being cost-effective.

> ### Reflective exercise
>
> Identify something in your practice/work environment that needs to be evaluated, and construct a research question that could be used to undertake the evaluation.

ARE ALL EVALUATIONS THE SAME?

Evaluation research can be divided into two types: formative and summative (Bowling, 2009). In formative evaluation, the aim is to enable improvements or develop a programme, intervention or service by collecting data whilst it is still active. Summative evaluations involve the collection of data about a programme, intervention or service with the aim of deciding whether it should continue or be repeated – for example, deciding if a smoking cessation programme should be repeated or whether discharge co-ordinators improve discharge procedures. In summative evaluations, the data collection can be active or inactive.

In healthcare and healthcare services, the collection of data usually focuses on the structure, process and outcome (Donabedian, 1980):

● Structure refers to the organisational framework for an activity or care-giving environment. These will include facilities, healthcare professionals and ancillary workers and resources available, such as the number of qualified nurses available at any one time.

● Process refers to the activities themselves and how services are organised and delivered. This can include the collection of quantitative data, such as the number of patients being treated and the waiting time to see a GP. It can also include the collection of qualitative data, such as details about the interactions between different professional groups and nurse–patient interactions.

● Outcome refers to the effectiveness or impact of any intervention in relation to individuals and communities, such as the reduction in the number of teenage pregnancies following the introduction of a new advisory service in schools. Health outcome refers to the impact of an intervention on a patient or, in other words, the effectiveness on the health status of the individual (Bowling, 2009).

The structure and process can influence effectiveness, and outcomes are identified as an effectiveness criterion that can be confidently attributed to antecedent care (Donabedian, 1988). In other words, the reasons for a change in practice, policy or service are directly linked to the structures and/or processes relating to that practice, policy or service. Donabedian's work has been frequently cited and is regarded as a valid model by which to evaluate a service (Moore et al., 2015).

WHAT APPROACHES CAN BE USED?

There have been numerous attempts to categorise or make sense of the possible approaches that could be used for evaluation. The type of approach used will depend not only on what is being evaluated (intervention, practice or policy), but also on the types of measurement that it will be possible to make; whether it is possible, or desirable, to have firm goals and objectives for the evaluation; the setting where the evaluation will be conducted; and the experience and, possibly, philosophical stance of the evaluator. Examples of some of the approaches that can be used are given below:

- Traditionally, a *goal-orientated approach* has been used in evaluation research. Here, the aim is to measure the extent to which an intervention has achieved specific goals and objectives. The goals need to be precise and measurable.

Experimental methods tend to be used in the goal-orientated approach. They will often be large scale, with expert evaluators being used to reduce the possibility of bias that may arise if healthcare professionals collect their own data. It may, however, be possible to avoid some of the risk of bias by ensuring, wherever possible, that the outcome measures are objective. An example of this type of approach is given below.

Research example 16.1

A goal-orientated and goal-free evaluation

An Advanced Nurse Practitioner (ANP) running a nurse-led continence clinic wishes to evaluate the effectiveness of the advice she provides. If she uses a *goal-orientated* approach, she will need to set out precise and measurable outcomes of effectiveness from the outset of the evaluation process.

Effectiveness could be defined as whether attendance improves continence, and one intended outcome could be a 25 per cent reduction in the number of incontinent episodes for patients with stress incontinence, measuring the number of incontinent episodes at the first and fifth advice sessions. She will need to ensure that improvement is the result of her advice and that it would not have been achieved by the usual advice/management. This could be done by randomly allocating patients to an intervention group (who get the ANP advice) or a control group (who receive the usual advice/management).

The evaluation will need to include a sufficient number of patients to permit a statistical calculation of significance, and advice on the sample size needed to meet this requirement should be sought. This demonstrates how like an experiment the goal-orientated approach is, and risk of bias is avoided or minimised by making the measure of effectiveness as objective as possible.

A *goal-free* approach to evaluating the nurse-led continence clinic would focus less on the impact of the ANP's advice on incontinence and consider the value of the clinic in terms of whether, or the extent to which, patients felt that their needs had been met. Patients' needs could be expressed in a number of ways, such as the impact incontinence

(Continued)

(Continued)

has on different aspects of their life. They may, therefore, see a value in the opportunities to discuss specific problems with the ANP or share experiences and coping strategies with other sufferers. These aspects of clinic attendance may be very important to some individuals, especially if they are unlikely to be able to achieve full continence due to the nature of their incontinence.

Unintended consequences like these could not be obtained by using an analytical approach; what is needed is a way of discovering or eliciting the feelings or perceptions of patients about attending the clinic. This could be done by conducting interviews or even focus groups and demonstrates the non-experimental nature of this approach and reliance on qualitative methods for this type of evaluation.

- The *experimental approach* to evaluation applies the principles of scientific experimentation. The aim is to be able to produce generalisable conclusions by controlling variables and simplifying the question being asked. The focus is on analytical methods and the data obtained will be quantifiable; for example, comparing outcomes of an intervention by random allocation to either the control group or intervention group (following procedures similar to those used for randomised controlled trials).
- *Goal-free approaches* to evaluation, as initially discussed by Scriven (1972), assume that the focus on goals can result in a narrow approach to evaluation and the possibility of missing unintended outcomes/consequences. A goal-free approach is similar to needs-based assessment where the actual needs being met are evaluated. This may mean that although an intervention does not achieve the specified goals, it is effective because it meets individual or local needs.

Here, there is a desire and/or need to probe aspects of the intervention that are not precise or easily measured. Data, therefore, will be qualitative, and it is likely that the researcher will interact closely with participants whilst collecting data, such as when conducting interviews. One consequence of this is that it becomes difficult for service providers to collect data about their own practice or service without serious risk of bias. It is common, therefore, to use an external evaluator (that is, external to the specific service provision or practice but not necessarily to the organisation) when this approach is employed. An example of this type of approach is given in the Research example 16.1.

- A *utilisation-focused approach* to evaluation is suggested, by Patton (2008), as being done for and with specific, intended primary users for specific, intended uses. Careful consideration of how every aspect of a project is used is central to a utilisation-focused approach. Therefore, the evaluator has to be involved from the outset and will assist users in deciding the exact nature and type of evaluation necessary. In other words, the evaluator will help users (of the evaluation research) to define the questions they want answered about an intervention, practice or policy. An example of this type of approach is given in the Research example 16.2 below.

Research example 16.2

Utilisation-focused and economic evaluations

A team of education facilitators want to implement and evaluate a new programme for mentoring student nurses.

A *utilisation-focused evaluation* of the mentoring programme would involve everyone connected with mentoring. This would require mentors, student nurses, practice educators and, possibly, ward managers, to work together in order to frame the questions that they want answered. For example: a student nurse might ask how the new programme will benefit his or her acquisition of clinical skills; a practice educator might ask if the new programme enables student nurses to work regularly with their mentor; and a mentor might ask what impact the new programme has for enabling students to achieve the competencies specific to a placement.

An *economic evaluation* of the mentoring programme would involve the evaluator calculating the resources used and benefits arising from them. Thus, the data collected would relate to things like: resources for training of mentors and other members of the ward team who have a role in the mentorship programme, and any additional time spent on mentoring compared with the previous programme; and outputs, such as the impact of the programme on student nurses' clinical practice in relation to patient care.

- *Economic evaluations* essentially involve the calculation of all resources used and the benefits arising from them (Patton, 2015). The research process in this type of evaluation will involve trying to quantify the resources used and putting a cost to them. Further calculations are then necessary to assess or quantify the benefits that are accrued by the input of these resources, meaning that a cost–benefit analysis will have to be undertaken. This may be an attractive form of evaluation for managers and service commissioners, but it will not always be possible to put a cost to the benefits of an intervention. For example, it will be relatively easy to evaluate a new dressing using a price comparison between the old and new dressing, time taken to apply the dressings, frequency of dressing changes needed and any change in healing time. However, a full evaluation should also include reference to patient comfort, and calculating the cost of this in terms of patient benefit will, inevitably, be difficult.

- *Mixed method evaluations* are similar to any other mixed method research and apply the same principles. In the example used above, it is easy to see that an economic evaluation of a new dressing will not provide a complete picture of the value or merit of the product in terms of patient care. Here, the addition of a comfort assessment may be an appropriate addition to the evaluation and means that the evaluation uses both qualitative and quantitative research designs. This could be done, for example, by developing a comfort scale from 1 to 10, and asking patients to indicate their level of comfort/discomfort during a dressing change and then compare responses for the old and new dressings. The addition of patients' perspectives may be particularly useful if there is minimal difference in the cost–benefit evaluation of the two dressings.

The mixed method approach highlights the fact that evaluation research makes use of a variety of research approaches and that it is important to use the approach that will best answer the question. This means that a good understanding of research designs and methods is necessary for anyone intending to undertake an evaluation research project.

WHAT OUTCOMES ARE USED IN EVALUATION RESEARCH?

In healthcare, outcomes are the impacts healthcare interventions have on patients' health as well as patients' evaluations of their healthcare. Outcomes refer to the effectiveness of the activities in relation to the achievement of the intended goal (Bowling, 2009). They often focus on things like survival, urgency and seriousness of healthcare needs, and measure 'health gains' and 'benefits' from specific interventions or programmes of care. However, these elements are not usually the main prompts for nursing care where considerations of interventions or ways of working that will improve an individual's quality of life or the quality of care delivery are the focus for an outcome. Outcomes that can measure the effectiveness of nursing will inevitably be complex and are likely to incorporate indicators such as comfort, satisfaction and sense of well-being, along-side more readily measurable physical and social indicators, such as number of pressure ulcers and number of nurses with a specialist nursing qualification.

The outcome measures used in any evaluation have to be appropriate to the question being asked. They can be qualitative or quantitative or a mixture of both. Outcome indicators can be classified as patient-, carer-, staff- and service-based. For example, patient-based outcomes could relate to symptom severity and be measured using a structured self-completion symptom checklist. This will give quantitative data and may enable comparison between different patients or groups of patients. A staff-based outcome could refer to satisfaction with the nature of the care delivered and be assessed by the use of interviews and questionnaires. This would provide a mixture of quantitative and qualitative data and might assist in reducing bias that is inevitable when individuals are assessing their own practice.

STEPS FOR CONDUCTING AN EVALUATION RESEARCH PROJECT

The steps for carrying out an evaluation are essentially the same as for any research project: setting and clarifying the aims and objectives, selecting an appropriate research design and dissemination of results. Evaluation research differs from a basic or 'pure' research project in that attention is directed towards practical problems or questions about an intervention, practice or policy rather than adding knowledge. It is characterised by a rigorous and systematic collection of evidence which is focused on finding out how well a practice, programme or policy is working (Connelly, 2015). The expectation for an evaluation research project is to use whichever research method is most appropriate, and a combination of methods is frequently used rather than a single methodological framework.

> **Reflective exercise**
>
> Consider a current need/problem in your own work/practice and decide how you would carry out an evaluation of it. Include a main aim, a set of objectives and what outcome measure you would employ.

Setting and clarifying aims and objectives

The first step of any evaluation is to decide on the over-riding purpose or overall aim of the evaluation – for example, to assess the effectiveness of Breast Care Nurse Specialists (BCNS) in breast-screening clinics.

Once the overall aim has been clarified, the objectives can be set. The objectives suggest how the evaluation can be realised – for example, to assess the effectiveness of the BCNS in relation to:

- patient support
- information giving
- quality of care.

This objective-setting process helps to establish, implicitly and explicitly, the criteria which will be used to judge whether the evaluation has achieved its purpose. For example, a pre-occupation with effectiveness and explicit outcomes rather than unintended outcomes/consequences may become apparent at this stage and will help influence the choice of research strategy. It is, therefore, important at this stage for the evaluator to confirm with the commissioners of the evaluation what type of effectiveness criteria they are interested in. For example, if the evaluation of the BCNS role is aimed at determining whether there is actually a role for BCNSs in screening clinics, the **evaluation outcomes** may include numbers of patients seen by the different professional groups working in breast-screening clinics. Alternatively, or in addition, the evaluation could investigate/identify the type of advice given by a BCNS and the benefit to patients' well-being compared with that given by other professionals. This latter evaluation will have very different effectiveness outcomes from the former and may help the decision-making process if quality of care is the criterion for determining whether BCNSs should continue to have a role in screening clinics.

Selecting an appropriate research design

The choice of research design will be driven by the aims and objectives of the evaluation and the resources available to carry it out. The selection of the most appropriate research design relies on having a good understanding of the aims of the evaluation and an awareness of the strengths and weaknesses of different research methods in being able to answer different types of question. For example, a survey which collects information in a standardised format (often via questionnaires) from groups of people could be used to evaluate the effectiveness of a healthy eating programme by asking participants to indicate what changes they have made in their eating habits. This type of approach may not, however, be appropriate if the evaluation focus was on the effectiveness of the healthy eating programme in reducing participants' weight or on reactions to the different elements of the programme.

Dissemination of results

All research results have to be reported, and this applies equally to evaluation research projects. The difference from other forms of research, however, is that evaluations are undertaken in a social and political context with multiple stakeholders. There is also the possibility that service providers could be sensitive about their own performances and may feel strongly about the content of the report and how the results are presented. For summative evaluations, in particular, where there is a risk of a service being terminated, it is very important that the results are reported with due care and attention to those on whom the report will have a direct impact.

There are, therefore, benefits in planning the dissemination strategy from the outset of the project. Similarly, developing a regular pattern of feedback and, where appropriate, interim reports will help maintain a rapport and ownership of the evaluation by those who are particularly involved with data collection and commissioners of the evaluation.

It is common to see recommendations for future practice, policy and programme development as an integral part of an evaluation. Recommendations should be clearly derived from the data collected and presented in the report. They are also more likely to be acted upon and implemented if they are practicable. Good practice when developing recommendations is to involve, wherever possible, those who will be making use of the results of the evaluation or the decision makers.

It is important to remember that evaluation research is not only concerned with the effectiveness of particular interventions that can be measured, but also with the processes that underpin the intervention, practice or policy.

CHAPTER SUMMARY

- Evaluation research is applied research that investigates the effectiveness of an intervention, practice or policy and, for nursing, the focus is often on patient care and delivery systems.
- Evaluation applies the scientific method of systematic and rigorous collection of research data.
- Evaluation research is different from audit because it aims to discover the reasons why changes have occurred, as well as what changes have actually occurred.
- Evaluation in healthcare and healthcare services is characterised by the collection of data about the structure, process, outcomes and appropriateness of services.
- Outcomes will usually include measurement of the impact of an intervention, practice or policy.
- Evaluation uses a variety of research methods, and different methods will be appropriate for different questions.

SUGGESTED FURTHER READING

Dahlberg, L. and McCaig, C. (2010) *Practical Research and Evaluation: A Start-to-Finish Guide for Practitioners*. London: Sage. This book is designed specifically for 'do-it-yourself' researchers working in health, social care and the community in either public or voluntary sectors. It is accessible and relevant to practitioners, uses non-technical language wherever possible and employs grounded examples, practical tips, checklists and reading lists throughout.

Examples of evaluation research

Cornish, J. and Jones, A. (2007) 'Evaluation of moving and handling training for pre-registration nurses and its application to practice', *Nurse Education in Practice*, 7: 128–34.

Cunningham, T., Geller, E. and Clarke, S. (2008) 'Impact of electronic prescribing in a hospital setting: A process-focused evaluation', *International Journal of Medical Informatics*, 77 (8): 546–54.

Farquhar, M., Preston, N., Evans, C.J., Grande, G., Short, V., Benalia, H., Higginson, I.J. and Todd, C. (2013) 'Mixed methods research in the development and evaluation of complex interventions in palliative and end-of-life care: Report on the MORECare consensus exercise', *Journal of Palliative Medicine*, 16 (12): 1550–60.

Hazra, A., Chanock, S., Giovannucci, E., Cox, D., Niu, T., Fuchs, C., et al. (2008) 'Large-scale evaluation of genetic variants in candidate genes for colorectal cancer risk in the Nurses' Health Study and Health Professionals' follow-up study', *Cancer, Epidemiology, Biomarkers and Prevention*, 17: 311–19.

Imhof, S., Kaskie, B. and Wyatt, M. (2007) 'Finding the way to a better death: An evaluation of palliative care referral tools', *Journal of Gerontological Nursing*, 33: 40–9.

Knowles, G., Hutchinson, C., Smith, G., Philip, I., McCormick, K. and Preston, E. (2008) 'Implementation and evaluation of a pilot education programme in colorectal cancer management for nurses in Scotland', *Nurse Education Today*, 28: 15–23.

Lee, L.-L., Hsu, N. and Chang, S.-C. (2007) 'An evaluation of the quality of nursing care in orthopaedic units', *Journal of Orthopaedic Nursing*, 11: 160–8.

Malin, N. (2000) 'Evaluation of clinical supervision in community homes and teams serving adults with learning disabilities', *Journal of Advanced Nursing*, 31: 548–57.

Manafi, M., McLeister, P., Cherry, A. and Wallis, M. (2008) 'Pilot process and outcome evaluation of the introduction of a clinical nutrition pathway in the care of in-hospital renal patients', *Journal of Renal Nutrition*, 18 (2): 223–9.

Murphy, J., Worswick, L., Pulman, A., Ford, G. and Jeffery, J (2015) 'Translating research into practice: Evaluation of an e-learning resource for healthcare professionals to provide nutrition advice and support for cancer survivors', *Nurse Education Today*, 35 (1): 271–6.

Potheini, P.T., Yildirim, V.E., Reichow, B. (2012) 'Interventions for toddlers with autism spectrum disorders: An evaluation of research evidence', *Journal of Early Intervention*, 34 (3): 166–89.

WEBSITES

Evaluation and the Health Professions: http://mmr.sagepub.com/

To access further resources related to this chapter, visit the companion website at https://study.sagepub.com/mouleaveyard3e

REFERENCES

Bowling, A. (2009) *Research Methods in Health: Investigating Health and Health Services*, 2nd edn. Buckingham: Open University Press.

Connelly, L.M. (2015) 'Evaluation research', *MEDSURG Nursing*, 24(1): 60, 34.

Department of Health (DH) (1996) *Towards an Evidence-based Health Service*. London: DH.

Department of Health (DH) (1997) *The New NHS: Modern and Dependable*. London: DH.

Department of Health (DH) (1999) *Making a Difference: Strengthening the Nursing, Midwifery and Health Visiting Contribution to Health and Healthcare*. London: DH.

Donabedian, A. (1980) *Explorations in Quality Assessment and Monitoring: The Definition of Quality and Approaches to its Assessment*. Ann Arbor, MI: Health Administration Press.

Donabedian, A. (1988) 'Quality assessment and assurance: Unity of purpose, diversity of means', *Inquiry*, 25: 173–92.

Gray, J. (2008) *Evidence-based Healthcare: How to Make Health Policy and Management Decisions*. London: Churchill Livingstone.

Lincoln, Y. and Guba, E. (1986) 'Research evaluation and policy analysis: Heuristics for disciplined enquiry', *Policy Studies Review*, 5: 546–65.

Moore, L., Lavoie, A., Bourgeois, G. and Lapointe, J. (2015) 'Donabedian's structure-process-outcome quality of care model: Validation in an integrated trauma system', *Journal of Trauma and Acute Care Surg*ery, 78(6): 1168–75.

Patton, M. (2008) *Utilisation-focused Evaluation: The New Century Text*. London: Sage.

Patton, M. (2015) *Qualitative Research and Evaluation Methods*. Thousand Oaks, CA: Sage.

Scriven, M. (1972) 'Pros and cons about goal-free evaluation: Evaluation comment', *Journal of Educational Evaluation*, 34: 1–7.

Wong, G., Greenhalgh, T. and Pawson, R. (2010) 'Internet based medical education: A realist review of what works, for whom and in what circumstances', *BMC Medical Education*, 10: 12.

17
CONSENSUS METHODS

Learning outcomes

This chapter will enable you to:

- Understand Delphi, nominal group and consensus techniques
- Appreciate when these techniques might be employed in data collection
- Understand the advantages and disadvantages of using the techniques

Consensus methods are used to try to establish common agreement in circumstances where there is a lack of understanding of a particular healthcare issue. The methods may be used, for example, when the healthcare team are trying to identify research priorities, are developing new roles or identifying competencies for practice. Consensus methods can be particularly helpful when the evidence base is lacking and the degree of effectiveness and appropriateness of care delivery is unknown. There are three main methods used in health: the Delphi technique, nominal group technique and consensus technique. Each is used to draw expert opinion together, collating the agreed views from those with experience. This is used to make care decisions and judgements. In this chapter we discuss the use of all three techniques.

Of the three, the Delphi technique is more commonly used in healthcare. It is used to gain expert views on a range of issues, such as setting care and research priorities. Nominal group techniques combine aspects of the Delphi technique with that of focus groups (discussed in Chapter 23). Finally, consensus methods draw experts from a range of professions to review particular aspects of care or policy. These methods can be used to develop clinical guidelines for practice. All three techniques can include professionals and service users (patients, carers, families) as experts and thus provide methods that can facilitate user involvement in healthcare development.

DELPHI TECHNIQUE

Whilst the **Delphi technique** has increasingly been used in healthcare to gain consensus opinion from a group of experts on a specific area of enquiry, it remains a generally under-used research approach. In healthcare settings the groups contributing to Delphi studies may include senior nurses, medical staff, members of the professions allied to medicine, and health service users. The Delphi technique involves trying to ascertain a consensus view amongst group members. The process of identifying consensus can involve returning to the group of experts at various stages of the research to draw agreement or obtain an overall view.

The Delphi technique starts with the research team identifying possible expert panel members. In some cases the nurse researcher may need to obtain ethical permission prior to approaching panel members. This can be the case if the research is to involve users of healthcare services, when the research team will need ethical approval from the local NHS Research Committee and possibly from the university ethics committee if the project involves university-based researchers (see Chapters 7 and 8).

Once the panel members have been identified and consent to take part is obtained, if necessary, the process of data collection can commence. This involves collecting data through a series of consecutive questionnaires. Using questionnaires can allow the researchers to collect data anonymously. These are usually posted to expert participants or can be emailed or made available for access on a password-protected website. Open-ended questions are used within the initial questionnaire to establish the general ideas, views and attitudes of the expert group towards the research issue. The questionnaires are returned and feedback is collated. To develop a further, more targeted questionnaire, the researchers use the initial findings. This second questionnaire will be focused on a number of specific issues. It is likely to be composed of a number of statements related to key topics. These are returned to the experts who are asked to rank their degree of agreement against the statements. Responses are again analysed before re-presenting a questionnaire that summarises the rankings. The experts are again asked to rank their level of agreement with the statements. Further analysis can establish the level of consensus or disagreement. If disparity remains, then the process of developing further statements in a questionnaire is revisited and further questionnaires are sent to experts to rank.

The approach is particularly helpful when attempting to establish research or care priorities, defining new roles or ways of working, and can be used to agree on resource priorities. It is suggested that the success of the Delphi technique relies on a number of factors. The initial questions must be formulated and structured to support the process; individual responses must be accurately recorded and transcribed; the response rates through successive rounds should be maintained; the data should be analysed after each round and the importance of feedback after each round should be understood (Keeney et al., 2010).

As a process of data collection, the Delphi technique has some advantages, including being less resource-intensive than many other methods. Additionally, the experts can remain anonymous. Providing a degree of anonymity means that the individual view is more likely to be achieved. Experts have an opportunity to be involved with the research process without having to attend face-to-face data collection sessions, which can support a wide geographical input. The process of data collection is less time-consuming and can be managed more flexibly, which may be more appealing to the participants and less inconvenient.

Whilst there are a number of advantages to using the Delphi technique, there are some potential disadvantages. The initial selection of experts may be ill-conceived and bias may be evident amongst some experts. Those using this methodology can experience difficulties maintaining commitment to the project by the expert group. Reducing response rates can indicate difficulties in trying to maintain enthusiasm. Difficulties of maintaining the group may also reflect the problems some experts can have in agreeing with the statements as they are developed and focused, perhaps in a direction that isn't consistent with their views. Additionally, it can be difficult to achieve consensus across the panel.

An example of using the Delphi technique is given in Research example 17.1.

Research example 17.1

The Delphi technique

Teo et al. (2015) used a two-stage Delphi online survey to gather information from men's health stakeholders across Asia. The first questionnaire included 107 items covering questions on 17 selected men's health issues. The 17 issues were based on the Asian Men's Health Report. The stakeholders included policy makers, clinicians, researchers and consumers. In total 128 stakeholders from 28 Asian countries responded to the first stage. The respondents were asked to indicate their concerns on men's health issues using a Likert scale (see Chapter 22). The stakeholders also provided some free text responses that were analysed thematically and used to develop the second stage questionnaire. This questionnaire consisted of 143 items on 15 key issues, again being scored using a Likert scale. The total 98 stakeholders responded from 19 countries. The stakeholders recommended that men's health policies and programmes should be developed.

We can see in the example from Teo et al. (2015) that the researchers employed the Delphi technique to draw on expert opinion. In this example, service users were not involved in the data collection process. The researchers started the process with an initial questionnaire and the responses were analysed and used to develop a second more focused questionnaire. The process has enabled the researchers to identify key priorities for policy and practice development in the field of men's health.

NOMINAL GROUP TECHNIQUE

Originally developed by Delbecq et al. (1975), the **nominal group technique (NGT)** was used in organisational planning. The technique uses some of the processes of the

Delphi technique and combines these with focus group methods (see Chapter 23). In contrast to the Delphi technique, the participants, or 'expert panel', meet face-to-face to try to achieve a consensus through a process of ranking and refining responses to key issues. The participants are invited to join the nominal group because they have some experience of the topics under discussion. The NGT may include clinical staff and/or service users and carers. The groups are around five to nine in number and are used to discuss a range of care or education issues. Examples of the types of issues considered might include how best to involve users in developing education programmes, the development of practice guidelines or how to identify problems experienced by patients living with chronic heart failure in the community.

Experts can be asked to prepare for the focus group discussions by reading materials and thinking through their views before a face-to-face meeting, so that they come prepared to enter into discussion and to vote on available options. They may also be asked to undertake an initial ranking of, for example, a healthcare intervention, before attending a meeting (Bowling, 2014). The NGT is a facilitated, structured and formal meeting that aims to generate a ranked list of views. The meetings can continue for some time to allow for agreement amongst the experts. The facilitator tries to involve all the participants in the meeting, drawing their opinions into the discussion and requiring them to record their views through ranking the options available. The experts can be asked to rank or rate their expert opinion on a scale 0 (not important) to 9 (very important). These ratings are collated and presented to the group. During the meeting the experts are asked to review the rankings and discuss their differences. Relevant literature may also be sourced to inform the discussions before the ranking is revisited and ratings changed.

The process therefore includes: the generation of ideas by the experts individually, the recording of ideas from around the group, a facilitated and time-limited discussion on each idea, and ranking of ideas through voting.

As with the Delphi technique, NGT provides a resource-effective way of bringing experts together to achieve a consensus view. The approach is quicker and cheaper to administer than many other data collection techniques, especially individual interviewing. However, as with focus group techniques, NGT can be affected if there are dominant characters in the group who sway the general discussion. Further limitations arise from the face-to-face nature of the meeting that means anonymity cannot be guaranteed and participant views may therefore be tempered in an open discussion forum.

See Research example 17.2 showing NGT in use.

Research example 17.2

The nominal group technique (NGT)

Harvey and Holmes (2012) used nominal group technique in four focus groups involving clinical experts from an emergency department and obstetric and midwifery areas of a regional hospital in Australia. The NGT was used to assess the triage (decisions about where to send for emergency treatment) and management of pregnant women in the emergency department. The protocol for running the NGT included five stages. The first stage was an initial introduction in the focus group, explanation of the purpose, and information giving (project information sheet and gaining consent). The second stage asked participants to respond alone to a series of questions by writing down ideas. Stage three included sharing ideas with participants stating their ideas to the group. Stage four allowed time for clarification and discussion, with the final stage including voting and ranking.

We can see from this example that the researchers started the process with initial questions to promote initial thinking. The 'experts' were asked to think about their responses to these questions alone, before sharing in a way that allowed everyone to state their views. This meant the approach was able to include all views at this early stage. Refinement of thinking and the development of consensus took place through clarification and discussions. A final vote and ranking enabled the researchers to achieve clinically relevant and focused ideas that they intended to base change on.

CONSENSUS TECHNIQUES

Consensus techniques can be called 'consensus development panels' (Bowling, 2014) or 'consensus knowledge-building forums' (Burns and Grove, 2014). They work on the same principles as the NGT, and bring experts together in one face-to-face forum to gain either further understanding or consensus in a particular field. The consensus method involves a panel of experts invited to take part. The panels are often multi-disciplinary in nature and may be composed entirely of professionals, healthcare users or a mixture of both. The panels are used to agree a consensus and develop clinical guidelines for practice (Burns and Grove, 2014). The process of developing guidelines can require the experts to include reference support to ensure that the practice developed is evidence-based. This means that an initial search and systematic review of the key literature may be undertaken to provide current evidence for the panel members. Scoping exercises might also be conducted, perhaps reviewing guidelines from a range of professional bodies or reviewing practice elsewhere. Information from both systematic reviews and scoping exercises could be given to panel members ahead of the meeting, providing the experts with current information to use in the discussions. The consensus panel will be able to draw on current knowledge in developing guidelines, and as part of the process of reviewing the existing evidence base they may identify gaps in knowledge. This means research priorities can also be identified as part of a consensus knowledge-building process.

Either an expert in the field or someone seen as a credible facilitator in the eyes of the expert panel members facilitates consensus techniques. Though only one meeting is involved, this can continue over a number of days. The nature of the process can make this a more costly data collection method, as there are costs attached in gathering background materials and in paying experts.

The method can facilitate multi-disciplinary healthcare team discussions, involving nurses and other healthcare professionals, in the development of new clinical guidelines for practice (see Research example 17.3). There is also scope to include healthcare users in the forums and enable their valuable input in the development of practice guidelines and statements.

Research example 17.3

A consensus technique

Bernatsky et al. (2013), conducting research in Canada, aimed to develop best-practice statements about the use of administrative data for rheumatic disease research and surveillance. They invited 52 staff to take part. This included epidemiologists, clinicians, managers and researchers, who formed working groups to examine three best-practice areas which were case definitions, epidemiology methods and comorbidity and outcome measures. Following this work, which included systematic and scoping reviews of key topics, the staff attended a two-day workshop. The focus of the workshop was to consider evidence of the reviews and develop best-practice statements through a process of presenting each statement, discussing and reviewing. Ultimately, 13 best-practice statements were developed and agreed by consensus. The statements provide guidance for practitioners.

DIFFERENCES BETWEEN THE CONSENSUS METHODS

Having explored the three main consensus methods, we have devised Table 17.1, which provides an overview of the main differences between Delphi technique, nominal group technique and consensus techniques. It particularly concentrates on those differences related to what the methods are used for, who might be involved, how data are collected and how consensus is achieved.

Table 17.1   Differences between consensus methods

Method	When is it used	Who is involved	How is data collected	How is consensus achieved
Delphi Technique	To identify research and care priorities; also can be used to determine new role composition.	Expert panel members	Experts complete a series of online or postal questionnaires.	Experts rank a series of statements. Through the process a level of agreement is achieved.
Nominal Group Technique	Organisational planning, assess management systems.	Clinical staff and the public who have had relevant experience	Undertake preparatory reading, panel meet and initially respond alone, then work as a focus group to discuss and debate.	Rank responses to key issues, refine and re-rank until consensus is achieved.

Method	When is it used	Who is involved	How is data collected	How is consensus achieved
Consensus methods	Developing practice guidelines.	Professionals, the public	Initial scoping and systematic review of evidence, one face-to-face forum facilitated by an expert in the field.	Consider evidence, develop best-practice statements, review and discuss these, rank/vote to achieve consensus.

CHAPTER SUMMARY

- Consensus techniques can be useful in cases where there is a lack of knowledge or understanding of a particular healthcare issue.
- Consensus techniques enable healthcare professionals to access the views of experts on aspects of practice, education and research.
- Consensus techniques can be used in developing clinical guidelines and in identifying agreement on health and research priorities.
- There are three main methods used in health: the Delphi technique, nominal group technique and consensus technique.
- The Delphi technique involves data collection via a series of consecutive questionnaires administered to the group of experts.
- One advantage is the anonymity provided to the participants, a second is the limited resources required to administer the technique.
- In the nominal group technique the participants meet face-to-face to try to achieve a consensus through a process of ranking and refining responses to key issues.
- The nominal group technique includes: generation of ideas by the experts individually, recording of ideas from around the group, discussion on each idea that is facilitated and time-limited, selection of group ideas and ranking of ideas through voting.
- Nurses and other healthcare professionals may be involved in consensus techniques as part of a multi-disciplinary healthcare team discussing the development of new clinical guidelines for practice.
- All three methods can include professionals and users (patients, carers, families) as experts and as such provide techniques that can facilitate user involvement in healthcare development.

SUGGESTED FURTHER READING

Bowling, A. (2014) *Research Methods in Health: Investigating Health and Health Services*, 4th edn. Buckingham: Open University Press. This book includes information on the use of consensus development methods in healthcare research. It discusses the approaches and how they can be applied, highlighting the strengths and limitations of use.

Keeney, S., Hasson, F. and McKenna, H. (2011) *The Delphi Technique in Nursing and Health Research*. Oxford: Wiley-Blackwell. This book provides a practical approach to using Delphi Technique in healthcare settings. It includes information on methodology, design, sampling, ethics, and reliability and validity. It also considers some of the limitations of the approach and how these might be addressed.

WEBSITES

To access further resources related to this chapter, visit the companion website at https://study.sagepub.com/mouleaveyard3e

REFERENCES

Bernatsky, S., Lix, L., O'Donnell, S. and Lacille, D. (2013) 'Consensus statements for the use of administrative health data in rheumatic disease research and surveillance', *Journal of Rheumatology*, 40 (1): 66–73.

Bowling, A. (2014) *Research Methods in Health: Investigating Health and Health Services*, 4th edn. Berkshire: Open University Press.

Burns, N. and Grove, S. (2014) *The Practice of Nursing Research:* Appraisal, synthesis, and generation of evidence, 7th edn. St Louis, MO: Saunders Elsevier.

Delbecq, A., Van de Ven, A. and Gustafson, D. (1975) *Group Techniques for Program Planning*. Glenview, IL: Scott, Foresman.

Harvey, N. and Holmes, C. (2012) 'Nominal group technique: An effective method for obtaining group consensus', *International Journal of Nursing Practice*, 18(2): 188–94.

Keeney, S., Hasson, F. and McKenna, H. (2011) *The Delphi Technique in Nursing and Health Research*. Oxford: Wiley-Blackwell.

Teo, C., Ng, C., Ho, C. and Tan, H. (2015) 'A consensus on men's health status and policy in Asia: A Delphi survey', *Public Health*, 129 (1): 60–7.

18
ACTION RESEARCH

Learning outcomes

This chapter will enable you to:

- understand action research
- be able to describe the action research process
- appreciate when action research can be utilised

Action research is an approach that is defined by its participatory nature and is usually associated with hands-on, small-scale projects. The aim is to gain knowledge whilst at the same time change or develop practice by engaging practitioners in the research process. The research is normally done at the same time as practice is being undertaken, and this can be in a full range of healthcare settings. Action research is practised under a variety of names other than action research, such as participatory action research (PAR), community-based research and collaborative enquiry. The emphasis on participation in action research has led it sometimes to be known as 'participatory action research'. Kemmis et al. (2014) suggest that the two terms – action research and participatory action research – are used interchangeably.

The actual process of action research is complex and requires that participants develop skills in research, practice, education and change management and implementation (Waterman, 2013).

The concept of action research came from the social psychologist Kurt Lewin and it was he who coined the phrase action research. Lewin described action research as: 'research leading to social action' *by use of* 'a spiral of steps, each of which is composed of a circle of planning, action, and fact-finding about the result of the action' (1946: 35).

This focuses on the key feature of action research, i.e. that it is a continuous process of observation, reflection and problem solving. Lewin also saw action research as a tool for the promotion of democracy; and more recently action research has been seen as a distillation of democratic principles into research (Robson, 2011). The actual merging of action and research has also been seen as a way of fighting oppression and social injustice (Stringer, 2007) and, to a lesser extent, of empowering women (Reinharz, 1992).

The emphasis for action research has now moved to become a method of community or organisational development by awareness-raising, the development of abilities to influence decision making and collaboration between healthcare practitioners, lay individuals and trained researchers. The very practical orientation and collaborative nature of action research can be very attractive in healthcare settings because it offers an opportunity for healthcare practitioners to gain first-hand experience of undertaking research, whilst at the same time implementing change, whatever the impetus/progenitor of the change is.

This chapter discusses the processes involved in action research, the ethical issues involved in undertaking action research, the issues associated with the practitioner/researcher role and the advantages and disadvantages associated with action research.

WHAT IS ACTION RESEARCH?

Stringer (2007) describes action research as 'look, think, act'. By *look*, Stringer means that participants should define and describe the problem to be investigated and its context. *Think* means reflecting, analysing and interpreting the situation in order to be able to develop more of an understanding of the problem, whilst *act* means that the solution to the problem should be formulated and actually put in place. This, in essence, is what action research is all about, but with this looking, thinking and acting process needing to be repeated until a solution to the problem that is satisfactory to all participants, is found.

Action research is different from other methods of research because it is not done on or with participants. Rather, it is designed, carried out and integrated into practice by practitioners (to whom the problem relates) in partnership with researchers (Lingard et al., 2008). This means that the research participants take an active part in carrying out the research themselves and are not being researched *on*, as is the case in conventional forms of research. This applies no matter who the participant is, although the actual extent of involvement will, of course, be dependent upon their role in the situation being investigated.

An action research study can be useful in investigating individuals with health problems and behaviours in an area with the aim of developing appropriate treatment and/or preventative programmes. For example, healthcare professionals working with individuals who have had an eating disorder and have relapsed may try to discover what the prompts are for relapse and go on to develop new programmes in order to reduce the likelihood of relapse in the future. Such an investigation using an action research method of study would mean that those individuals with a relapsed eating disorder would have as much involvement in the development of new preventative programmes as the healthcare professionals. Action research can equally be used to investigate or learn about practice – see, for example, Mander et al. (2010) who used action research to investigate the feasibility of a midwife-led normal birthing unit in China and Lorhan et al.'s (2015) study on the role of volunteers at an outpatient cancer centre.

From the outset, action research has been involved with practical issues, i.e. the types of issues and problems, concerns and needs that arise in daily practice. It is also seen as research that is specifically concerned with change. This means that action research is not only about gaining a better understanding of the problems being investigated or increasing knowledge, but actually sets out to change things as an integral part of the research process (Denscombe, 2010). Action research is, therefore, more likely to be situation-specific and less easily generalised. However, if you identify a problem in your work area, it is equally possible that other practitioners may have similar problems if they work in related areas and may find the solution(s) you develop utilising action research can be adapted to their own particular situation. An example of action research demonstrating change that could be useful in other care settings is the Allan et al. (2015) study 'Supporting staff to respond effectively to informal complaints: Findings from an action research study.' The study used an action research approach to understand how nurses and midwives manage informal complaints at ward level.

The purposes of action research in healthcare are concerned with practitioners looking for ways in which the quality of care can be enhanced (Koshy et al., 2011). This links, according to Hughes (2008), with the World Health Organization's 1946 definition of health that identifies it as a state of complete physical, mental and social well-being and not merely the absence of disease or infirmity. An assumption from this definition of health is that the health of individuals and communities is dependent on environmental factors, the quality of relationships, beliefs and attitudes as well as biomedical factors. This implies that we see ourselves as being interdependent, and hence a holistic approach is required in order to understand health. Action research is able to facilitate this by developing in-depth understandings whereby it is possible to produce practical knowledge that is useful for individuals in everyday life and within their specific environments.

Bradbury (2015) further explains that the purpose of action research is to work towards practical outcomes and develop new ways of understanding things because reflection and the application of theory are both part of the action research process. The participatory nature of action research requires the researcher to work with all stakeholders involved in the area of research, whilst also working for them (Bradbury, 2015).

Action research is a process. The aim of this process is to change an existing situation for the better through the involvement of individuals that are part of that particular situation. All research is about generating knowledge and action research is no different in this respect. However, the knowledge generated by action research is of a specific nature and predominantly within a practical context with the aim of making a change in that specific situation. The practical context for you as a practitioner and researcher will be the healthcare setting in which you work and the change will relate to any aspect of your practice that you identify as being problematic. For example, in the Allan et al. (2015) study, the prompt was robust systems are required to support staff to improve their response to informal complaints and improve the patient experience.

In addition, action research has a learning component. This means that whilst you are actively participating in the project, you will be gaining knowledge about your work situation and learning about the process of research, including data analysis and writing up.

DEFINITIONS

Actually defining action research can be problematic because there are a number of different models. The following definitions may go some way in helping to clarify what action research is all about:

> AR [action research] is social research carried out by a team that encompasses a professional action researcher and the members of an organization, community, or network ('stakeholders') who are seeking to improve the participants' situation. AR promotes broad participation in the research process and supports action leading to a more just, sustainable, or satisfying situation for the stakeholders. (Greenwood and Levin, 2007: 3)

> [Action research] involves healthcare practitioners conducting systematic enquiries in order to help them improve their own practices, which in turn can enhance their working environment and the working environments of those who are part of it – clients, patients and users. (Koshy et al., 2011)

> Action research is a process by which change is achieved and new knowledge about a situation is generated. … it is difficult to change a situation without working to understand it more fully, and in trying better to understand things, the possibilities for change often emerge. (Williamson, 2012: 7)

These definitions show that action research is not readily described in straightforward terms as is more usual in other research methodologies. They do, however, demonstrate why action research is such an attractive research methodology in healthcare settings, because the aim from the outset is to bring about change that is practically (clinically) orientated. More importantly, they demonstrate the key features or concepts associated with action research. In their seminal text, Carr and Kemmis (1986) note that the main principles of action research include its:

- participatory character
- democratic impulse
- simultaneous contribution to knowledge (social science) and practice (change).

The *participatory character* is usually regarded as fundamental in action research since there is an expectation that the participants have identified a need for change and have agreed to take an active part in bringing this about. This does not, however, mean that every participant will have the same sense of need or willingness to be involved with the process. There is also the possibility that conflict will arise during the process, but if facilitators (internal or external) gain the trust of participants they should be able to set out ground rules for resolution of any conflicts that arise.

The *democratic impulse* refers to the need for all participants to be seen as equals within the research process. This should mean that everyone is actively engaged in the activity, and hence the outcome(s) are more meaningful to the participants. It should also make the implementation of any change, developed by the research process, acceptable and meaningful to practitioners, thus making it more readily rooted in the reality of day-to-day practice (Meyer, 2000).

The *simultaneous contribution to knowledge and practice* of action research, according to Meyer (2000), is one way of dealing with the theory–practice gap by making the process fit directly with practitioners' own problems and unique situations. In action research, you are made very aware of your own situation and experience, and can therefore generate findings that mean something to you. It does, however, highlight that knowledge contribution is context-specific and any generalisation will be different from that of more conventional forms of research.

The actual core of action research has been described by Thomas (2013) as:

- done by practitioners on their own initiative
- being primarily about developing practice and empowering practitioners
- involving a commitment to change and action based on reflection
- using the process of planning, reflection and re-planning to keep the process moving forward until the problem is resolved to the satisfaction of the participants.

This final point of planning, reflection and re-planning highlights the cyclical nature of action research which seeks to ensure that the research actually feeds directly into practice and that the process is ongoing until a satisfactory resolution of the problem identified at the outset has been achieved.

TYPES OF ACTION RESEARCH

Action research is similar to evaluation research (see Chapter 16) in that it utilises conventional research designs, so that qualitative, quantitative or mixed methods can be employed in order to achieve the desired goals. There are, however, according to Whitelaw et al. (2003), three broad types of action research that span the methodological continuum from positivist to interpretivist (see Chapter 11). These are:

- technical–scientific
- mutual–collaborative
- critical and emancipatory.

In the *technical–scientific* approach, the researcher is the expert who plans and conducts the research with practitioners in the field and gives advice on the actions that should be taken. This means that the researcher, although acting as a facilitator, actually leads the project. This type of approach is often used when the research aims to 'test' an intervention and will use methods that are akin to scientific research, such as a quasi-experimental design with a control and experimental group.

In the *mutual–collaborative* approach, the researcher and practitioners work together to identify the research problem. This collaboration continues throughout the project to develop the intervention and change together. In this type of approach, other stakeholders, such as service users, are much more likely to be involved as participants.

This approach is useful for exploring more practical issues and the changes that lead on from the results can be rapidly implemented. The researcher may still take on the facilitator role during the research but this will be directed by the needs of the project rather than by the researcher being an active leader.

In the *critical and emancipatory* approach, action research not only aims to improve outcomes and promote a change in practice, but also to help practitioners to critique their work settings and practices. There is a focus on helping professionals to develop critical understanding of the situation they are in; the practice, practitioner and practice settings are all considered.

Whichever type of action research approach is utilised, it will be cyclical.

ACTION RESEARCH AS A CYCLICAL PROCESS

As we have already seen, action research involves a number of stages that enable a continuous process of planning, reflection and re-planning. Thus, there is a cycle of enquiry in which the research feeds directly back into practice and where the process is ongoing until an effective change has been achieved. Lewin (1946) described this as a spiral of steps and these have been interpreted in diagrammatic form by many authors. Figure 18.1 demonstrates not only the cyclical nature of action research but also the continuous nature of action research. Note that it refers to continual improvement which implies that once improvement stops or the desired outcome has been reached, the process of research is at an end.

An alternative **action research cycle** is shown in Figure 18.2 and highlights what happens in each stage research of the action research process. These two diagrammatic representations of the action research process are simply given as examples but not all action research projects will follow these patterns. The flexibility of action research means that the constant evaluation and reflection may lead to the cycles being truncated as new ways to proceed become apparent. Each stage of the cycle can overlap with other stages, so do not expect it to be a smooth process. It is more than likely that there will be forward and backward movements within the process, rather than a continual forward movement as implied in Figure 18.1.

The first cycle of action research is essentially:

1. Having an idea or seeing a problem.
2. Examining the idea/problem and then gathering more information about it by observations and reviewing the literature.
3. Planning actions that will resolve the problem or working out how to make the idea applicable for practice.
4. Putting the plan into action.
5. Reflecting on the outcomes of the implemented plan.

This last reflective process will lead to a revision of the original idea and lead on to another cycle of activity.

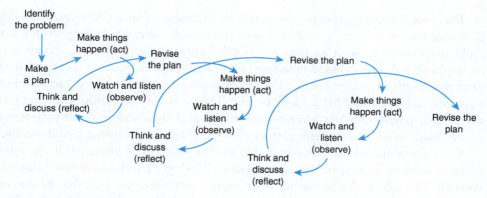

Figure 18.1   Action research cycle

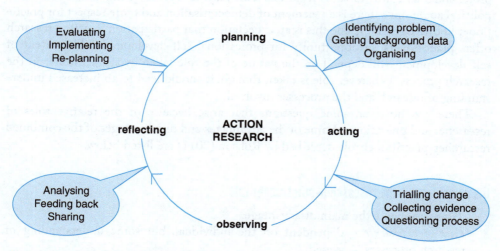

Figure 18.2   A single action research cycle

PARTICIPATING IN THE RESEARCH PROCESS

The most distinguishing feature of action research is commonly regarded as its partici-patory nature. Traditionally, an expert undertakes research, with the researcher initiating the process, determining the research question, designing the means of data collection and analysis. Once the research has been completed, the researcher will write a report and results may be fed back in some form to those who were involved in the research. These individuals may, or may not, implement changes, if appropriate, in practice on the basis of the findings. Action research is very different where the imperative is for practitioners to be active participants in the sense of being a 'partner in the research' (Denscombe, 2010), rather than just taking part as you would if you were completing a questionnaire or being interviewed for a conventional study.

There are different forms of partnership or participation in action research. It can be you as the professional practitioner who initiates the research, having identified a problem or come up with an idea which will improve care quality if a change can be implemented. This 'insider' initiation of the action research process is regarded as practitioner-driven and means that the practitioner is not simply an equal partner but a sponsor and director of the research process. This does not necessarily mean that you would have to have all of the research knowledge and skills to undertake the project but you are likely to be the dominant partner with the researcher following your direction.

Even if practitioners do not initiate the research, there is an alteration in the relationship between participant and researcher to it being a collaborative one in action research. The role of the researcher as an expert continues, but will often be one of a facilitator of the project and a resource that can be drawn upon when needed. The rationale for this different relationship relates to the way practitioner knowledge, both professional and situational, is regarded. This may be seen as giving action research a political angle since there is an element of democratisation and more respect for practitioner knowledge. Alongside this is an expectation that participation in action research offers practitioners an opportunity for professional self-development. The extent of self-development will depend on the nature of the role taken by a practitioner in the research process. Whatever role is taken though, it should lead to an increased understanding of research and the processes involved.

There are, however, some questions that arise because of the relative roles of researcher and practitioner. Some of the advantages and disadvantages of the combined researcher-practitioner role described by Robson (2011) are listed below.

Disadvantages of the researcher-practitioner role

1. *Time* – probably the main disadvantage.
2. *Lack of experience* – dependent on the individual, but some understanding of research processes is needed.
3. *Lack of confidence* – lack of experience in doing research leads to a lack of confidence.
4. *'Insider' problems* – an insider may have preconceptions about issues and/or solutions. Hierarchy difficulties may arise (i.e. high-status and low-status possibilities of the researcher-practitioner), along with the possibility of outsider advice being more highly valued than that of the insider.

Advantages of the researcher-practitioner role

1. *'Insider' opportunities* – having pre-existing knowledge and experience about the situation and individuals involved.
2. *'Practitioner' opportunities* – there is likely to be a substantial reduction in implementation problems.
3. *'Researcher-practitioner' synergy* – practitioner insights and role help in the design, carrying out and analysis of useful and appropriate studies.

STAGES OF ACTION RESEARCH

The stages of action research are more or less the stages already identified in the cyclical process; though in an actual action research project they may overlap or be interlinked. It is, however, important to recognise from the outset that reflection should really be part of each stage, as it is the key component of the action research process (Koshy et al., 2011).

The stages may be described as:

- planning
- acting
- observing
- reflecting.

Each of these stages will involve a number of elements and are likely to be different in each cycle of an action research project.

Planning

Planning is the stage where the issue to be investigated is identified and the project is set up. Also, because action research is about individuals in a given situation attempting to change something, there is a need from the outset to get them involved in the research process. This is often where the researcher can take the lead by taking on the role of facilitator. At the beginning of the project, it is essential that stakeholders (e.g. nurses, healthcare assistants, patients, managers, doctors, physiotherapists) are identified, and to make sure that they are all aware who else is involved in the project, as well as its aims and likely events. A facilitator will also be very useful in helping to promote a positive climate of interaction and the activity that participants are going to be involved in (Bowling, 2009). Getting everyone involved and 'on-side' may not be easy, but making regular contact and having meetings with all of those involved will go a long way to maintaining their sense of continuous involvement and feeling some sort of ownership of the project.

You can see from this that any action research facilitator needs to have considerable skills in communication, negotiation and networking. It is important that the facilitator, whoever takes on the role, must be legitimised in that role by being knowledgeable, neutral and non-threatening to all involved, and have their role carefully agreed with each of the relevant social groups. Additionally, ground rules should be established with the facilitator so that no group of practitioners feels that their input is less relevant than those of another group, and that confidences will be respected between the different group participants.

The main aim for this stage of the process is to discuss and identify the specific concern or issue to be resolved or how a new idea can be implemented. This is usually initiated by investigating individual interpretations of the situation and issue/concern/idea. Other practical details that may need to be considered and discussed at this time include justifying the investment of time and effort into the project and expectations for the project outcomes. It may also be possible to determine, or at least have an idea of, what the changed situation may look like at the end of the project (Koshy et al., 2011).

There are also, according to Koshy et al. (2011), a number of practical issues that need to be addressed during this stage of an action research project, such as:

- Motivation and interest

Because the issue for the project arises from the researcher's experience and context, it is anticipated that motivation can be maintained provided there is sufficient workplace interest. Lack of interest at the outset of a project by a significant proportion of practitioners should act as a warning that the process is likely to be problematic and may stall before it really gets going. This means that time and effort has to be devoted to informing all potential participants and ensuring that they are committed to the whole project from the outset to reduce the risk of non-completion.

- The research topic or question

The same issues around determining the research question arise in action research as with any other research methodology. This also applies to the nature of data collection and analysis. The important thing is to remain open-minded and let the question lead, rather than having pre-determined ideas about modes of data collection and remaining tentative and speculative about the outcomes.

- Scope and resources

Being realistic about the scope of an action research project is just like any other research study. Many action research projects are small-scale, but the impact of even small changes in practice can have a significant impact on care quality. You also need to consider what resources you have available for the project. Will participants have sufficient time and any necessary equipment made available? Are there other changes happening/planned within the organisation that may interfere with the project, and are facilities available for data analysis?

- Design

This is a very important aspect of the planning stage. As with any research study, there must be a clear aim and objectives and activities that will relate to the achievement of the objectives. Methods of data collection and analysis will also need to be determined, and at this time a literature review may be useful in helping to define the question and deciding the best methods to employ for data collection. It is possible to use almost any research methodology in action research – quantitative, qualitative or mixed methods – the choice being dependent on the situation and research question. For example, Ma Jesusa (2015) used a mixed methods approach in a study that aimed to improve the sexual and reproductive health of women with disability in the Philippines, and Allan et al. (2015) used focus groups to enable a group of nurses to provide information on responses to informal complaints.

- Working collaboratively

A key feature of action research is its collaborative nature. It therefore should go without saying that it is important for everyone participating in such a project to feel 'ownership' and be willing to change practice. Whatever the role of the researcher (whether one of a group of action researchers, leader, facilitator or contributor), it is important that everyone's contributions are valued and respected. There is a need for a trusting relationship between colleagues to be established as part of the research process if the project is to be successful, and will require that researchers are able to accept critical comments and respond positively to them. This means that there is a need for action research participants to agree ground rules for behaviour in meetings.

- Consider dissemination

Finally, as with all research, in action research projects consideration must be given to how findings will be disseminated. It may be that supporters and/or funders of the project will expect a formal written report. Will it be appropriate to report on findings within the wider workplace, in a conference presentation, as part of a professional development activity or to write it up for publication? Although action research projects may be small-scale, it is important that the findings are disseminated so that other practitioners can gain from your experience of undertaking a project whatever the outcomes. Action research projects are not usually expected to be generalisable; however, outcomes may be useful for similar practice situations. For example, the study by Allan et al. (2015) may offer insight for other acute NHS trusts that may have problems supporting informal complaints.

Acting

The acting stage of action research is all about trying out the change in practice, following the plan that you developed in the *planning* stage. This also includes collecting and compiling data or evidence about the impact of the change. The type of data to be collected will of course depend on the research question and the most appropriate way for it to be answered. Data collection may be relatively straightforward in the sense of getting participants to complete questionnaires, although it is likely that a study-specific questionnaire will have to be designed prior to this (see Chapter 22). Or it may be that interviews and/or focus groups may give more appropriate data. Time and effort are essential for data collection activities; otherwise there will be insufficient evidence about the impact of change.

Throughout this stage of the project, you should be questioning the process (reflecting) and making changes as required. As stated before, action research is a flexible process, so that when unexpected difficulties arise, perhaps as the change is being put into practice, adaptations can be made and the plan modified in the light of experience and relevant evidence.

Observing

Obviously, any data collected will need to be analysed and this may need specialist expertise, especially if it is complex data or the type of data that participants have little experience of analysing. This may also provide an excellent opportunity for you to develop your own data analysis skills by working with an experienced researcher/ data analyst (quantitative or qualitative or mixed data). The findings should then be discussed with participants for their interpretation. Here, you may feel that some of the findings may not be of interest to some participants or groups of participants, but they should still be offered the opportunity to consider all of the data and allowed to decide for themselves. Once there is a consensus on how the findings should be interpreted, they can be reported and then shared with others.

The who, how and purpose of data analysis require discussion between participants and need to be actively managed by the researcher/facilitator. This should also take into account the experience, abilities and development of participants involved and that the data continues to be owned by them. For example, an experienced researcher may do the detailed analysis of a set of interviews but, in order to develop the qualitative data analysis skills of a participant(s) a portion of the data is analysed by some participants, possibly those who initiated the action research process.

As with a conventional research project, there is not only a need to write up your research but to remember that the perspective of an action researcher in presenting findings will be different. In an action research project, the researcher is not detached from the research setting and does not have sole responsibility for data collection and analysis (Waterman, 2013).

You should also consider who your report audience will be. This means that you may have to adapt your report to accommodate the wants of your colleagues, your tutor, your boss, for a qualification or for publication. However, as with all other aspects of action research there is a need to be participative, and all those who have been involved with the project should have the opportunity to comment on any report that comes out and to actually be involved in the preparation of the report if they wish.

Reflecting

Reflection is the central tenet of action research and as such should be an ongoing exercise throughout the process. However, reflection at this stage in the cycle has as its primary role evaluation of the first cycle of the process. This reflective exercise will lead to better understanding of the problem/issue and identification of those areas requiring more investigation and how practice can be developed further.

Reflection in action research is similar to reflective practices in healthcare generally. However, in action research reflection is centred on one group problem which all participants are focusing upon rather than individual professional groups considering a series of problems (Koshy et al., 2011). Additionally, there is the possibility that outcomes from reflective sessions may be published in the research report so confidential issues need to be considered and discussed. Because practitioners are used to reflective practice, it is possible to assume that they will find the reflective activities easy, but additional training and practice in moderating reflective action research meetings should be given before any one individual takes on the role.

There are a number of options for reflecting, such as using reflective models or an open format with or without some questions to act as prompts, and individual or group reflection. Group reflection allows for wide discussion and may also enhance the collaborative nature of the research. Lee (2009) explains how group reflection was used in an action research study evaluating a nurse-led unit in a community hospital. She describes how group reflection helped to affirm that practice of participation, as well as being a good way for:

> reviewing the quality of the research, its match with the methods and outcome. It also helped illuminate the team members' research development and learning concerning the themes explored previously. It affirmed that involvement in the research process is a way of learning by practice and helps to demystify the process of research. Group reflection demonstrates the value of participation in that those most directly involved with the unit, professionals and ex-service users alike, were able to identify their own priorities for the study and shape the research for themselves. It suggests participation helped development of personal and professional skills particularly in relation to research and professional practice. It also helped clarify and explore values and beliefs about practice, especially about the user experience during healthcare. (Lee, 2009: 40)

Reflective exercise

Now you have read about the purpose and stages of action research, you should be able to identify the type of issue/problem that is suitable for investigation using action research.

Look at the following list of research questions. Which most suits the action research approach?

1. Does the restricted use of restraint lead to an increase in falls in the elderly in nursing homes?
2. What are teenagers' experiences of transition from care homes to independent living?
3. Is there a relationship between joint nursing and physiotherapy manual handling training programmes and safer manual handing practice?
4. How do patients react when asked to walk to the operating room?
5. Why do patients ask for antibiotics for sore throats?
6. Does more discussion about lifestyle preferences improve the transition of older people from hospital to care homes?

How did you do? See the Appendix at the end of this chapter.

ETHICAL ISSUES IN ACTION RESEARCH

The participatory nature of action research means that there is a need to respect the sensitivities and rights of colleagues and patients who become involved in the research. Ethical approval is required because:

- during action research observations and/or medical documents are used for purposes other than direct care
- researchers need to confirm that they will respect the confidentiality of participants
- change and development emanating from the research must be visible and open to suggestions from others.

Waterman (2013) suggests that confidentiality and anonymity are likely to be an ethical issue that needs to be negotiated in advance. It cannot be assumed that everyone will want the content of their interview shared with other participants. Similarly, the use of anonymous quotations will not necessarily ensure that a participant's identity is hidden. However, some participants may want to be identified because doing so may give recognition and status, though they may not want to be identified by individual quotations. This reaction is exemplified in Waterman et al.'s 2006 study, 'Intervening in the process of stigmatisation: Challenging social inequalities in the context of HIV/AIDS home-based care in Kenya'.

ADVANTAGES AND DISADVANTAGES OF ACTION RESEARCH

As with any research, there are both advantages and disadvantages of action research, and these need to be taken into account before embarking on an action research process.

Advantages

- *Practicality* – action research is able to address very practical problems in a positive way by being able to give feedback on findings throughout the research process and into the practice environment. This should enable developments and improvements to be more readily owned by the practitioners involved.
- *Participation* – enables practitioners to be actively involved in research and improve understanding of research practice. Participants can direct the research process and may improve appreciation of, and respect for, practitioner knowledge and expertise.
- *Continuity* – the continuous cycle of development and change in the practice setting should provide benefits because it is aimed at improving healthcare.
- *Professional development* – it may contribute to professional self-development, depending on individual involvement and commitment to the action research project.

Disadvantages

- *Workload* – inevitably, action research involves some extra work for practitioners even if anticipated outcomes will lead to more effective/efficient practice.
- *Control* – the actual practice setting of the research means that the possibility of having control over factors of relevance is limited. Research that is done as part of normal practice does not readily allow for variables to be manipulated or controls to be put in place.
- *Scope and scale* – the actual work-site approach and involvement of practitioners means that there will inevitably be limitations to the scope and scale of the research, as well as making generalisation of findings problematic.
- *Impartiality* – the nature of action research means that researchers are almost guaranteed to be partial and connected. This is different from other researchers and not concurrent with the traditional view of science, and leads to a risk that findings are not regarded as being 'good' research.

CONTEXTS FOR ACTION RESEARCH

The literature shows that there are many contexts where action research can be used. In their systematic review and guidance for assessment, Waterman et al. (2001) listed the main issues addressed in a review of 47 projects as:

- professional education and skills training (30 per cent), including issues around professional development
- inappropriate or conflicting practices (27 per cent) relating to education, clinical supervision, core nursing skills, clinical care and policy
- lack of evidence (26 per cent) to support current practices and innovations, particularly in relation to change and development
- professional roles (21 per cent) relating to the need for clarification of new and existing roles
- health service provision (17 per cent) relating to issues around the lack of provision between institutions and to particular patient groups, and management underperformance
- communication and/or involvement (15 per cent) relating to a lack of communication between different practitioners; practitioners and managers; and practitioners and their patients, and to a lack of involvement of these different groups
- targets, standards and guidelines (13 per cent) relating to a lack of clear targets or standards not met – these include situations where managers were unable to implement the necessary change
- implementation of research in practice (6 per cent)
- power (2 per cent).

There are, however, contexts where action research is inappropriate and these include:

- pushing through an unpopular policy or initiative
- persuading practitioners that they have contributed to thinking and participated in a policy decision when it has already been made
- as a means of trying to bring a dysfunctional team together
- when a significant number of staff or organisational changes are anticipated
- when an organisation or specific setting within an organisation is averse to change
- when there are insufficient resources or too many other competing priorities.

CHAPTER SUMMARY

- Action research is research in a clinical setting that involves a period of inquiry to bring about a change intervention aimed at improvement by involving, describing, interpreting and explaining a specific social situation.
- Action research is a critical social activity that relies on participative and collaborative working in order to generate change and new knowledge.
- A cyclical framework of planning, acting, observing and reflecting is used.
- The cyclical process should be used flexibly to allow participants and researchers to move between stages as directed by the project findings and experiences.
- Action research is participatory and democratic with the aim of improving care quality.
- In nursing, action research is primarily about improving professional practice, raising standards and generating new knowledge grounded in the reality of practice.

SUGGESTED FURTHER READING

Koshy, E., Koshy, V. and Waterman, H. (2011) *Action Research in Healthcare*. London: Sage. This book explains action research in detail, giving many examples, and seeks to answer queries a reader may have before they arise. It is practically orientated, taking you through the process step by step.

Waterman, H. (2013) 'Action research and health', in M. Saks and J. Allsop (eds), *Researching Health: Qualitative, Quantitative and Mixed Methods*, 2nd edn. London: Sage. pp. 148–68. Waterman explains how to carry out an action research project, with good explanations of the processes involved given in a clear and coherent way. She highlights the associated challenges and shows how action research can have a positive impact on healthcare practice.

WEBSITES

Center for Collaborative Action Research: http://cadres.pepperdine.edu/ccar/define.html
Participatory Action Research Toolkit: www.dur.ac.uk/resources/beacon/PARtoolkit.pdf

 To access further resources related to this chapter, visit the companion website at https://study.sagepub.com/mouleaveyard3e

REFERENCES

Allan, H., Odelius, A., Hunter, B., Bryan, K., Knibb, W., Sahne, J. and Gallagher, A. (2015) 'Supporting staff to respond to effectively to informal complaints: Findings from an action research study', *Journal of Clinical Nursing*, 24 (15/16): 2106–14.

Bowling, A. (2009) *Research Methods in Health*, 3rd edn. Maidenhead: Open University Press.

Bradbury, H. (2015) *The Sage Handbook of Action Research*, 3rd edn. London: Sage.

Carr, W. and Kemmis, S. (1986) *Becoming Critical: Education, Knowledge and Action Research*. London: Falmer.

Denscombe, M. (2010) *The Good Research Guide for Small Scale Research Projects*, 4th edn. Maidenhead: Open University Press.

Greenwood, D. and Levin, M. (2007) *An Introduction to Action Research: Social Research for Social Change*, 2nd edn. Thousand Oaks: Sage.

Hughes, I. (2008) 'Action research in healthcare', in P. Reason and H. Bradbury (eds), *The SAGE Handbook of Action Research: Participative Inquiry and Practice*. London: Sage. pp. 381–93.

Kemmis, K., McTaggart, R. and Nixon, R. (2014) *The Action Research Planner: Doing Critical Participatory Action Research*. Singapore: Springer.

Koshy, E., Koshy, V. and Waterman, H. (2011) *Action Research in Healthcare*. London: Sage.

Lee, N.J. (2009) 'Using group reflection in an action research study', *Nurse Researcher*, 16 (2): 30–42.

Lewin, K. (1946) 'Action research and minority problems', *Journal of Social Issues*, 2: 34–46.

Lingard, L., Albert, M. and Levinson, W. (2008) 'Grounded theory, mixed methods, and action research', *British Medical Journal*, 337: 459–61.

Lorhan, S., van der Westhuizen, M. and Gossman, S. (2015) 'The role of volunteers at an outpatient cancer center: How do volunteers enhance the patient experience?', *Supportive Care in Cancer*, 23 (6): 1597–1605.

Ma Jesusa, M. (2015) 'W-DARE: A three year program of participatory action research to improve the sexual and reproductive health of women with disabilities in the Philippines', *BMC Public Health*, 15 (1): 1–7.

Mander, R., Cheung, N.F., Wang, X., Fu, W. and Zhu, J. (2010) 'Beginning an action research project to investigate the feasibility of a midwife-led normal birthing unit in China', *Journal of Clinical Nursing*, 19 (3/4): 517–26.

Meyer, J. (2000) 'Using qualitative methods in health related action research', *British Medical Journal*, 320: 178–81.

Mitchell, A., Conlon, A., Armstrong, M. and Ryan, A. (2005) 'Towards rehabilitative handling in caring for patients following stroke: A participatory action research project', *International Journal for Older People Nursing*, 14 (3a): 3–12.

Reed, J. (2005) 'Using action research in nursing practice with older people: Democratising knowledge', *Journal of Clinical Nursing*, 14: 594–600.

Reinharz, S. (1992) *Feminist Methods in Social Research*. Oxford: Oxford University Press.

Robson, C. (2011) *Real World Research*, 3rd edn. Oxford: Blackwell.

Stringer, E.T. (2007) *Action Research*, 3rd edn. London: Sage.

Thomas, G. (2013) *How to Do Your Research Project*, 2nd edn. London: Sage.

Waterman, H. (2013) 'Action research and health', in M. Saks and J. Allsop (eds), *Researching Health: Qualitative, Quantitative and Mixed Methods*, 2nd edn. London: Sage. pp. 148–68.

Waterman, H., Tillen, D., Dickson, R. and de Koning, K. (2001) 'Action research: A systematic review and guidance for assessment', *Health Technology Assessment*, 5 (23): iii–157.

Waterman, H., Griffiths, J., Gellard, L., O'Keeffe, C., Olang, G., Obwanda, E., et al. (2006) 'Intervening in the process of stigmatisation: Challenging social inequalities in the context of

HIV/AIDS home-based care in Kenya', in M. Saks and J. Allsop (eds), *Researching Health: Qualitative, Quantitative and Mixed Methods*. London: Sage.

Whitelaw, S., Beattie, A., Balogh, R. and Watson, J. (2003) *A Review of the Nature of Action Research*. Cardiff: Welsh Assembly Government, Sustainable Health Action.

Williamson, R. (2012) 'What is action research?', in R. Williamson, L. Bellman and J. Webster, *Action Research in Nursing and Healthcare*. London: Sage.

World Health Organization (WHO) (1946) 'Preamble to the Constitution of the World Health Organization as adopted by the International Health Conference, New York, 19–22 June 1946', *Official Records of the World Health Organization*, 2 (100).

APPENDIX

It is possible for the third and sixth questions to be explored by action research projects:

● Is there a relationship between joint nursing and physiotherapy manual handling training programmes held on the ward and safer manual handling practice?

By involving a multi-disciplinary team, the impact of joint training could be evaluated by assessing the quality of manual handling practised on the ward as measured by a reduction in inappropriate manual handling techniques and injury.

This question is loosely based on Mitchell et al.'s 2005 study, 'Towards rehabilitative handling in caring for patients following stroke: A participatory action research project', in the *International Journal for Older People Nursing*.

● Does more discussion about lifestyle preferences improve the transition of older people from hospital to care homes?

By involving patients and a multi-disciplinary team, a 'daily living plan' that specifies patient preferences could be developed and implemented in practice.

This question is loosely based on Reed's 2005 study, 'Using action research in nursing practice with older people: Democratising knowledge', in the *Journal of Clinical Nursing*.

19

CASE STUDIES AND OTHER RESEARCH APPROACHES

Learning outcomes

This chapter will enable you to:

- understand case study research
- appreciate when case studies might be employed
- understand historical research and its use
- appreciate feminist inquiry as a research approach

In order to answer the research question or hypothesis, the nurse researcher needs to identify an appropriate research approach. In Chapter 11, we discussed the different qualitative, quantitative and mixed methods approaches available to researchers and related the selection of design to the need to address the research question. In this chapter we discuss case study research which is used to explore a particular practice or approach and can draw on both qualitative and quantitative methods of data collection. This design can help us to understand the particular and specific, but also to draw implications that can be more broadly applicable. We also consider historical research. This approach draws on data from the past and interprets this to help understand and develop practice. Researchers may be working with different oral and documentary sources to inform knowledge development. Finally, we refer to feminist inquiry as research that focuses on the experiences of women, which can be particularly appropriate for nurse researchers, who are often women researching women. Feminist researchers adopt a gender perspective, viewing research as being for and with women rather than about them.

CASE STUDIES

The **case study** approach allows the nurse researcher to conduct an investigation into single or multiple cases in their 'real life' context, though often just one case is researched to considerable depth. The approach therefore appeals to practitioners who work with individual service users or 'cases' in their practice roles. For research purposes, the case may be a patient, a family, a group, a hospital ward or an entire hospital or community.

Case study design

Case study research is often the preferred method when the following three factors exist;

1. the main research questions ask 'How' or 'Why',
2. the data collection events cannot be controlled and,
3. the study has a contemporary focus (Yin, 2014).

When designing case study research it is suggested that five main factors need to be considered which include case study questions, the propositions, units of analysis and logical linking of the data to the propositions and criteria for interpretation (Yin, 2014).

Case study questions

The types of research questions that might be asked include descriptive questions that seek to explore 'What is happening', and inferential questions which seek to explore 'How things are linked' (Clarke and Reed, 2010: 240). Case study research is a useful approach in evaluation studies (see Chapter 16), where the types of research questions could be asking 'How?' or 'Why?'. These evaluation questions will review what is working well and what isn't and how things are working. Case study research will also support evaluation studies as they enable the research team to consider current practice and can support the collected data for current events that cannot be controlled. Examples of case study research questions might include:

- 'How are specialist cancer nurses receiving educational updates?'
- 'How has the new protocol for taking patients to X-ray saved ward staff time?'
- 'How is the newly implemented admission service working?'
- 'How is public involvement working to support research activity in a particular caring organisation?'

Propositions

It is desirable to state propositions within case study research, though it is acknowledged that this is not always possible. For example, taking the question about public involvement in research above, you may think that the organisation involves the public in research activities because this is beneficial for them. If this proposition is stated it will help the researcher to think about what to collect data about. The researcher will need to collect data that explores the benefits of public involvement in research for the organisation, and look at how the benefits are manifest. The researcher may also propose that there are benefits for the public through such involvement. The public may feel they are making a meaningful contribution to the research agenda of the organisation through their involvement and could perceive that through involvement they have an impact on a wider public. To explore this proposition the researcher will need to collect data that explores the potential benefits of involvement for the public.

Units of analysis

In case study research it is imperative that the extent and scope of the case is defined and that the boundaries of the research are set. This is important to ensure that appropriate cases are included, so as to allow the researcher to collect and analyse data that is focused on addressing the research question(s). To define the scope of the case, the researcher needs to have a degree of insight into the context and issues in order to identify specific research questions and the sampling framework. When the research aims and questions are known, and the propositions are understood, the researcher can specify the case characteristics for the study.

Though the amount of cases in a study is usually small, the number of variables considered in the case study can be great, as the researcher aims to include all the factors thought to influence the case in the study. Depending on the focus of the study, researchers may be involved in collecting data about current behaviours and practices, and can also review the effect of the past, considering the history and previous behaviour patterns of the case subjects.

As the researcher is interested in obtaining detailed information from the cases or subjects, they may spend some time engaged with each case. Yin (2014) suggests that the case study approach can be used to explore, describe or give explanation about the case. For example, case studies can be used to generate a hypothesis for testing, provide descriptive information about a group or give evidence to support theory or practice development. A case study design can allow researchers to demonstrate the effectiveness of a particular care approach or practice, through looking at how an intervention impacts on the case. In order to provide description and/or explanation, case studies can include qualitative or quantitative research methods and often incorporate both. The range of data collection techniques used can include observations, interviewing, written data collection or physiological and psychological measurement (see Chapters 22–25).

Linking the data to propositions

Data analysis may include dealing with large amounts of qualitative material and quantitative results. Data analysis is linked to the initial study propositions. Difference techniques for analysis can be used such as pattern matching, where the findings of the case study are compared with the propositions (Yin, 2014). Using the public involvement in research example above, the major propositions were related to the benefits to both the organisation and to the members of the public themselves. Data would be collected to assess the propositions and if the results obtained support and are matched to the predictions, this allows conclusions to be drawn and the propositions to be affirmed or challenged.

Criteria for interpretation

Yin (2014) refers to the need to ensure the robustness of the findings. He suggests this can be achieved through, 'identifying and addressing rival explanations for your findings' (Yin, 2014: 36). Rival explanations should be identified at the development stages of the case study design and plans to collect data to explore the rival explanations should be made. Taking the public involvement in research example above, a cynical rival explanation could suggest that the organisation is engaging with the public as this is a requirement to secure research funding. Collecting data relating to the reasons for engagement with the public would help the researcher to explore this rival explanation.

Case study use

Case studies are being used more frequently in healthcare research, despite the concerns expressed by some researchers that the method often relies on presenting data from a single case that may not be generalised more widely (Gomm et al., 2000). For example, a particular relationship may be peculiar to the group of patients studied as the case and may not be generally evident in other, similar groups.

Those involved in case study research work need to ensure rigour through the research process to help address such concerns. The researchers will need to clearly identify the initial research question(s), explain the sampling of cases and collect multiple data, fusing different data collection methods. Most case study research will collect data from different stakeholders and can employ a range of data collection techniques in one study (see Research example 19.1). The researchers need to show how the data was analysed to address the propositions and discuss issues of generalisability to a wider audience (see Stake, 1995; Yin, 2014). In providing detailed description of the research process and findings, the researcher allows readers of the research to consider whether the results can be generalised to a wider population.

Presentation

The presentation of a case study requires detailed contextual description and this can raise ethical issues. For example, whilst it is possible to avoid using names, the depth of description of the case can impact on the maintenance of confidentiality. This should be identified as part of ethical approval processes and participants should consent to engagement in the project knowing confidentiality may be compromised. Researchers can offer to show the participants draft reports for comment and can write the reports in such a way as to try and avoid any association between individuals and organisations. An example of a case study is given in Research example 19.1.

Reflective exercise

You could think about a case study exploring the question, 'How do carers experience a new support service?' To answer this question, you would need to be clear who would be included in the case. Who do you think the sample might be? What will the researcher need to know about the new service in order to work out what data to collect?

In the above exercise, the case will draw a sample from carers who have received the new service, though as data are collected the scope of the case may develop to include collection from a wider group of stakeholders. Such stakeholders could include staff delivering the service, the commissioners of the service and members of the carers' extended family. The sampling framework can be identified when developing the project proposal, though when the sample composition is initially unclear, further scoping work may be required before this can be completed. For example, the researchers may want to undertake a local survey or scoping exercise; this can include having conversations with funders, commissioners, service providers and service users, in order to determine the scope of the case.

Research example 19.1

Example of a single embedded case study

Al Awaisi et al. (2015) explored the experiences of new graduate nurses in the Sultanate of Oman using an embedded single case design. The researcher used Yin's case study approach, employing qualitative case study research to explore the complexity of transition from a new graduate to practitioner for nursing students in Oman. The case included new graduate nurses working at a local hospital who were graduates in 2009 and 2010. The design explored the single case with multiple units of analysis embedded within. Purposive sampling was used to recruit the new graduates and other key informants such as the preceptors, managers and head nurses. Data was collected using three main methods: interviews (with the students and key informants), observations (field notes were taken of the interviews and at other related events, e.g. meetings) and documentary analysis (of guidelines/policies/competency assessment/course documents, etc.). The data was analysed thematically focusing on addressing the aims of the study. The data from all three sources were analysed and grouped into codes that were then built into themes.

We can see in this example that the case study was a single individual case. The data collection included three different methods. This meant there was some triangulation to the data (see Chapter 11). Al Awaisi et al. (2015) also discussed the application of processes of trustworthiness in the study to improve credibility (see Chapter 13).

HISTORICAL RESEARCH

Historical researchers examine past events to increase understanding and gain new knowledge. They believe that by studying data and materials related to the past, we can inform current and future practice (Lewenson and Herrmann, 2008).

Those undertaking **historical research** need to identify research questions to address and consider the sources of material that may be available to answer them. A number of sources can be used, including oral or documentary recordings. The types of sources available could include photographs, tape recordings, video and written documents such as letters, diaries, memoranda and formal written records. These might be held in libraries or private collections. In the future, such sources could also include digitalised and web-based materials.

Many of the sources used will not have been collected for research purposes and therefore the quality could be questionable. The historical researcher will need to ensure the originality of materials used, as they must be confident of the reliability and validity of the source. External and internal criticism is used to determine the accuracy and authenticity of a source. The origins of the source need to be known to satisfy external criticism and establish validity. To review the validity of a source, the researcher will need to establish who produced the material, when, where and how. These questions can be applied to any historical source, be it a written, visual or an oral account. Internal criticism seeks to establish the reliability of the material. In order to achieve this, a second piece of evidence related to the same event and recorded by an independent source is needed. This allows comparisons of materials to establish reliability. Thus, the diary account of one person may be compared with that of another to establish reliability.

The sources available to historians are described as primary and secondary. A primary source is an eyewitness account, which may be recorded as visual, verbal or written data. For example, photographs and letters produced by nurses on a particular ward at a certain time provide primary data about the ward. This is seen as the most valid and reliable source. Those who did not experience the event produce secondary sources. Thus, someone looking at a set of documents and photographs of a ward can produce their interpretation of it as a secondary source. Research example 19.2 gives an illustration.

Research example 19.2

Example of historical research

Thaweeboon et al. (2011) examined the history and development of the first nursing school in Thailand, founded in 1896. The historical study collected data through reviewing relevant literature and interviewing senior nurses to capture their views. The data were subjected to content analysis and were reviewed through a historical lens and revealed that the school development had included three key phases resulting in the professionalisation of nursing and the preparation of graduate nurses. At this stage the school had transformed into a Faculty of Nursing.

This example shows the importance of **historical data** in informing our understanding of the development of nursing as a profession in Thailand and how its evolution has been shaped by policy and other changes.

FEMINIST RESEARCH

There are many variations in **feminist research**, though put simply it is research undertaken without social restraint. It is emancipatory, asking new questions, particularly in relation to marginalised groups in society. Feminist research arose from a discontent with research studies that were thought to be male-focused and hid the voice of women and other vulnerable groups in society, as men conducted research on women, identifying topics for research that may have limited relevance for women. Kitzinger wrote:

> Feminist social scientists argued that men define reality on their own terms, to legitimate *their* experience, *their* own particular version of events, while women's experience, not fitting the male model, is trivialised and denied or distorted. (2004: 125)

Kitzinger (2004) identified the second wave of feminism in the 1970s as focusing on reclaiming and naming women's experiences and challenging male dominance in establishing truth. Feminist researchers attempted to address the male monopoly on truth through undertaking research from a position that ensured women's views and experiences were researched and heard. The research methods used to access women's experiences were often qualitative, such as interviews or focus groups, which allow researchers to record and listen to women. The characteristics of feminist research were seen as women researching women, focusing on women's experiences, researching in a collaborative and non-exploitative way that focused on research with and for women rather than about them. The researcher and participant relationship aimed to create mutual knowledge as part of the research process and worked in a reciprocal way, so that both parties benefitted from the research.

It is suggested that feminist research has gone beyond this 'qualitative' position and is using a wide range of research methods to conduct research for women (Olesen, 2000). For example, Oakley (1989) suggests that experimental research, such as randomised controlled trials, can be conducted in an emancipatory way to draw benefits for women. Variations in feminist research can consider the views and experiences of individual women through more qualitative approaches or can take a perspective on how policy and structures within society affect women more generally. Beckman (2014) presents eight key principles of feminist research, which include power imbalances, listening to the voices of women, reflexivity and social relationships during the research process. Beckman also comments on the use of multi-disciplinary and mixed methods research. There is no correct method and Beckman suggests that mixed methods are often most appropriate that combine before qualitative and quantitative approaches to answer research questions.

Within nursing, the large body of the profession are women, and therefore feminist studies have been able to explore the nature of women's work within healthcare and the experience of women patients, and to examine women's health. See Research example 19.3.

Research example 19.3

Example of feminist enquiry

Jefford and Fahy (2015) recruited 26 practising midwives in Australia to explore clinical reasoning during second stage labour using a feminist approach. The authors believed that midwives were not prepared sufficiently or supported to use clinical reasoning skills. Interviews were conducted using open-ended questions to allow the participants to provide full and open comment. The interview transcripts were analysed through a feminist lens, using the research question to guide the interpretative process. The findings were sent to a sub-group of participants for verification. Key emergent themes included analytical decision making, particle analytical decision-making but failure to act, and non-analytical decision making. Over half of the participants had the ability to use clinical reasoning but less than half of these followed the process to the end.

We can see in this example that the researchers took an approach which allowed the women to participate in the collection and interpretation of data. An interview approach was used to capture in-depth data on the process of clinical decision making. Female midwives conducted the interviews using a feminist approach, which valued the relationship between female researchers and participants.

Reflective exercise

Which vulnerable groups do you think might be involved in feminist research? What questions might be explored using the approach? Who might be involved in data collection? What type of data collection approach could be used?

CHAPTER SUMMARY

- The case study approach allows the nurse researcher to conduct an investigation into single or multiple cases in their 'real life' context. Case study design can be used to explore, describe or give explanation about a case, which might be a patient, ward or wider community. A case study design can allow researchers to demonstrate the effectiveness of a particular care approach or practice. Historical researchers believe that by studying data and materials related to the past we can inform current and future practice. The historical researcher will need to ensure the originality of materials used, as they need to be confident of the reliability and validity of the source.
- There are many variations in feminist research that can be carried out by women, for women. Research problems considered are relevant for women and can be investigated through qualitative or quantitative methods.

SUGGESTED FURTHER READING

Hesse-Biber, S-N. (ed.) (2011) *The Handbook of Feminist Research. Theory and Praxis*, 2nd edn. Thousand Oaks: Sage. A guide to conducting social science research on, for and about women. The text introduces a number of feminist epistemologies, methodologies and methods.

Lewenson, S. and Herrmann, E. (eds) (2008) *Capturing Nursing History: A Guide to Historical Methods in Research*. New York: Springer. The text offers tools for conducting historical research and includes case studies on how to conduct research.

Thomas, G. (2011) *How to do your Case Study. A Guide for Students and Researchers*. London: Sage. This publication covers what a case study is, how to do one and disseminating the results.

Yin, R. (2014) *Case Study Research: Design and Methods* (Applied Social Research Methods). Thousand Oaks: Sage. Presents a guide as to how to set up and execute case study research. Includes a number of examples to help with understanding.

WEBSITES

Historical Research: http://onlinelibrary.wiley.com/journal/10.1111/%28ISSN%291468-2281 – this journal includes articles in the field of health and nursing research and covers the application of different historical research methods.

To access further resources related to this chapter, visit the companion website at https://study.sagepub.com/mouleaveyard3e

REFERENCES

Al Awaisi, H., Cooke, H. and Pryjmachuk, S. (2015) 'The experiences of newly graduated nurses during their first year of practice in the Sultanate of Oman – A Case Study', *International Journal of Nursing Studies*, 52 (11): 1723–34.

Beckman, L. (2014) 'Training in feminist research methodology: Doing research on the margins', *Women and Therapy*, 37 (1-2): 164–77.

Clarke, C. and Reed, J. (2010) 'Case study research', in K. Gerrish and A. Lacey (eds), *The Research Process in Nursing*, 6th edn. Oxford: Wiley-Blackwell. pp. 237–47.

Gomm, R., Hammersley, M. and Foster, P. (2000) 'Case study and generalisation', in R. Gomm, M. Hammersley and P. Foster (eds), *Case Study Method*. London: Sage. pp. 98–116.

Jefford, E. and Fahy, K. (2015) 'Midwives' clinical reasoning during second stage labour: Report on an interpretative study', *Midwifery*, 31 (5): 519–25.

Kitzinger, C. (2004) 'Feminist approaches', in C. Seale, G. Gobo, J. Gubrium and D. Silverman (eds), *Qualitative Research Practice*. London: Sage. pp. 125–40.

Lewenson, S. and Herrmann, E. (eds) (2008) *Capturing Nursing History: A Guide to Historical Methods in Research*. New York: Springer.

Oakley, A. (1989) 'Who's afraid of the randomised controlled trial? Some dilemmas of the scientific method and "good" research', *Women & Health*, 15: 25.

Olesen, V. (2000) 'Feminisms and qualitative research at and into the millennium', in N. Denzin and Y. Lincoln (eds), *Handbook of Qualitative Research*, 2nd edn. Thousand Oaks, CA: Sage. pp. 215–55.

Stake, R. (1995) *The Art of Case Study Research*. London: Sage.

Thaweeboon, T., Peachpansri, S., Pochanapan, S., Senachack, P. and Pinyopasakul, W. (2011) 'Development of the School of Nursing, Midwifery, and Public Health at Siriraj, Thailand 1896–1971: A historical study', *Nursing and Health Sciences*, 13 (4): 440–6.

Yin, R. (2014) *Case Study Research: Design and Methods*, 5th edn. London: Sage.

20

SYSTEMATIC LITERATURE REVIEWS

Learning outcomes

This chapter will enable you to:

- understand the nature and purpose of systematic reviews
- recognise the processes involved in conducting a systematic review
- have a basic understanding of meta-analysis and thematic analysis in a systematic review
- appreciate the value and role systematic reviews play in establishing an evidence base for practice

All healthcare professionals are expected to deliver, and patients expect, care that is based on up-to-date clinically relevant knowledge – in other words, to practise evidence-based care. The notion underpinning evidence-based practice is that it closes the gap between clinical research and the real world, and provides tools to interpret and apply research findings. There is, however, an increasing volume of research evidence in the healthcare literature that is of variable quality and sometimes difficult to access. Systematic reviews provide a means of summarising the literature on a specific topic that helps in assessing the value for practice of some of this research evidence. In essence, systematic reviews synthesise the best evidence that can help inform practice decisions by providing a quality filter and précis of large amounts of evidence, as well as being able to provide a basis for the development of clinical practice guidelines.

In Chapter 6, we described literature reviews which justify the need for a research proposal or report. These literature reviews are useful for providing a general perspective on a topic and are appropriate for describing the history of a problem or its management. They generally demonstrate the gaps in the literature but do not necessarily answer a specific question. They should be carried out systematically, with a clearly stated method for searching, appraising and analysing the literature. There is a fine line dividing a literature review from a systematic review. Systematic reviews use a very explicit and detailed method to systematically search, critically appraise and synthesise the evidence from clinical research. They aim to find *every* piece of published and unpublished literature on a topic and then employ clear inclusion criteria and quality measures to determine what is included in the review. Systematic reviews provide an overview that summarises the world literature on a specific topic and are recognised as providing good quality research evidence. Literature reviews which precede a research project also need to be done systematically; they might however be undertaken in less detail than a full systematic review.

Students often question whether they are doing a systematic review when they undertake their dissertation. Again, there can be a fine line between a student project and a full systematic review. It is unusual for a student to have the resources and team available to undertake a systematic review; however all students should follow the process for undertaking a systematic review with the understanding that they are unlikely to be able to complete the review in the detail required for a full systematic review.

This chapter discusses systematic reviews, thematic and meta-analysis and the techniques for undertaking a systematic review.

WHY ARE SYSTEMATIC REVIEWS NEEDED?

The imperative for all healthcare to be **evidence-based** has been one of the drivers for having good quality evidence in the form of **systematic reviews**. The idea of systematically reviewing the literature is not new and goes back to the earliest medical researchers. For example, Pearson, in 1904, synthesised the data from several studies on the efficacy of typhoid vaccination (Egger et al., 1998). He justified the aggregation of data because many of the studies were far too small to allow for any definitive opinion to be formed when note was taken of the probability of error involved.

The 1950s and 1960s then saw rapid developments in healthcare that were not always supported by research evidence. Cochrane (1972) estimated that less than 10 per cent of medical interventions were supported by objective evidence and that they actually did more harm than good. He also noted that many randomised controlled trials (RCTs) had been done but that the results were not readily accessible to practitioners: 'It is surely a great criticism of our profession that we have not organised a critical summary, by speciality or subspecialty, adapted periodically, of all relevant randomised controlled trials' (1972: 1).

The challenge issued by Cochrane eventually led to the establishment of the Cochrane Collaboration. This is a worldwide network of healthcare professionals and research methodologists that has the aim of building up and maintaining a database of up-to-date systematic reviews that can be readily accessed by healthcare professionals and the general public. The Cochrane Collaboration is now just one of a number of organisations that exist to support the undertaking and dissemination of systematic reviews, and further demonstrates the role of systematic reviews in current healthcare practice.

WHAT IS A SYSTEMATIC REVIEW?

A systematic review is defined as:

> a review of the evidence on a clearly formulated question that uses systematic and explicit methods to identify, select and critically appraise relevant primary research, and to extract and analyse data from the studies that are included in the review. (CRD, 2009: 3)

The expectation is that a systematic review is undertaken with the same diligence as primary research, and when two or more study results can be combined statistically the review may include a **meta-analysis**. Where the results of the studies cannot be combined statistically, a **thematic analysis** can be undertaken. A systematic review is regarded as secondary research because it does not collect new data (primary research) but makes use of previously published literature. The aim is to assess all of the available research on a particular topic. It is systematic because a rigorous approach to selection criteria, appraisal, synthesis and the summary of findings is used.

Good examples of systematic reviews can be found at the Cochrane Collaboration (http://uk/cochrane.org) and the Campbell Collaboration (www.campbellcollaboration .org). The Cochrane Collaboration systematic reviews focus on systematic reviews of effectiveness of treatment and interventions whilst the Campbell Collaboration are more focused on social care situations.

What evidence is included in a systematic review?

The evidence included in a systematic review depends on the research question. Hierarchies of evidence have already been discussed in Chapter 1. Many systematic reviews contain predominantly randomised controlled trials. This is because, as described above, the original systematic reviews were concerned with determining the effectiveness of interventions – a process which can best be determined through randomised controlled trials. Thus systematic reviews originated from a positivist research paradigm. The positivist perspective assumes that data and their analysis are value-free and can be controlled in a way that data regarding cause and effect can be obtained. There is also an expectation that research aims to provide information that will help to predict what will happen in the future, for example, a randomised controlled trial might demonstrate which drug is better than another. These results can then be inferred to the wider population. Given the level of control applied in a randomised controlled trial compared to a cohort study, for example, most researchers agree that randomised controlled trials provide stronger evidence for assessing the effectiveness of a drug or other intervention than other research methods, for example case control or cohort studies. This gives rise to the notion that it is possible to have a hierarchy or league table of research designs where some types of research are classed as being of better quality than others. These positivist **research hierarchies** vary, but they are all essentially in agreement; a suggested hierarchy is given in Figure 20.1. These hierarchies are useful

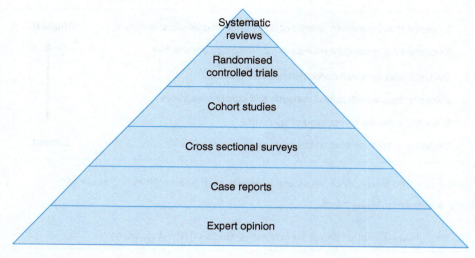

Figure 20.1 A positivist hierarchy of research evidence

for those undertaking which research methods should be included within a systematic review, as in some circumstances it is possible to state with some certainty which research methods will be most helpful in answering the research question. For example, for a systematic review aimed at determining effectiveness, researchers will search for randomised controlled trials in the first instance. If no good quality randomised controlled trials are identified, researchers will search for the 'next best' type of research which is likely to be cohort or case control studies.

However not all research questions consider questions of effectiveness. This means that systematic reviews will not necessarily follow the positivist approach which suggests that RCTs are the gold standard evidence for inclusion. For example, many systematic reviews address research questions which require the combination of a broad range of research designs. This makes the concept of a hierarchy of evidence complex. Rather than refer to hierarchies of evidence that are inappropriate for the research question, it is important for researchers to identify the types of research that will be relevant for answering the particular research question. Aveyard (2014) advocates that those undertaking a literature review develop their own 'hierarchy of evidence' in which researchers consider their research question carefully in order to determine the research methods that might produce research that contributes to answering that question. Researchers need to bear in mind that this 'hierarchy' is not likely to be definitive and they should remain open to other relevant research encountered.

Until recently, the notion of a hierarchy of research methodologies has not been considered relevant by researchers who use a naturalistic approach where most of the data obtained will be qualitative. A naturalist approach assumes that the research method chosen reflects the question, and as such a hierarchy is irrelevant and different methods are seen as being on a continuum. However there is now discussion that different qualitative approaches are more appropriate for different research questions (Noyes, 2010)

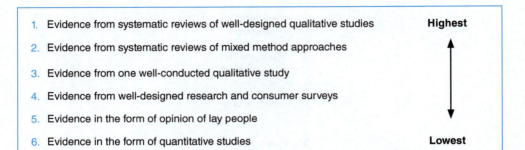

1. Evidence from systematic reviews of well-designed qualitative studies   **Highest**

2. Evidence from systematic reviews of mixed method approaches

3. Evidence from one well-conducted qualitative study

4. Evidence from well-designed research and consumer surveys

5. Evidence in the form of opinion of lay people

6. Evidence in the form of quantitative studies   **Lowest**

Figure 20.2   The hierarchy of 'views and experiences of interventions and services'

Source: Adapted from Noyes (2010)

Table 20.1   Hierarchy of evidence for qualitative studies (Daly et al., 2007)

Level I – Generalisable studies	Sampling focused by theory and the literature, extended as a result of analysis to capture a diversity of experience; analytic procedures comprehensive and clear.
Level II – Conceptual studies	Theoretical concepts guide sample selection, based on analysis of literature. Analysis recognises diversity in participants' views.
Level III – Descriptive studies	Sample selected to illustrate practical rather than theoretical issues. Record a range of illustrative quotes including themes from the accounts of 'many', 'most' or 'some'.
Level IV – Single case study	Provides rich data on the views or experiences of one person. Can provide insights in unexplored contexts.

and some qualitative hierarchies of evidence have been developed, depending on the research question.

Noyes (2010: 530) gives an example of a hierarchy of evidence that could help us understand client or patient experience. The hierarchy of 'views and experiences of interventions and services' is given in Figure 20.2.

Daly et al. (2007) also provide a hierarchy of evidence for understanding the impact of qualitative studies. This hierarchy clearly also depends on the relevance of the research to the research question.

WHAT ARE THE ADVANTAGES AND DISADVANTAGES OF SYSTEMATIC REVIEWS?

Systematic reviews are generally considered to provide very high-quality results and therefore beneficial in guiding practice because they use justified and explicit methods in the identification and analysis of studies included. This should also result in any conclusions and/or recommendations being reliable and accurate. One major advantage of systematic reviews is that healthcare providers, researchers and policy makers can assimilate large amounts of information quickly.

It should also be noted that the outcomes and recommendations of a systematic review will depend on the amount of evidence available. This highlights the fact that, although systematic reviews are often seen to provide the best possible evidence on which to base recommendations for practice, care must be taken to ensure that there is sufficient evidence upon which to undertake the review; otherwise it will be limited in value. Remember that there has to be a sufficiency of research available for a review to be able to offer sensible and appropriate recommendations. This is quite apart from the need to ensure that other aspects important to the topic, such as quality of life and patient preference, are included if the evidence is to be used to guide practice.

STAGES IN THE SYSTEMATIC REVIEW PROCESS

In this section, the eight stages involved in a systematic review are explained, and the box below gives a list of some of the online resources available to help guide you through the process. You will be able to see from the number of stages involved, and from what is expected at each stage, that doing a systematic review is a lengthy and involved piece of research. Most systematic reviews will be undertaken by a group of researchers (or reviewers) and will often be reviewed by specialists (i.e. peer reviewed) before being submitted for publication.

Stage 1: Determine the question

Just like any other type of research, a systematic review needs a well-formulated question or focus. The question needs to be stated very clearly so that there is no risk of misunderstanding the purpose of the review. Quite often, and particularly in Cochrane systematic reviews, the question is set out as a brief statement – for example, 'A review to compare the efficacy of two different interventions (A and B) in the management of a specific problem (X)'. The title of the review could be 'A or B in the treatment of X'.

In the example which we will refer to throughout this chapter, Luangasanatip et al. (2015) undertook a systematic review to compare the efficacy of interventions to promote hand hygiene. The authors state their main objective was to evaluate the relative efficacy of the World Health Organization's 2005 campaign, and other interventions to promote hand hygiene among hospital workers

In addition to the question guiding reviewers' assessments of the relevance of studies, a review's question and objectives are used by readers in their initial assessment of the relevance of a review in their search for evidence (Cochrane Centre, 2011).

Stage 2: Define terms or concepts

The question and objectives are used to determine the key components for the initial searching strategies. As discussed in Chapter 4, it is essential that the terms used are clearly defined and not ambiguous. For example, if you are reviewing studies on the efficacy of handwashing, you need to decide which handwashing interventions you will consider and how their efficacy has been evaluated. This process of defining terms and concepts also assists in the development of terms that will be used later to search for studies.

Stage 3: Set inclusion and exclusion criteria

Decisions about which studies to include in, and about the scope of, a review often involve judgements. Therefore, inclusion and exclusion criteria are set to define the boundaries of the review, as discussed in Chapter 4. These criteria have to be justified and able to withstand critical appraisal by experts and readers of the review. The expectation is that any limitations are relevant and appropriate for reducing the possibility of any significant evidence being missed.

For example, in Luangasanatip et al.'s study (2015), the following inclusion criteria were set: studies should evaluate more than one intervention that intended to promote hand hygiene compliance; they were randomised controlled trials, non-randomised controlled trials, controlled before-and-after studies, or used an interrupted time series design.

The types of study to be included in the review can also depend on reviewers' definitions of evidence, so that, for example, it is not uncommon for systematic reviews only to include RCTs because, as has already been discussed, many systematic review questions are concerned with the effectiveness of treatments or interventions where RCTs will provide the most robust evidence.

Stage 4: Search for and collect studies that seem relevant to the question/focus of the review

A comprehensive, unbiased search is an essential requirement for any systematic review, and every attempt should be made to retrieve all relevant studies. Most research reports will be published in journals, but findings can also be presented at conferences (which may or may not be followed by publication) and in theses and dissertations. This requires a reviewer to make every effort to find unpublished works as well as searching all the appropriate databases. This is important as there is evidence that many studies with non-significant results remain unpublished (Goldacre, 2015). A checklist of data sources for systematic reviews is given below:

Checklist of data sources for a systematic review

- CINAHL
- MEDLINE
- BNI
- Other medical and paramedical databases, e.g. AMED, CANCERLIT

- Cochrane controlled clinical trial register
- 'Grey literature' (theses, internal reports, non-peer-reviewed journals, pharmaceutical industry files)
- References (and references of references) listed in primary sources
- Other unpublished sources known to experts – find by personal communication
- Foreign language literature.

A systematic review usually involves a team of researchers who agree on search terms, databases to be searched and inclusion/exclusion criteria. From a nursing perspective, perhaps the most relevant databases are the Cumulative Index of Nursing and Allied Health Literature (CINAHL), the British Nursing Index (BNI) and MEDLINE – all of which can be accessed via the NHS National Library for Health. In addition to database searches, researchers will also hand-search journals to locate relevant articles. For example, some nursing special interest journals may not be linked to the databases or may be indexed under key terms which are not included in the database search.

Searching successfully is a skill that requires training and experience, and is considered in detail in Chapter 4. The expectation is that the search strategy will be as comprehensive as possible. This means that the terms used in the search have to be as inclusive as possible but should be sufficiently exact to avoid the search locating large numbers of irrelevant articles. It is also very important to keep and record the search strategy so that the process can be repeated, as well as keeping a record of all the search results. There are now a variety of specially designed reference management software packages available to assist with this, such as Endnote, ProCite and Reference Manager. An example of a comprehensive search strategy and the search terms used in Luangasanatip et al.'s (2015) review is provided in the Appendix at the end of this chapter.

Remember, though, that searching is only part of the process; it is just as important to review all of the articles found by the search to determine whether they are relevant to the research question (this is discussed in Chapter 5). Even the most appropriate search strategy is likely to identify irrelevant articles, such as discussion or opinion-based articles, rather than research reports.

The results of the search strategy and the final inclusion of studies in the review is often presented using a PRISMA diagram, which records all the results of the searches and how these are checked against the inclusion and exclusion criteria, and how many are in the final review. The Prisma Diagram displayed in Luangasanatip et al.'s (2015) review is shown below.

Stage 5: Consider the studies against inclusion criteria and assessment of the quality

Before any synthesis of the retrieved relevant studies can be undertaken, the studies must be checked against the inclusion and exclusion criteria to check their eligibility.

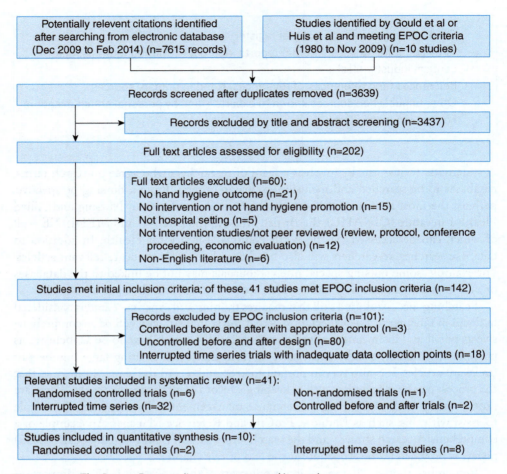

Figure 20.3   The Prisma Diagram (Luangasanatip et al.'s, 2015)

To help with this process, it is usual to develop a data extraction form specifically for the review. The form enables the reviewer to check the study details against the inclusion and exclusion criteria and to document the relevant findings. The information is then tabulated to give researchers information about each of the studies retrieved and ensures that only studies which meet the criteria set are included in the next stage of the review process.

In Luangasanatip et al.'s (2015) study two reviewers independently reviewed the titles and abstracts of each citation to assess eligibility. Consensus was reached by discussion of how initial assessments differed. The reviewers extracted data about the study design, duration, population and activities to promote hand hygiene, clinical and microbiological outcomes, measurements and settings.

Once the eligibility and content of the studies has been confirmed, the quality of them must be assessed. In Chapter 5, we discussed the principles of critical appraisal and the tools that are available to help with this. Some systematic reviews will exclude research papers because of considerations of quality whilst others will include them but take into consideration quality issues within the analysis.

The overall aim for the assessment of the quality of a study is to avoid subjectivity. One way of doing this is to get two or more researchers/reviewers to undertake the assessment independently and to resolve any differences of opinion by discussion, or with the assistance of a third reviewer.

Stage 6: Synthesise the evidence – aggregate statistical results (meta-analysis) where appropriate

Most literature reviews focus on evidence from primary sources, that is, research that has used original data or generated/collected its own data. This means that the original researchers will have carried out a primary analysis of the data and this will be published in the paper. Data analysis in a literature review is concerned with a **secondary analysis** of data, the synthesis of a number of research studies, and the aggregation of the data sets within them. The aim of synthesis is to collate and summarise the data extracted from the primary studies included in the review (CRD, 2009).

There are different ways in which this can be done, depending on the type of studies included in the review. If the primary research studies are sufficiently similar and data has been collected and analysed in a similar way, a **meta-analysis** can be undertaken. The aim of a meta-analysis is to find out if there is a difference between the intervention groups and control groups when the results of all the studies are merged, rather than looking at the results of studies individually.

A meta-analysis is a statistical amalgam of the findings of a number of research studies that have been carried out on a specific topic (an example of a meta-analysis is given in Figure 20.4). The term was first used by Glass (1976) and is sometimes referred to as an 'analysis of analyses'. It is, however, really a synthesis or bringing together of the analysis of individual investigations of the same general topic. A systematic review that incorporates a meta-analysis refers back to the original data provided by the published (and sometimes unpublished) studies. This data is then combined in a statistical calculation. The aim is to provide a more precise and, therefore, a more trustworthy estimate of the true effect of an intervention that is obtained by looking at the results of many studies within one statistical test. Meta-analysis can be a very useful tool when the findings from a number of individual studies have insufficient statistical power to provide credible information but where bringing together the results of many studies will enable more meaningful conclusions to be drawn. The amalgamation of findings may also facilitate the generalisability of findings which again would not be possible from the conclusion of individual studies.

There are a variety of ways of undertaking a meta-analysis. Most commonly, some sort of determination of 'average effect size' is made (Glass, 1976). It is expected that data from published RCTs can be extracted and pooled with those from other RCTs, providing that there is commonality between the studies. The findings of the individual studies are not simply added up and averaged; weightings can be given according to the size and quality of individual studies, with larger studies and those with a good quality rating being accorded a greater weighting.

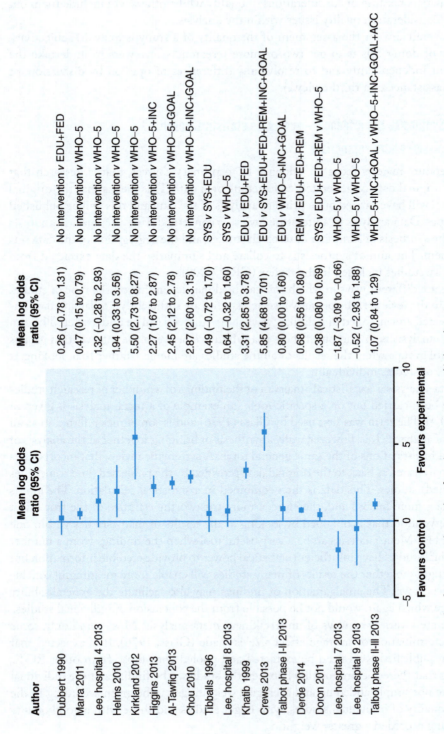

Author	Mean log odds ratio (95% CI)		Mean log odds ratio (95% CI)	
Dubbert 1990		0.26 (−0.78 to 1.31)	No intervention v EDU+FED	
Marra 2011		0.47 (0.15 to 0.79)	No intervention v WHO−5	
Lee, hospital 4 2013		1.32 (−0.28 to 2.93)	No intervention v WHO−5	
Helms 2010		1.94 (0.33 to 3.56)	No intervention v WHO−5	
Kirkland 2012		5.50 (2.73 to 8.27)	No intervention v WHO−5	
Higgins 2013		2.27 (1.67 to 2.87)	No intervention v WHO−5+INC	
Al-Tawfiq 2013		2.45 (2.12 to 2.78)	No intervention v WHO−5+GOAL	
Chou 2010		2.87 (2.60 to 3.15)	No intervention v WHO−5+INC+GOAL	
Tibballs 1996		0.49 (−0.72 to 1.70)	SYS v SYS+EDU	
Lee, hospital 8 2013		0.64 (−0.32 to 1.60)	SYS v WHO−5	
Khatib 1999		3.31 (2.85 to 3.78)	EDU v EDU+FED	
Crews 2013		5.85 (4.68 to 7.01)	EDU v SYS+EDU+FED+REM+INC+GOAL	
Talbot phase I-II 2013		0.80 (0.00 to 1.60)	EDU v WHO−5+INC+GOAL	
Derde 2014		0.68 (0.56 to 0.80)	REM v EDU+FED+REM	
Doron 2011		0.38 (0.080 to 0.69)	SYS v EDU+FED+REM v WHO−5	
Lee, hospital 7 2013		−1.87 (−3.09 to −0.66)	WHO−5 v WHO−5	
Lee, hospital 9 2013		−0.52 (−2.93 to 1.88)	WHO−5 v WHO−5	
Talbot phase II-III 2013		1.07 (0.84 to 1.29)	WHO−5+INC+GOAL v WHO−5+INC+GOAL+ACC	

Figure 20.4 An example of a meta-analysis taken from Luangasanatip et al.'s (2015) review

Sometimes meta-analysis will not be appropriate. There is a risk that reviewers and users of reviews lose sight of the importance of reflection and judgement in the analysis (CRD, 2009). It must also be remembered that studies can be very heterogeneous (inconsistent) in their design, quality and patient populations, and therefore the pooling of data may not be a valid activity.

The analysis of qualitative studies in a systematic review is generally a form of thematic analysis (Aveyard et al., 2016). This can be complex if the study characteristics are very diverse and will require considerable judgement, according to the NHS Centre for Reviews and Dissemination (CRD, 2009). It is, however, essential that the process is transparent, as would be expected of every other type of synthesis in a systematic review.

Stage 7: Compare analysis with other reviewers

One way of reducing the potential for subjectivity is for reviewers to compare their independent analyses and syntheses and then present a consensus. This will not completely avoid subjectivity and the possibility of bias, but it will add a level of transparency and increase the validity in a systematic review.

Stage 8: Prepare a critical summary and make recommendations

The reason for undertaking a systematic review is to appraise and synthesise the evidence currently available in order to answer a specific question. It is expected that recommendations will be made on the basis of the evidence appraised. The experience of collecting, appraising and synthesising the research that has been conducted means that researchers/reviewers are also able to comment on the quality of that research and make recommendations for future research. For example, the conclusions from Luangasanatip et al.'s (2015) study were that there is evidence that the WHO campaign is effective at increasing hand hygiene compliance and that additional interventions including goal setting, reward incentives and accountability can lead to further improvements.

Reflective exercise

Download a systematic review from the Cochrane Library, on a topic that interests you, and read through it to see how it differs from a literature review you would find in a nursing journal.

CHAPTER SUMMARY

- A systematic review is a mode of literature review that aims to summarise the world literature on a specific topic using explicit methods to systematically search, critically appraise and synthesise the evidence from clinical research.

- Systematic literature reviews are central to evidence-based practice because they synthesise the best evidence, can help to inform practice decisions by providing a quality filter and synthesis of large amounts of evidence, and provide a basis for clinical practice guidelines.
- Meta-analysis is the use of statistical methods to summarise the results of individual studies, with the aim of providing more precise estimates of the effects of healthcare interventions than those derived from the individual studies included in a review.
- A systematic review and meta-analysis are termed as secondary research because no new data are collected.
- A systematic review answers a specific question using a rigorous process of search, selection, appraisal, synthesis and summarisation of findings of primary research that is analogous to procedures that would be used in a randomised controlled trial.
- It is expected that all possible sources of literature are searched (electronically and by hand) in order to provide as comprehensive as possible a review of existing research to answer a specific question.
- Recommendations are made on the basis of the evidence appraised but may not be sufficient to guide practice and/or inform decision making unless they are based on a large body of good quality research, and particularly from RCTs.
- Data from systematic reviews can provide evidence for the development of clinical guidelines.
- Care has to be taken to ensure that findings from systematic reviews are used appropriately, and that evidence from research that includes accounts of things like quality of life and patient preferences are considered alongside that of 'scientific' research.

SUGGESTED FURTHER READING

Aveyard, H., Payne, S. and Preston, N. (2016) *A Postgraduate's Guide to Doing a Literature Review in Health and Social Care*. Maidenhead: Open University Press. This book provides an in-depth but accessible guide to doing a literature review.

Bettany-Saltikov, J. (2012) *How to Do a Systematic Literature Review in Nursing: A Step-by-Step Guide*. Milton Keynes: RCN Publishing and Open University Press. This book does what it says on the label and walks the reader through the entire process, breaking the task down into manageable steps, and making it useful for anyone undertaking their first literature review for study or clinical practice improvement.

WEBSITES

Cochrane reviews: www.cochranelibrary.com
Health Technology Assessment (HTA) programme: www.ncchta.org

To access further resources related to this chapter, visit the companion website at https://study.sagepub.com/mouleaveyard3e

REFERENCES

Aveyard H (2014) *Doing a Literature Review in Health and Social Care.* Maidenhead: Open University Press.

Aveyard, H., Payne, S. and Preston, N. (2016) *A Postgraduate's Guide to Doing a Literature Review in Health and Social Care.* Maidenhead: Open University Press.

Centre for Reviews and Dissemination (CRD) (2009) *Undertaking Systematic Reviews of Research and Effectiveness: CRD Guidelines for those Carrying out or Commissioning Reviews.* York: NHS Centre for Reviews and Dissemination, University of York.

Cochrane, A. (1972) *Effectiveness and Efficiency: Random Reflections on Health Services.* London: Nuffield Provincial Hospitals Trust.

Cochrane Centre (2011) *Cochrane Collaboration Handbook for Systematic Reviews.* Oxford: Cochrane Collaboration.

Daly, J., Willis, K., Small, R., Green, J., Welch, N., Kealy, M. et al. (2007) 'A hierarchy of evidence for assessing qualitative health research', *Journal of Clinical Epidemiology*, 60: 43–9.

Egger, M., Schneider, M. and Smith, G. (1998) 'Meta-analysis: Spurious precision? Meta-analysis of observational studies', *British Medical Journal*, 316: 140–4.

Glass, G. (1976) 'Primary, secondary, and meta-analysis of research', *Educational Researcher*, 5: 3–8.

Goldacre, B. (2015) 'How to get all trials reported: audit, better data, and individual accountability',. *PLoS Med*, 12(4): e1001821. Available at: https://www.researchgate.net/publication/275046407_How_to_Get_All_Trials_Reported_Audit_Better_Data_and_Individual_Accountability (accessed May 9 2016).

Luangasanatip, N., Hongsuwan, M., Limmathurotsakul, D., Lubell, Y., Lee, A., Harbarth, S., Day, N.P.J., Graves, N. and Cooper, B.S. (2015) 'Comparative efficacy of interventions to promote hand hygiene in hospital: Systematic review and network meta-analysis', *British Medical Journal*, 351, doi: 10.1136/bmj.h3728.

Noyes, J. (2010) 'Never mind the quality, feel the depth! The evolving role of qualitative research in Cochrane intervention reviews', *Journal of Research in Nursing*, 15: 525–34.

APPENDIX

Electronic search strategy (Search terms taken from the systematic review undertaken by Luangasanatip (2015))

Databases	Adapted from Gould et al.		Adapted from Huis et al.	
MEDLINE	1	Handwashing/	1	Randomized controlled trial/
	2	(hand antisepsis or handwash$ or hand wash$ or hand disinfection or hand hygiene or surgical scrub$).tw.	2	random$.tw.
			3	experiment$.tw.
			4	(time adj series).tw.
	3	1 or 2	5	(pre test or pretest or post test or posttest).tw.
	4	exp Hand/		
	5	exp Sterilization/	6	impact.tw.
	6	4 and 5	7	intervention$.tw.
	7	3 or 6	8	chang$.tw.
	8	randomized controlled trial.pt.	9	evaluat$.tw.
	9	controlled clinical trial.pt.	10	effect?.tw.
	10	intervention studies/	11	compar$.tw.
	11	experiment$.tw.	12	control$.tw.
	12	(time adj series).tw.	13	or/1-12
	13	(pre test or pretest or (posttest or post test)).tw.	14	limit 13 to humans
			15	(hand washing or handwashing or hand hygiene)
	14	random allocation/	16	14 and 15
	15	impact.tw.	17	limit 16 to yr="2009 - Current"
	16	intervention?.tw.	18	exp hospitals/
	17	chang$.tw.	19	hospital$.tw.
	18	evaluation studies/	20	exp inpatients/
	19	evaluat$.tw.	21	inpatient$.tw.
	20	effect?.tw.	22	exp health care/
	21	comparative study/	23	health care$.tw.
	22	animal/	24	healthcare$.tw.
	23	human/	25	infirmary$.tw.
	24	22 not 23	26	nosocomial$.tw.
	25	or/8-21	27	intensive care unit$.tw.
	26	25 not 24	28	ward$.tw.
	27	7 and 26	29	OR/18-28
	28	limit 27 to yr="2009 -Current"	30	17 and 29
	29	exp hospitals/		
	30	hospital$.tw.		
	31	exp inpatients/		
	32	inpatient$.tw.		
	33	exp health care/		
	34	health care$.tw.		
	35	healthcare$.tw.		
	36	infirmary$.tw.		
	37	nosocomial$.tw.		
	38	intensive care unit$.tw.		
	39	ward$.tw.		
	40	OR/29-39		
	41	28 and 40		

*EPOC Methodological filter Randomized Controlled Trial [publication type] OR Controlled Clinical Trial [publication type] OR Comparative Study OR Evaluation Studies OR 'comparative study' OR 'effects' OR 'effect' OR 'evaluations' OR 'evaluating' OR 'evaluation' OR 'evaluates' OR 'changing' OR 'changes' OR 'change' OR 'interventions' OR 'intervention' OR 'impact' OR 'random allocation' OR 'post test' OR 'posttest' OR 'pre test' OR 'pretest' OR 'time series' OR 'experimental' OR 'experiments' OR 'experiment' OR 'intervention studies' OR 'intervention study' OR 'controlled clinical trial' OR 'randomised controlled trial' OR 'randomized controlled trial'

Databases	Adapted from Gould et al.		Adapted from Huis et al.	
EMBASE	1	Handwashing/	1	Randomized controlled trial/
	2	(hand antisepsis or handwash$ or hand wash$ or hand disinfection or hand hygiene or surgical scrub$).tw.	2	random$.tw.
			3	experiment$.tw.
			4	(time adj series).tw.
	3	1 or 2	5	(pre test or pretest or post test or posttest).tw.
	4	exp Hand/	6	impact.tw.
	5	exp Sterilization/	7	intervention$.tw.
	6	4 and 5	8	chang$.tw.
	7	3 or 6	9	evaluat$.tw.
	8	randomized controlled trial/	10	effect?.tw.
	9	randomi$.tw.	11	compar$.tw.
	10	exp controlled clinical trial/	12	control$.tw.
	11	controlled clinical trial$.tw.	13	or/1-12
	12	intervention studies/	14	limit 13 to humans
	13	experiment$.tw.	15	(hand washing or handwashing or hand hygiene).
	14	(time adj series).tw.		
	15	(pre test or pretest or (posttest or post test)).tw.	16	14 and 15
	16	random allocation/	17	limit 16 to yr="2009 - Current"
	17	impact.tw.	18	exp hospital/
	18	intervention?.tw.	19	hospital$.tw.
	19	chang$.tw.	20	exp hospital patient/
	20	evaluation studies/	21	inpatient$.tw.
	21	evaluat$.tw.	22	exp health care/
	22	effect?.tw.	23	health care$.tw.
	23	comparative study/	24	healthcare$.tw.
	24	animal/	25	infirmary$.tw.
	25	human/	26	nosocomial$.tw.
	26	24 not 25	27	intensive care unit$.tw.
	27	or/8-23	28	ward$.tw.
	28	27 not 26	29	or/18-28
	29	7 and 28	30	17 and 29
	30	limit 29 to yr="2009 -Current"		
	31	exp hospitals/		
	32	hospital$.tw.		
	33	exp hospital patient/		
	34	inpatient$.tw.		
	35	exp health care/		
	36	health care$.tw.		
	37	healthcare$.tw.		
	38	infirmary$.tw.		
	39	nosocomial$.tw.		
	40	intensive care unit$.tw.		
	41	ward$.tw.		
	42	or/31-41		
	43	30 and 42		
CINAHL	1	(MH "Handwashing+")	1	(MH "Clinical Trials+")
	2	(hand antisepsis OR handwash* OR hand wash* OR hand disinfection OR hand hygiene OR surgical scrub*)	2	clinical trial*
			3	"comparative studies"
			4	"experimental studies"
	3	1 OR 2	5	"time series"
	4	Hand*	6	impact*
	5	Sterilization*	7	evaluat*
	6	4 AND 5	8	effect*
	7	3 OR 6	9	(MH "Pretest-Posttest Design+")
	8	(MH "Clinical Trials+")	10	(MH "Quasi-Experimental Studies+")
	9	clinical trial*		
	10	randomi*	11	or/1-10
	11	controlled clinical trial*	12	(MH "Handwashing+")

(Continued)

Appendix (Continued)

Databases	Adapted from Gould et al.		Adapted from Huis et al.	
	12	intervention studies*	13	(handwashing OR hand hygiene)
	13	experiment*	14	or/12-13
	14	"time series"	15	11 and 14
	15	(MH "Pretest-Posttest Design+")	16	limit 15 to yr="2009 – Current"
	16	random allocation*	17	(MH "Hospitals+")
	17	impact*	18	(MH "Hospital Units+")
	18	intervention?	19	Intensive Care Units
	19	chang*	20	(MH "Inpatients")
	20	(MH "Evaluation Research+")	21	(MH "Child, Hospitalized")
	21	evaluat*	22	(MH "Adolescent, Hospitalized")
	22	effect?	23	(MH "Aged, Hospitalized")
	23	comparative study*	24	(hospitalized OR hospitalised)
	24	(MH "Animals+")	25	(health care OR healthcare)
	25	(MH "Human+")	24	healthcare$.tw.
	26	24 NOT 25	25	infirmary$.tw.
	27	OR/8-23	26	nosocomial$.tw.
	28	27 NOT 26	27	intensive care unit$.tw.
	29	7 and 28	28	ward$.tw.
	30	limit 29 to yr="2009 -Current"	26	or/17-25
	31	(MH "Hospitals+")	27	16 AND 26
	32	(MH "Hospital Units+")		
	33	hospital*		
	34	Intensive Care Units		
	35	(MH "Inpatients")		
	36	(MH "Child, Hospitalized")		
	37	(MH "Adolescent, Hospitalized")		
	38	(MH "Aged, Hospitalized")		
	39	(hospitalized OR hospitalised)		
	40	(health care OR healthcare)		
	24	healthcare$.tw.		
	25	infirmary$.tw.		
	26	nosocomial$.tw.		
	27	intensive care unit$.tw.		
	28	ward$.tw.		
	41	or/31-40		
	42	30 AND 41		
BNI	1	handwash* (137)	n/a	
	2	hand wash* (170)		
	3	hand antisep* (22)		
	4	hand disinfection (39)		
	5	hand hygiene (369)		
	6	hand decontamination (43)		
	7	hand cleansing (29)		
	8	hand cleaning (27)		
	9	1 OR 2 OR 3 OR 4 OR 5 OR 6 OR 7 OR 8 (599)		
	10	hand (1438)		
	11	sterilization (106)		
	12	9 OR 11 (702)		
	13	limit 12 to "2009 to Current"		
CRD Database	n/a		1	MeSH DESCRIPTOR Clinical Trial EXPLODE ALL TREES
			2	Clinical Trial*
			3	control*
			4	random*
			5	comparative stud*
			6	experimental stud*
			7	time series*
			8	impact*

Databases	Adapted from Gould et al.		Adapted from Huis et al.	
			9	intervention*
			10	evaluat*
			11	effect*
			12	Chang*
			13	Compar*
			14	Experiment*
			15	(pretest OR pre test OR posttest OR post test)
			16	#1 OR #2 OR #3 OR #4 OR #5 OR #6 OR #7 OR #8 OR #9 OR #10 OR #11 OR #12 OR #13 OR #14 OR #15
			17	MeSH DESCRIPTOR Handwashing EXPLODE ALL TREES
			18	(hand washing OR handwashing OR hand hygiene)
			19	#17 OR #18
			20	#15 AND #19
			21	(#20) FROM 2009 TO 2013
			22	MeSH DESCRIPTOR Hospitals EXPLODE ALL TREES (MH
			23	MeSH DESCRIPTOR Hospital Units EXPLODE ALL TREES (MH
			24	hospital*
			25	Intensive Care Unit*
			26	MeSH DESCRIPTOR Inpatients EXPLODE ALL TREES
			27	MeSH DESCRIPTOR Adolescent, Hospitalized EXPLODE ALL TREES
			28	MeSH DESCRIPTOR Adolescent, Institutionalized EXPLODE ALL TREES
			29	MeSH DESCRIPTOR Child, Hospitalized EXPLODE ALL TREES
			30	MeSH DESCRIPTOR Child, Institutionalized EXPLODE ALL TREES
			31	(hospitalised OR hospitalized OR healthcare OR health care)
			32	#22 OR #23 OR #24 OR #25 OR #26 OR #27 OR #28 OR #29 OR #30 OR #31
			33	#21 AND #32
Cochrane Library	1	MeSH descriptor: [Hand hygiene] explode all trees	1	MeSH descriptor: [Clinical Trial] explode all trees
	2	(hand antisepsis OR handwash* OR hand wash* OR hand disinfection OR hand hygiene OR surgical scrub*)	2	Clinical Trial*
			3	control*
	3	1 OR 2	4	random*
	4	Hand*	5	comparative stud*
	5	Sterilization*	6	experimental stud*
	6	4 AND 5	7	time series*
	7	3 OR 6	8	impact*
	8	MeSH descriptor: [Clinical Trial] explode all trees	9	intervention*
			10	evaluat*
	9	clinical trial*	11	effect*
	10	randomi*	12	Chang*
	11	controlled clinical trial*	13	Compar*
	12	intervention studies*	14	Experiment*
	13	experiment*	15	(pretest OR pre test OR posttest OR post test)

(Continued)

Appendix (Continued)

Databases	Adapted from Gould et al.	Adapted from Huis et al.
	14 time series*	16 #1 OR #2 OR #3 OR #4 OR #5 OR #6 OR #7 OR #8 OR #9 OR #10 OR #11 OR #12 OR #13 OR #14 OR #15
	15 (pretest OR pre test OR posttest OR post test)	
	16 random allocation*	17 MeSH descriptor: [Hand hygiene] explode all trees
	17 impact*	
	18 intervention?	18 (hand washing OR handwashing OR hand hygiene)
	19 chang*	
	20 evaluat*	19 #17 OR #18
	21 effect*	20 #16 AND #19
	22 comparative study*	21 (#20) FROM 2009 TO 2013
	23 OR/8-22	22 MeSH descriptor: [Hospitals] explode all trees
	24 7 and 23	
	25 limit 24 to yr="2009 -Current"	23 MeSH descriptor: [Hospital Units] explode all trees
	26 MeSH descriptor: [Hospitals] explode all trees	
	27 MeSH descriptor: [Hospital Units] explode all trees	24 hospital*
	28 hospital*	25 Intensive Care Unit*
	29 Intensive Care Unit*	26 MeSH descriptor: [Inpatients] explode all trees
	30 MeSH descriptor: [Inpatients] explode all trees	
	31 MeSH descriptor: [Adolescent, Hospitalized] explode all trees	27 MeSH descriptor: [Adolescent, Hospitalized] explode all trees
	32 MeSH descriptor: [Adolescent, Institutionalized] explode all trees	28 MeSH descriptor: [Adolescent, Institutionalized] explode all trees
	33 MeSH descriptor: [Child, Hospitalized] explode all trees	29 MeSH descriptor: [Child, Hospitalized] explode all trees
	34 MeSH descriptor: [Child, Institutionalized] explode all trees	30 MeSH descriptor: [Child, Institutionalized] explode all trees
	35 (hospitalised OR hospitalized OR healthcare OR health care)	31 (hospitalised OR hospitalized OR healthcare OR health care)
	36 #26 OR #27 OR #28 OR #29 OR #30 OR #31 OR #32 OR #33 OR #34 OR #35	32 #22 OR #23 OR #24 OR #25 OR #26 OR #27 OR #28 OR #29 OR #30 OR #31 32 #21 AND #32
	37 #25 AND #36	
Current Clinical Control Trial	n/a	("hand hygiene" OR "hand washing" OR "handwashing" OR "hand sanitizer" OR "hand rubbing" OR "hand rubs") AND ("hospital" OR "healthcare" OR "inpatients" OR "intensive care unit" OR "hospitalised" OR "hospitalized" OR "nosocomial")
ACP journal	("hand hygiene" OR "hand washing" OR "handwashing" OR "hand sanitizer" OR "hand rubbing" OR "hand rubs") AND ("hospital" OR "healthcare" OR "inpatients" OR "intensive care unit" OR "hospitalised" OR "hospitalized" OR "nosocomial")	n/a
Evidence-Based Medicine Reviews	1 handwashing.sh. 2 handwash$.tx. 3 hand wash$.tx. 4 hand disinfection.tx. 5 hand hygiene.tx. 6 surgical scrub$.tx. 7 hand decontamination.mp. [mp=ti, to, ab, tx, kw, ct, sh, hw] 8 hand cleansing.mp. [mp=ti, to, ab, tx, kw, ct, sh, hw] 9 hand cleaning.mp. [mp=ti, to, ab, tx, kw, ct, sh, hw] 10 1or2or3or4or5or6or7or8or9 11 from 10 keep 1-249 12 10 13 limit 12 to yr="2005 Current"	n/a

21
MIXED METHODS

Learning outcomes

This chapter will enable you to:

- understand the rationale for using mixed methods in nursing research
- appreciate when mixed methods might be employed
- understand the implications of using mixed methods

Nurse researchers are increasingly using a number of data collection methods in a single research project and combining both qualitative and quantitative approaches to address research questions. In this chapter, we present a review of the reasons why a mixed methods approach is proving popular in nursing research. The ways in which mixed methods can be applied within a research design are reviewed and the implications of combining research methods within one research project are considered.

RATIONALE FOR THE USE OF MIXED METHODS

Denzin (2009) is a strong advocate of the use of **mixed methods** in social research. He suggests that researchers should seek to employ as many methodological perspectives as practical when investigating research problems. One of the main reasons for combining methods in research is the scope offered for **triangulation**, where the results of either a qualitative or quantitative method can be reviewed alongside the results generated by an alternative method (Robson, 2011; Cresswell, 2013). For example, the results of an attitude measure to, say, the use of computers in healthcare could be explored in interviews. Denzin (2009) suggests that there are four possible types of triangulation that can be achieved in social research (see Table 21.1).

Accessing multiple data sources might involve interviewing student nurses and lecturers about curriculum design, or including healthcare professionals, patients and relatives as participants in research. Combining different research methods in one design can be achieved through using a survey tool with staff, followed by conducting interviews and observations of practice.

Table 21.1　Denzin's types of triangulation

Types of triangulation	Explanation
Data	Using a number of data sources with a similar focus to obtain a range of views about a question or topic, thus aiming to achieve validation through comparing diverse opinion.
Method	Combining more than one research method, such as qualitative and quantitative methods.
Researcher	Using researchers from diverse backgrounds, such as a psychologist, nurse and social scientist, who bring different viewpoints to a research team.
Theory	Comparing the usefulness of competing theories or hypotheses.

Here we concentrate on the rationale for the use of mixed methods in nursing research. It should be remembered that nurses draw on a number of data sources in their daily practice in order to make judgements. For example, in the assessment of a patient the nurse will take quantitative measurements of blood pressure, pulse, temperature and respirations. Additionally, observational data will be used, gained from looking at the patient; furthermore interviewing the patient will reveal additional information about their health. Information will also be available through other physiological measures, such as the results of blood tests and from investigations including scans and invasive procedures. Given the range of information used in clinical practice, it is unsurprising that researchers investigating complex research problems should engage with a range of methods.

A review of the range of research methods available (see Chapters 22 to 25) highlights the strengths and weaknesses of each. Observations can introduce the **Hawthorne effect** through the intrusion of the researcher and can affect participant behaviour, whereas interview discussion can reflect power differences seen between the researcher and interviewee. No one method is perfect, though using a combination of methods can, it is argued, limit the potential deficits and biases of one particular method (Curry and Nunez-Smith, 2015). Thus, combining methods from **qualitative** and **quantitative research** can enhance the reliability, validity and trustworthiness of a research study and its overall quality (see Chapter 13). See Research example 21.1.

Research example 21.1

Example of methodological triangulation in nursing practice

Verweij et al. (2014) drew on three different methods to limit the weaknesses in the study and address the research aim and questions. The research aimed to evaluate the use of tabards to reduce interruptions and minimise drug administration errors. The study was conducted at a Dutch university hospital, involving three 60-bed wards. The methods employed included pre-intervention observations, where staff were observed undertaking drug rounds and interruptions were recorded. This pre-observation period was followed by the introduction of the tabards and a post-intervention observation period.

This included asking the staff one question about their experience of tabard use after each observation. Finally, staff were invited to take part in focus groups where more in-depth qualitative data was collected.

Having a range of results collected through different methods in one study allows the researcher to compare findings and make conclusions based on a variety of data. This improves confidence in the validity and accuracy of the results.

APPLICATIONS OF MIXED METHODS

Healthcare researchers use mixed methods to address a variety of research problems. Bryman (2004) suggests 11 different ways in which mixed methods are employed in social research and challenges readers to identify more. Bryman (2004) suggests mixed methods are used at different stages of the research process to access both the researcher and participant perspective and to gain views of both the institution or organisation and the individual. In healthcare research, mixed methods are also used in a number of different ways:

- to compare findings through triangulation
- to research different perspectives of the same issue
- to generate data from different approaches, often combining qualitative and quantitative methods
- to support the development, implementation and evaluation of interventions.

Comparing research findings through triangulation

As mentioned earlier, there are various ways of achieving triangulation in a research study. In this section, we will concentrate on the triangulation of research methods, the potential for combining qualitative and quantitative methods or triangulating different qualitative or quantitative methods in one research design (Denzin, 2009). More commonly, triangulation would involve the researcher using two or more different methods of data collection in a study (Denzin, 2009). This would enable the researcher to access a range of data, which can be compared to try to present a more accurate or complete view. Triangulation of methods can improve the validity and accuracy of the findings and confirm results, or can add to the scope of the findings. There is the potential for mixed methods to achieve both increased accuracy and scope of a study.

A number of researchers are using a mixed methods approach to address complex research questions, employing a range of methods in the pursuit of knowledge. Whilst there are potential benefits to using mixed methods, it should be remembered that designs employing a triangulation of methods incur greater research costs and require additional resources. Triangulation should therefore be employed when a mixed methods approach is thought necessary to answer the research question(s) posed (see Research example 21.2).

Research example 21.2

The use of triangulation

Lee et al. (2013) used methodological triangulation in a study, which aimed to explore the experiences of horizontal violence in an intensive care unit (ICU) in Korea. That is, violence received from colleagues and other staff members. The researchers worked with five participating hospitals in Korea as part of the study. Triangulation of methods was employed to generate more complete data. Two approaches to data collection were involved: a survey and focus group interviews. In total, 134 ICU nurses participated in the survey. This provided some quantitative data. Three focus groups provided qualitative data and allowed the researchers to explore some of the issues emerging from the survey. The survey data highlighted the problem of horizontal violence, confirming 94.0 per cent of the participants had experienced this at some time in the previous six months. The qualitative data revealed 17 themes describing the types and influence of violence. Obviously, the triangulation of data provided richness and informed the study findings. The use of interviewing has provided important supporting data and allowed the nurses to provide explanations of the survey data.

Using research methods to explore different perspectives of the same issue

Nursing practice can generate broad and complex research areas for study, often identifying several different approaches that can be taken to consider one area of practice. In these cases, mixed methods could be used to address different research questions or aspects of one issue.

For example, a number of research questions could be asked about cardiac rehabilitation services provided to patients following a myocardial infarction. In taking different perspectives on this issue, researchers might explore a variety of aspects that would require the use of different research methods, such as:

- patient experiences of the service
- relatives' views of the service
- measurement of the effectiveness of cardiac rehabilitation programmes for those involved.

To address the first two issues, in-depth interviews could be conducted with patients and relatives who have experience of cardiac rehabilitation services. Data collected here would enable the research team to develop some understanding of patient and relative perspectives of cardiac rehabilitation services. A third component of the study centring on the effectiveness of cardiac rehabilitation programmes would measure, perhaps through a survey of physiological measures, the impact of the service on lifestyle and health. This could explore whether the service had any long-term benefit for the patient. In exploring different aspects of one area, a fuller picture can be gained to inform the further development of services.

Generating data from different approaches combining qualitative and quantitative methods

Given the complexity of nursing research questions and issues, there will be occasions when a research design will include both qualitative and quantitative methods, using one approach to support and enhance the other (see Research example 21.3). Each research method has its limitations (see Chapters 22 to 25), and therefore combining methods within one study can achieve a more comprehensive view of the research subject.

A questionnaire survey can be used to obtain data from a large population on a particular subject. Analysis of the data will provide useful information, though may leave unanswered questions about context and a range of issues that could usefully be explored through conversation. Focus group or individual interviews would give scope to explore understandings, experiences and interpretations, and add a quality dimension to the research. Through a more in-depth discussion, the researcher can explore the survey results more fully and has the potential to gain wider and deeper understanding. Alternatively, research collecting qualitative data initially through diaries or interviews could usefully gain a broader view of issues and employ a follow-up survey. The results of qualitative data may also enable researchers to generate a research hypothesis that can be tested through quantitative methods (see Chapter 9).

Research example 21.3

Combining quantitative and qualitative research methods

Moule et al. (2007) used both quantitative and qualitative methods in research that explored the use and development of e-learning in health sciences and practice disciplines. The initial phase of the project included a survey of higher education institutes. Using a database from the funder (Higher Education Academy), a survey tool was distributed for completion online. This allowed the researcher to capture data from a broad geographical area and from a large number of institutions. The results of the survey provided detailed information about the use of e-learning in the different health disciplines across the higher education sector. These results were used to identify a sample for the second phase of the research, allowing the researcher to identify the particular characteristics of 'early adopter' and 'late adopter' for inclusion in the second phase of the study. During the second phase, four case study sites were engaged, including those describing themselves as early and late adopters of e-learning. Within the case study sites, qualitative data were collected through interviews with staff and focus groups with students, and a review of e-learning provision, and teaching and learning policies was conducted. This phase of the project enabled the researchers to explore in greater detail some of the aspects raised in the survey and to examine issues such as the barriers to e-learning and enabling factors. In this example, we can see that the combination of both quantitative and qualitative methods enabled the researchers to access broad scoping data needed to address the research questions, but also to inform the second phase which sought to collect more in-depth data and understand the barriers and enablers to using e-learning in higher education settings.

Developing, implementing and evaluating interventions

Nursing and healthcare interventions are often guided by policy and practice guidance that are based on the best available evidence. Chapter 1 described the place of research in nursing and the hierarchy of evidence that informs practice and policy development. Often, those developing practice guidance prefer to use the 'best' form of evidence, the 'gold standard' being seen as research evidence developed through the randomised control trial method (see Chapter 14).

The current resuscitation guidelines (Resuscitation Council (UK), 2015) are based on different levels of evidence and on the best current knowledge, and are updated regularly as that evidence base is developed through research and practice. Resuscitation policy reflects a range of underpinning knowledge, from across the levels of evidence (see Chapters 1 and 20), though would ideally be developed from evidence positioned at level 1, a systematic review of several randomised controlled trials. There are other aspects of care delivery, however, that can be supported by evidence developed at level 6, from personal and professional expertise, including patient views and opinions. Thus, a range of research methods might be employed to develop, implement and evaluate the broad spectrum of care that nurses are involved with (see Research example 21.4). What is of prime importance is the need to ensure that the methods used will enable the research team to address the research questions posed. Certain questions looking at patient satisfaction and experiences of interventions require a qualitative method.

Research example 21.4

Research using mixed methods to implement and evaluate a nursing intervention

Saurman et al. (2011) evaluated a Mental Health Emergency Care Rural Access project, designed to provide 24-hour access to mental health specialists in remote areas of Australia using video-conferencing equipment. The initial service development was informed by a review of existing models supporting remote access and through consultation with a range of stakeholders over a prolonged period. The new service aimed to improve access to expert mental health assessment and advice for more generalist staff in remote rural areas through tele-health links. Staff in the emergency department were offered training about the new service and in the use of technology. A triangulation design was used to evaluate the impact of the services and data were collected in the following ways:

1. A researcher was located with the service delivery team to understand team working and monitor routine data collection.
2. Data were collected on each contact telephone call.
3. Semi-structured interviews were conducted with 20 staff at baseline and 6 months, to explore the accessibility and acceptability of the service.
4. 31 patients were asked to rate their experience with video assessment.

The mixed methods evaluation was designed to measure service processes and effects, and whilst it included some patient outcome measures it was not specifically aiming to assess this. The overall outcomes were positive and the team concluded the service was effective. In the UK, service evaluation is important in informing the commissioning of services and resource expenditure. Often, evaluation is conducted to include data collected from a range of stakeholders and will include quantitative data about the effectiveness of the service and whether or not it is achieving its intended outcomes. Consequently, a range of data collection approaches will be used, including both qualitative and quantitative data.

IMPLICATIONS OF USING MIXED METHODS

Readers of research employing a mixed methods approach to data collection should be aware of the need to understand the strengths and weaknesses of each individual method (see Chapters 23 to 25), as well as being able to review how the methods were used to answer specific research question(s). They should also be cognisant of the additional time and resource demands placed on a team employing a mixed methods approach.

CHAPTER SUMMARY

- Mixed methods are commonly used in nursing research.
- Using a number of data sources in one study, combining research methods and using researchers from diverse backgrounds can achieve triangulation.
- The perceived strengths of mixed methods offer the potential to increase the scope of the study and the validity and accuracy of the findings.
- Mixed methods enable researchers to address complex research questions.
- If different methods achieve conflicting results, this can be problematic.

SUGGESTED FURTHER READING

Andrew, S. and Halcomb, E. (eds) (2009) *Mixed Methods Research for Nursing and the Health Sciences*. Oxford: Wiley-Blackwell. The book considers a range of issues that might emerge in undertaking mixed methods research; it explains how to conduct research using mixed methods and provides some examples of application.

WEBSITES

Journal of Mixed Methods Research: http://mmr.sagepub.com/ – this journal is an interdisciplinary publication that covers epidemiological, methodological and theoretical articles about the use of mixed methods research in a range of disciplines.

To access further resources related to this chapter, visit the companion website at http://study.sagepub.com/mouleaveyard3e

REFERENCES

Bryman, A. (2004) *Quantity and Quality in Social Research*. London: Routledge.

Cresswell, J. (2013) *Research Design: Qualitative, Quantitative and Mixed Methods Approaches*, 4th edn. Newbury Park, CA: Sage.

Curry, L. and Nunez-Smith, M. (2015) *Mixed Methods in Health Sciences Research. A Practical Primer*. Thousand Oaks, CA: Sage.

Denzin, N. (2009) *The Research Act: A Theoretical Introduction to Sociological Methods*, 4th edn. Somerset, NJ: Transaction.

Lee, Y-O., Kang, J., Seonyoung, Y., Lee, Y. and Kim, B-J. (2013) 'A methodological triangulation study on the experience of horizontal violence in intensive care nurses', *Journal of Korean Critical Care Nursing*, 6 (2): 37–50.

Moule, P., Ward, R., Shepherd, K., Lockyer, L. and Almeida, C. (2007) *Scoping E-learning in Health Sciences and Practice*. Bristol: Faculty of Health and Social Care, University of the West of England.

Resuscitation Council (UK) (2015) *Guidelines for Adult Basic Life Support*. Available at: www.resus.org.uk/resuscitation-guidelines/ (accessed 26 October 2015).

Robson, C. (2011) *Real World Research*, 3rd edn. Oxford: Wiley.

Saurman, E., Perkins, D., Roberts, R., Roberts, A., Patfield, M. and Lyle, D. (2011) 'Responding to mental health emergencies: Implementation of an innovative tele health service in rural and remote New South Wales, Australia', *Journal of Emergency Nursing*, 37 (5): 453–9.

Verweij, L., Smeulers, M., Maaskant, J. and Vermeulen, H. (2014) 'Quiet please! Drug round tabards: Are they effective and accepted? A mixed methods study', *Journal of Nursing Scholarship*, 46 (5): 340–8.

22
SURVEY DESIGN AND QUESTIONNAIRES

Learning outcomes

This chapter will enable you to:

- explain the characteristics of surveys and the stages involved in carrying out a sample survey
- describe the advantages and disadvantages of surveys
- critically appraise the main features of questionnaires
- describe the development of a questionnaire
- critically appraise the design aspects of questionnaires
- list the basic stages in the development of measurement tools
- discuss the use of epidemiological research in healthcare

A **survey** is non-experimental research that aims to gain data from a sample of the population (large or small) of interest, by direct questioning using questionnaires, interviews or, less frequently, by observations.

Surveys are common and it is likely that you will have been asked at some time to complete one. They are one of the oldest means of obtaining information about populations. For example, the Doomsday Book compiled around 1066 gives information about the English population at the time of the Norman invasion. Modern social surveys originated in Victorian Britain (Bowling, 2009) and were often concerned with obtaining information about poverty. Nowadays, surveys are likely to be associated with politics, especially at the time of national elections, or marketing and attempting to find out what is happening in society today, such as the British Social Attitudes Survey. These are large-scale surveys and take considerable amounts of time, effort, personnel and cost to carry them out. Even relatively small-scale surveys take a significant amount of time and effort if they are to be successfully carried out.

In this chapter, the main features of surveys and questionnaires are discussed, along with their advantages and disadvantages. The stages for conducting a survey and how to develop questionnaires are explained.

Questionnaires and measurement scales are used extensively as data collection tools in surveys and frequently in experimental designs. A cautionary note: researchers often underestimate the time required to develop a sound questionnaire or a measurement tool with acceptable properties.

WHAT IS A SURVEY?

According to de Vaus (2014) the distinguishing features of a survey are the structured form of the data collected and the methods of analysis used. Surveys generally collect a structured and systematic set of data; data is collected in the same way from each participant so that the findings are directly comparable.

The use of surveys in health is common and they are used in health technology assessment, health needs assessment, epidemiological research (see later), audit and other quality assessment issues. Questionnaire surveys, in particular, are a frequently used method of gathering primary quantitative data from patients and healthcare practitioners. Such surveys do, however, need to provide valid, unbiased and reliable data from a sample of the population being studied. When data are collected from a sample of the population of interest to the researcher, it is known as a 'sample survey'. Sometimes it may be possible to survey an entire population – for example, all registered nurses working in a health trust. However usually a representative sample from a wider population is taken.

The unit of analysis in a survey is the individual, although this 'individual' can also be an organisation in a multi-level study. For example, questions could be asked of individuals attending a family planning clinic; all of the family planning clinics in a health district could be questioned, or individuals and clinics could be questioned as part of a survey about access to family planning services.

SURVEY DESIGNS

Social surveys are used to measure attitudes, knowledge and behaviour and there are two main types: descriptive and longitudinal surveys.

Descriptive surveys aim to describe populations, to study associations between variables within populations and to establish trends (Bowling, 2009). They are referred to as descriptive or cross-sectional because the information is collected at one point in time and the respondents are ordinarily reporting on past events, feelings and behaviour, for example within the last week or month. They actually describe the phenomenon of interest and observed associations in order to estimate population parameters, such as the prevalence of falls in hospitals; to test hypotheses, for example that falls are more common in hospitals when bedrails are used without risk assessment; and to

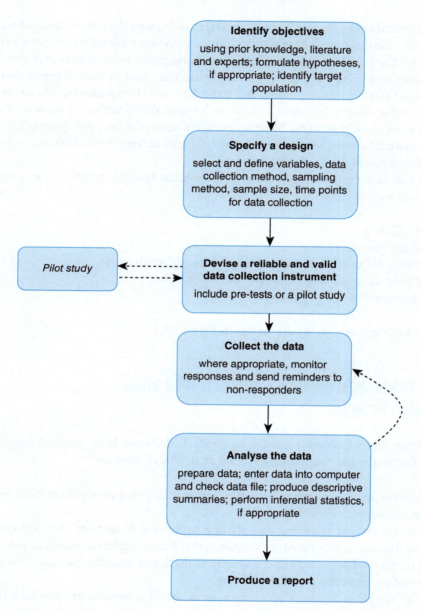

Figure 22.1   Basic stages in a survey

generate hypotheses about the possible cause-and-effect associations between variables. Descriptive surveys are often referred to as cross-sectional because data are collected from the population of interest at one point in time. The notion of 'one point in time' should not be taken literally; it is probably more realistic to think of it as data being collected over a set number of weeks or months (depending on the practicalities of actually collecting the data), but being treated as if it were collected simultaneously.

Analytical or *longitudinal* surveys are different because they are conducted on more than one point in time. These surveys aim to investigate causal associations between variables. They are known as longitudinal because they analyse events over time, with the survey tool being administered at more than one point in time. Because they analyse events at more than one point, and if the data collection points have been carefully timed, unlike descriptive surveys they can suggest the direction of cause-and-effect associations (Bowling, 2009). Most longitudinal surveys collect data prospectively and tend to either follow up the same population (panel survey) or use different samples at each data collection period (trend survey).

The focus for any survey is dependent upon the research question(s) and research objectives and is:

- fact finding
- asking questions
- gaining information about attitudes/opinions/health status
- helping us to understand/predict health/behaviour
- representative of a population.

The basic stages of a survey are set out in Figure 22.1.

WHAT MAKES SURVEY RESEARCH DIFFERENT FROM OTHER RESEARCH METHODS?

Whatever type of survey you wish to conduct, the same basic principles apply, and according to the seminal work of McColl et al. (2001) these are:

- Surveys involve collecting new data, rather than being purely theoretical or based on information already available.
- Surveys involve collecting data about a population of units of some defined type, but they are usually based on samples, rather than complete censuses, of these units.
- The method for selecting the sample is fixed and objective; ideally, it should be based on statistical probability theory.
- The sample of units for which data are collected is often large (hundreds or even thousands).
- The procedures for sampling these units and for collecting information are explicit, systematic and standardised.
- There is careful prior definition of the information to be collected from each sampled unit.
- The data collected and the results are quantitative (counts, rates, etc.); measurements are applied in a standardised way to each sample unit in order to achieve objective measurement of concepts, attributes and so on, and thereby yield comparable results across the entire sample.

- The data collected are such that they can be handled purely arithmetically (quantified); qualities or attributes (e.g. gender, strength of opinion) are assigned a numerical code so that they can be more readily manipulated in statistical analyses.
- The results from measurements made on the sample are summarised statistically.
- Conclusions about the population are drawn within confidence limits defined by using sampling theory (i.e. inferences are made from the sample to the underlying population).
- Conclusions may be descriptive of the population or based on the testing of specified hypotheses.
- Surveys are conducted in the 'real world', under circumstances that cannot be fully controlled, rather than in the more rarefied laboratory setting of biomedical research.
- Surveys use a wide range of human skills and other resources and require much planning and teamwork. (2001: 1)

In essence, the above list explains the processes involved in conducting a survey, and from this it becomes very obvious that the data will be quantitative. There may be some parts which appear to provide qualitative data but, as has already been explained, data are explicit, systematic and standardised. Hence, there is no expectation that the responses of individuals can be explored further because this would mean that the data are not standardised. This does not mean that responses to a questionnaire may not be in 'free form' but they are not truly qualitative data (see Chapter 15). The key features of survey research are set out in Table 22.1.

Table 22.1   Key features of survey research

No manipulation	• No deliberate manipulation of any attribute/variable
	• Study conducted in a natural setting
Some control of the conduct of the study	For example:
	• same measurement tool
	• specified point in time
	• same environmental setting
	• participants satisfy same inclusion and exclusion criteria
Random selection of cases/participants	This is essential for generalisation
No random allocation of participants to groups	
Pilot study	• small-scale
	Provides:
	• clarity
	• understanding
	• comprehensibility
	• face validity
	• content validity
	• data for sample size calculation

Reflective exercise

By now, you should be able to recognise the differences between survey and experimental research. Try drawing a chart/table to compare and contrast the main features of a survey with those of an experiment.

An example is given at the end of this chapter in Table 22.5, but try not to refer to it until you have completed your own table.

ASSUMPTIONS OF SURVEY METHODS

There are a number of assumptions that can be made about survey research, including:

- Generality of data is more important than individuality.
- Data are summarised over all participants or pre-specified subgroups.
- Individuals are not identified or reported.
- Participants share a frame of reference – for example, any question has exactly the same meaning to all participants.
- A common framework allows concepts to be quantified.
- Responses provide an accurate description of attitudes, attributes, behaviour, beliefs, health status, knowledge or psychological traits/status.
- Data are non-contextual.
- The context in which the data were collected has no effect on the data.

DATA COLLECTION METHODS

There are a number of data collection methods that can be used in surveys, although questionnaires tend to be the most commonly used:

- Questionnaires – discussed in much more detail later.
- Structured interviews – here an interviewer/researcher will ask a set of questions and note your responses, often from a list of options. These can be conducted face-to-face or on the telephone.
- Structured diaries – where the individual keeps a record of relevant activities over a set period of time. The diary may be prescriptive or the individual may be able to record the information in their own way.
- Structured observations – such as observing the activities of care assistants when escorting patients to the X-ray department.
- Extracting data from records or documents – this type of survey is frequently used in **epidemiological surveys** (see later in this chapter).

Each data collection method will have its own advantages and disadvantages. This means that you have to determine which method will best fit with your research question and population sample in order to get as good a response rate as possible.

THE ROLE OF SAMPLING IN SURVEYS

Sampling is important and necessary in survey research methodology because it will be impacted on by the resources and time available to conduct the survey, as well as affecting the generalisability of its findings. If the sample of a survey is insufficient to make it statistically reliable, then the results will not be generalisable.

The general considerations that underlie sampling in surveys relate to how the research population is defined; being able to obtain a list of possible cases/participants; how the sampling method is selected; and deciding on the sample size. These considerations are also closely related to each other and to the selected method for data collection. There are statistical tables/websites that can calculate sample sizes to give a statistically significant result based on results from a pilot study, or, of course, you could ask the advice of a statistician or experienced researcher.

A number of issues concerning the ability to generalise findings are closely linked with the availability of a list of potential cases or participants. Such a list may:

- *match* the population of interest
  - ideal but unrealistic
- *include* cases that are not members of the population of interest
  - screen cases for eligibility
- *omit* cases that are members of the population of interest
  - inaccessibility of cases, behaviour, contexts, situations of interest
  - potential bias, hard to detect.

Reflective exercise

Think about how you would design a survey to answer one of the following research questions:

- What are the characteristic patterns and modes of practice of therapists in respect of clients with rheumatoid arthritis?
- What is the prevalence of anorexia nervosa among school-age children?
- Do nurses' attitudes towards performing certain routine tasks for patients with AIDS differ in respect of the extent of their knowledge about this condition and how this knowledge was acquired?

ETHICAL IMPLICATIONS

An important issue that needs to be considered is the need for informed consent. It is often assumed that the completion of a survey questionnaire, which can be sent by post or online, is equivalent to consent. However, it is always necessary to ensure that potential participants are aware of the purpose of the study and what will happen to the data. Privacy, confidentially and anonymity must be assured. In addition, the potential effects of any sensitive or personal questions need to be thought through at the design stage – in particular, with regard to psychological harm. Finally, don't forget the implications of the Data Protection Act 1998. Response rates may be influenced by participants' uncertainty about confidentiality and anonymity and may be exacerbated in online surveys, especially if the questionnaire is an email attachment rather than web-based.

WHAT IS A QUESTIONNAIRE?

Questionnaires are often, but not exclusively, used to collect data for a survey. A questionnaire consists of a formalised series of questions. The actual information required from a questionnaire will depend on the research question, and a list of information requirements will inform the question content. Questionnaires are usually associated with quantifiable data. Complex concepts such as behaviours and attitudes are measured by the construction of **rating scales**, which effectively converts what is ordinarily seen as qualitative data into a quantitative format that will more readily allow for comparison between individuals. Furthermore, the inclusion of open-ended questions allows respondents an opportunity to respond in their own words. The open-ended question, although providing qualitative-type data, still does not pass questionnaires into the qualitative research domain because there is no opportunity to unravel the real meaning of each response (Parahoo, 2014). Equally, responses to questions may be conditional. Individuals may respond to structured response categories but in reality their 'correct' answer is 'it depends'. This reflects the notion that individuals do not necessarily have only one view in answer to a question, but the questionnaire may force them to choose one response.

A basic assumption underlying the use of questionnaires is that there is a shared understanding of the words, phrases and concepts used. This means that care must be taken when designing questions to avoid misinterpretation of questions and to minimise any influence word or question ordering may have on responses.

The word *questionnaire* has several common usages (Oppenheim, 2000):

1. A collection of written items or questions that are posted (either as 'snail mail', email attachment or online) to participants for them to provide written answers (this might comprise ticking selected responses) before return to the researchers.

2.   A collection of written items or questions that are handed to individuals (perhaps in a group) by a researcher; the participant(s) complete(s) the answers and give(s) the completed questionnaire back to the researcher.

3.   A collection of written items or questions that the researcher asks participants (either face-to-face or by telephone), recording their responses.

4.   A collection of items that comprise different perspectives on one underlying construct, the answers to which are pooled to produce a 'measure of that construct'. Such items may be included in a questionnaire as defined by (1), (2) and (3) above.

In this chapter, *questionnaire* will refer to (1), (2) or (3) above; option (4) will be referred to as a *tool, scale* or *instrument* – for example, *measurement scale, rating scale, attitude scale*.

Option (3) is usually referred to as a *structured interview*, since the wording and ordering of questions is the same (or standardised) for all respondents.

FUNCTION OF A QUESTIONNAIRE

The function of a questionnaire is to provide measures of aspects such as:

*   attitudes (towards, e.g., drink-driving, vulnerable groups in society)
*   attributes (e.g. demographics, the duration of some conditions)
*   behaviours (self-reported actions or activities)
*   beliefs (acceptance of a statement or proposition)
*   health status (perceived physical or functional ability)
*   knowledge (e.g. on the dangers of taking drugs)
*   psychological traits or states (e.g. stress, depression).

These aspects can be implicit or explicit in the research question. The aim is to develop a set of questions that will enable you to get answers to your research question.

DESIGNING AND DEVELOPING QUESTIONNAIRES

The following key stages are involved in the design and development of a questionnaire:

1.   *Specify the research question*: this forms the starting point of the entire research process, and is no different from any other research methodology.

2.   *Identify broad categories of interest/information*: the design of a questionnaire cannot begin until the researcher has determined what aspects or issues are to be investigated. In general, *every* question or item in the questionnaire should provide some useful information towards answering the research question.

Demographic and biographical data (for example, age, gender, education) are useful for contextualising results and limiting the potential generalisation of findings.

3. *Identify the respondents*: the characteristics of potential respondents will influence decisions made at each stage in the development of a questionnaire.

4. *Decide on the mode of administration and completion*: the questionnaire may be posted to potential respondents for self-completion, handed to them (individually or as a group) by the researcher on a convenient occasion, or web-based methods may be used to distribute the questionnaire. Alternatively, the researcher might use the questionnaire as an interview schedule (either face-to-face or by telephone), completing the responses provided by the respondents.

Online data collection is becoming increasingly common and raises issues other than those associated with paper-based questionnaires. The reported disadvantages of online questionnaires include sample bias, psychometric distortions, 'technophobia' and lower response rates (Hunter, 2012). However, they can be an inexpensive, quick and convenient way of collecting data, and it is possible to capture the data directly into a database. How you actually distribute your questionnaire and arrange for its return will have an impact on your response rate (see later in the chapter).

5. *Determine questionnaire content*: this comprises several stages. Specific topics are identified within each broad category or theme that was identified under Step 2. This detail may be informed by theoretical considerations, literature searches, a review of previous research studies, focus group interviews, and input from professionals and peers. The search strategy should cover existing questionnaires and/or measurement scales/tools/instruments.

   Some specific topics may require more than one question to be asked to elicit a complete answer. Use of an existing measurement scale/tool/instrument may be appropriate in some instances – issues of reliability and validity must be addressed (see later in the chapter). In addition, permission should be sought to use the scale, copyright checked, and payment made as appropriate.

6. *Appraise the length of the questionnaire*: it is important to remember that a long questionnaire imposes a higher burden on respondents, which may adversely affect response rates. There is also a higher administrative burden – photocopying, data inputting, etc. You need to query the role and importance of each item/question and exclude any that have been included for 'fringe interest', i.e. interesting but not necessary to be able to answer the research question.

7. *Choose types of questions:*

   i. Open questions allow respondents to answer in their own choice of words, whereas closed questions specify the options from which respondents must answer, i.e. respondents choose from the same pre-specified list of responses.

      Open questions allow spontaneity and expression of aspects/issues of importance or perceived salience to the respondents. They are useful when little is known about the research topic, but may be time-consuming to analyse. For example:

Question (a) Why are you studying for a postgraduate qualification?

When open questions are used in questionnaires, the responses obtained are frequently described as providing qualitative data. This data cannot, however, be accurately called qualitative data because the responses are static and there is not usually any opportunity for the researcher to confirm meaning or probe further.

ii.   Closed questions restrict the amount and breadth of information being collected. They enable more questions to be answered in a fixed period of time, require less writing (since they usually entail ticking or crossing an option or a box), are useful when there is a fair amount of prior knowledge on the research topic and are easy to analyse. For example:

Question (b) A postgraduate qualification will enhance my professional practice.

Answer: Yes ☐   No ☐   Don't know ☐

8. *Choose response options*

An alternative wording to question (b) might be:

Question (c) A postgraduate qualification will change my professional practice.

The response options might be presented as a:

i.   Numerical rating scale

1	2	3	4	5	6	7
'no change'			'change definitely'			for the better'

The respondent would be asked to circle the number between 1 and 7 that represented their opinion.

In this instance, the above may represent a 'biased' set of response options in that it excludes the possibility that attainment of a postgraduate qualification might have a negative impact on professional practice. We would hope that the latter is very highly improbable, but if it is not impossible then perhaps a less 'biased' set of response options might be:

1	2	3	4	5	6	7
'change definitely					'change definitely	
for the worse'					for the better'	

Here, response option 4 would indicate 'no change' in professional practice. Some researchers advocate the use of an even number of responses so that there is no 'middle' option that, in many instances, may be viewed as a safe or neutral response. An even number of responses would force a respondent to declare a negative or positive opinion on the issue/aspect in question. There is no consensus on the optimum number of response options – there are 7 in the illustration, but 4, 5, 6 and a maximum of 11 are also recommended.

ii. Visual Analogue Scale (VAS)

'worst imaginable'   'no change'   'most beneficial change'

The respondent is asked to place a vertical line on the line to indicate their expected change in practice.

The 'scale' line should be exactly 100mm in length. It is represented horizontally in our illustration, but some authors believe that it should be drawn vertically with the 'worst' or 'lowest' response at the bottom and the 'best' or 'highest' response at the top – this simulates a ladder. A score is taken as the distance from the left (or bottom) of the line to a respondent's vertical line. The distance is usually measured in millimetres (although it is often expressed in cm). The literature contains much debate about VASs (see, for example, Knapp, 1990; Sim and Wright, 2000; Streiner and Norman, 2008). VASs have been used with some success to measure self-rated levels of pain (McDowell and Newell, 1996).

iii. Adjectival or adverbial rating scale

Not at all   Somewhat   Moderately   Very much   Extremely

This is a series of adjectives or adverbs, arranged hierarchically, in which the ordering is unambiguous (hence, there is a need to choose the words very carefully).

Other examples include:

Very often   Often   Sometimes   Seldom   Never or almost never

Without ANY   With SOME   With MUCH   UNABLE
difficulty   difficulty   difficulty   to do

A few minutes   Several minutes in an hour   Several hours   A day
or two More than two days

(for example, with regard to the usual duration of some specific event/ activity during the previous four weeks)

In general, the adverbs/adjectives have different meanings in different contexts. For example, what we perceive to be 'frequent' visits to a dentist may be viewed as 'extremely infrequent' when referred to shopping for clothes, or 'very frequent' when referred to buying a house.

iv. Other response options include checklists and ranking procedures.

Checklists involve listing a set or series of questions and asking respondents to select those that apply (Table 22.2 gives an example of a checklist).

Ranking asks respondents to rate the importance or strength of agreement relative to the way other items in the set have been rated (de Vaus, 2014), such as from least to most important (Table 22.3 gives an example of a ranking scale).

Table 22.2   Example of a checklist

The next question is about things that may have happened to you personally in your place of work. Please indicate how recently, if ever, these things have happened to you.

	Yes, within the past 12months	Yes, within the past 2–3 years	Yes, more than 3 years ago	No, never
1. Has a patient/visitor threatened you with physical harm in your workplace?				
2. Has a patient/visitor ever hit, slapped, kicked or physically harmed you in your workplace?				
3. Has a patient/visitor verbally abused you in your workplace?				

Table 22.3   Example of a ranking question

Question 1

What are the most important factors in choosing a General Practitioner? Please rank from the list below by putting 1 to 4 in the boxes (1 = most important, 4 = least important)

Distance from home

Parking spaces available

Availability of appointments

Female doctor available

v.   Specialised scales have been developed to measure respondents' attitudes or beliefs on one or more topics. These are called Likert scales, Guttman scales, Thurstone scales and the Semantic differential scale.

The Likert scale is a very common means of attitude measurement. It asks the respondent to indicate their agreement/approval or disagreement/disapproval with one or more statements, for example:

Strongly agree   Agree   Neither   Disagree   Strongly disagree

The term 'Likert' is often misused to describe an adverbial/adjectival scale. As mentioned above, the 'Neither' option is often omitted so that the respondent is forced to make a decision. You might like to think through the advantages and disadvantages of this approach as a general strategy.

9.   *Check the timeframe for questions:* questions may refer to the past, present or future. The point in time or period of time should be stated explicitly and unambiguously at the beginning of questions. For example:

- Tick the one statement in each group that best describes your opinion *today* on each issue.
- In the following question, put a cross against the one option that best describes the way that you have been feeling over the *past week, including today.*
- From the following words, tick all those that describe your general behaviour to friends over the *past four weeks.*

The previous six months is usually recommended as the maximum period over which respondents' memories are reliable. It is more difficult to give advice about the usefulness of responses for the future. These are the respondents' thoughts, beliefs, feelings and attitudes for that future point in time as perceived at the time of completion of the questionnaire.

10. *Consider the wording of questions/items:* the actual words you use in your questionnaire will have a major impact on your respondents. If your questions are ambiguous or unclear, then it is likely that your questionnaire will not properly answer your research question.

Look at a published questionnaire and consider how well the questions are worded. For example, the EORTC QLQ-BIL21 is a disease-specific module for patients with gallbladder cancer, looking specifically at health quality of life, and has questions such as the following:

During the past week:

   i. Have you had trouble with eating?
  ii. Have you felt full up too quickly after beginning to eat?
 iii. Have you had problems with your sense of taste?
  iv. Were you restricted in the types of food you could eat as a result of your disease or treatment?
   v. Have your skin or eyes been yellow (jaundiced)?

11. *Questionnaire layout and presentation*: good layout and presentation can help to:

- ensure that questions are clear and unambiguous
- ensure that the questionnaire, and any subsections within it, are filled in correctly
- maximise response rate
- minimise bias between responders and non-responders. (Sim and Wright, 2000: 264)

There are some obvious practical aspects to consider. Self-completed questionnaires should be word-processed using Arial typeface with a font size of 12 (or larger if this is appropriate for the potential respondent population). There should be a title and return address on the front page, and a 'Thank you' message with space for comments on the back page.

Research has demonstrated that, in general, capitals are more difficult to read than lower case and, therefore, capitals should not be used for emphasis. The questionnaire should have an attractive appearance with adequate space for responses, and not look too cluttered, i.e. ensure that the questions are well spaced or arranged to give the appearance of free space on each page. In addition, it is sound practice to ensure that a question does not straddle different pages and similarly for items within a measurement tool. Respondents must be given clear, explicit instructions on what questions to answer and when it is appropriate to 'skip' a question or questions.

Response rate is improved when a postal/online questionnaire is accompanied by an introductory letter. This letter, written in a friendly but not patronising style, should clearly explain the purpose of and potential benefit from the study, why the recipient has been selected as a potential respondent, and what he/she has to do if they agree to participate in the study (including approximately how long it will take to complete the questionnaire). It is important to provide assurances of anonymity and confidentiality, and to give a name and contact details for further information. Many people now expect to see some statement about the Data Protection Act 1998 and which ethics committee has approved the research study. It is advisable to indicate a return-by date and to include a self-addressed, stamped envelope (which will encourage a return). Other strategies, such as marking questionnaires to enable identification of non-returns, colour of paper used, and printing on single/double-sided paper also help to improve response rates.

12. *Sequencing*: There are different schools of thought here. Some authors (e.g. Moser and Kalton, 1993) advise that the first questions should be non-threatening and easy to answer (e.g. demographic information), so that respondents feel confident about being able to answer the questionnaire. However, others (e.g. Babbie, 2011) disagree with this practice, saying that mundane items may put off potential respondents as they are uninteresting. A compromise might be to have questions at the beginning that do not require much effort to answer but which stimulate the respondent's interest – a challenge!

There is general agreement that sensitive and/or more personal questions should appear later in a questionnaire rather than near the beginning. In any event, respondents ought to be able to discern some logical sequencing of questions. This may be through grouping questions of similar content or form, or the same timeframe.

Once you have developed a questionnaire, you should conduct a pilot study. A **pilot study** is a small-scale replica of the proposed study and is essential in any research. It uses a small sample of participants who are representative of the study population. Its purpose is to identify ambiguities and/or difficulties with the questionnaire, including comprehension, ease of use and completion time. It also serves to identify problems with administration, recruitment strategy, data inputting and data analysis, and provides a crude estimate of the expected response rate. A second pilot may be necessary if major changes are made.

> ### Reflective exercise
>
> Make a list of the potential strengths and weaknesses/disadvantages of question-naires when used as a data collection tool in survey research.

DESIGNING AND DEVELOPING MEASUREMENT TOOLS OR RATING SCALES

The basic principle of scaling is used every day. The picture we try to build up of people when we first meet them is a composite formed from a number of clues which help us gain an impression of their friendliness, reliability, intelligence, and so on.

In research, and survey research in particular, a scale is essentially a formalised and systematic version of this everyday happening. A scale is a measure composed of infor-mation derived from several questions or indicators (de Vaus, 2014). By converting the information contained in several relatively specific indicators, a single new and more abstract variable is constructed. This is useful in helping to get at the complexity of a concept. Thus, instead of measuring whether someone supports the death penalty by asking if they would be prepared to act as state executioner, we would ask about a range of issues which we think link to support for the death penalty.

The development of measurement tools or rating scales is covered in detail in texts such as Streiner and Norman (2008) and de Vaus (2014). Only a listing of the key stages is given here:

1. Clarify the 'construct' to be measured.
2. Devise a pool of items considered relevant:

    - based on theory
    - literature search, other instruments/tools
    - interviews/focus groups/Delphi with 'experts' in the field
    - interviews/focus groups with a representative sample from the target population.

3. Choose the response format – see earlier sections on open/closed questions, types of response option, etc.
4. Check content validity and wording of items – the validity of a questionnaire relates to its ability to measure what it is expected to measure. To establish con-tent or face validity, you could submit your questionnaire to an expert panel for review. Criterion-validity is established by comparing the results obtained from the questionnaire with other research data collected. For example, a question-naire about confidence in computer use could be compared with observational data that recorded actual use.
5. Select existing scales that can be used to validate the new scale.
6. Perform a pilot study evaluation of the instrument's performance:

    - examine ambiguities, endorsement frequencies, etc.
    - revise the instrument in light of the pilot study.

7. Conduct a study on a large sample to check:

- reliability
- validity within a specific context.

WAYS TO IMPROVE RESPONSE RATES

Reference has already been made to some ways that response rates to questionnaires may be improved. An actual response rate is calculated out of the number of eligible respondents able to be included in the study as a percentage of the total study population.

$$\text{Response rate} = \frac{\text{Number returned}}{\text{N in sample} - (\text{ineligible} + \text{unreachable})} \times 100$$

For example, if the number of eligible questionnaires returned is 45 and the sample size is 60, the response rate is:

$$\frac{45}{60} \times 100 = 75\%$$

There is no agreed standard for an acceptable response rate (Bowling, 2009), but obviously any researcher will want to get as many responses as possible. A response rate of 75 per cent and above is commonly regarded as being good, but this will still give 25 per cent of non-responders and it is possible that these individuals may differ in some important way from the responders. Thus, the survey may be biased because the differences between responders and non-responders cannot be properly accounted for in estimates.

There are a number of ways in which to increase your survey response rate, and inevitably the response rate will depend on the nature of the survey.

Improving response rates in interviews (face-to-face or telephone)

- Advance notification of your intention to call will help to allay suspicion of your visit and explain the purpose of the survey beforehand.
- Arrange a suitable time and place for the interview.
- Look neat and tidy and use a confident approach that assumes co-operation but avoids argumentativeness (de Vaus, 2014).
- Introduce yourself carefully, giving the name of your organisation as well as your own name; and have a photographic identification card at hand to show if requested.
- Give the interviewee a copy of the survey information sheet for them to read before you start the interview and for them to keep as a record to explain the survey.
- Confirm the interviewee's informed consent before starting the interview.

Improving response rates for postal surveys

- Include a covering letter with the questionnaire. This gives the main opportunity for you to motivate the respondent to complete the survey. The letter should:
  - have an official letterhead
  - contain the date of mailing
  - include the full name and address of the respondent
  - explain the purpose of the survey in clear and unambiguous terms
  - explain why and how the respondent has been selected for participation in the survey
  - offer an assurance of confidentiality
  - give some indication of how the results will be used, and how and when the recipient may obtain a copy of the results if they wish
  - include an offer to answer any questions that they might have about the survey and the questionnaire, ideally providing a free telephone number
  - mention use of a translator who understands the nature of the survey and can modify the questions if necessary without changing their original meaning. (de Vaus, 2014)
- Personalise envelopes so that they don't look like circulars and include a self-addressed stamped envelope for the return of the questionnaire.
- Think about the timing of the questionnaire delivery – try to avoid busy times of the year such as the Christmas and Easter holidays.
- Follow up on non-responders – you may need to do this two or three times. You should try and vary the way respondents are contacted to increase the opportunity of getting a completed questionnaire.
- Have questionnaires available in other languages.

Improving response rates for online surveys

Differing results from online surveys may reflect different levels of computer use and confidence in using computers. However, there are some things that will probably increase response rates, such as:

- sending invitations to participate via email
- advertising for participants online, e.g. via an appropriate information website
- developing a specific website and advertising this on relevant web forums
- online 'snowballing' – so that respondents forward the questionnaire link to friends and colleagues who they know will be interested
- using a questionnaire link – this avoids respondents having to download the questionnaire, complete it and then return it to the researcher
- incorporating videos/graphics to increase understanding of the purpose of the questionnaire and make completion more active

- making sure that there is sufficient space for respondents answering open-ended questions
- piloting the questionnaire to ensure that each full page is visible on standard computers.

ADVANTAGES AND DISADVANTAGES OF SURVEYS

Surveys are frequently used within nursing and healthcare research. It must be remembered, however, that asking and answering questions in the 'unreal' setting of a questionnaire or interview is not the same as discussing an issue naturally. From a very practical perspective, surveys can allow for massive amounts of quantitative data to be collected and if data are collected with technical proficiency, with internal reliability and a statistically appropriate sample, then they may be regarded as valid and able to provide generalisable results.

There are some advantages and disadvantages that apply to all questionnaire-based surveys and others that relate specifically to certain types of questionnaire-based surveys.

Disadvantages

- General

Data are affected by the characteristics of respondents – for example, their knowledge of the issue, memory (an especially important factor to be considered when surveying older people), experience, personality and motivation. Respondents may not always give 'true' responses – they may attempt to give answers that show them in 'the best light', even when they know that the questionnaire is anonymous, or respond in the way that they feel the researcher wants them to.

- Self-administered questionnaires

These frequently have a low response rate and it is difficult to be sure that the sample is representative because it is impossible to identify the characteristics of non-responders. Ambiguities and misinterpretations of the questions are difficult to detect, and it is impossible to be sure that respondents have responded reliably or have taken the survey seriously. These apply whether the survey is completed in the presence of the researcher, online or as a postal survey.

- Interview surveys

Interviewers may influence respondents via their personal characteristics and/or motivation, as well as their experience and skills of conducting research interviews. This influence may also affect the development of a relationship between interviewer and interviewee, thus inhibiting the interviewee's responses. Further, because there is a direct interaction, it is possible that the interviewee may be less sure about anonymity and be less open with their responses.

Advantages

- General

Questionnaire surveys can provide a relatively simple and straightforward means of studying attitudes, values, beliefs and motives. They are readily adapted which can make it possible to collect generalisable data from across most populations. Much of the data can be standardised.

- Self-administered questionnaires

Surveys can be very efficient at providing large amounts of data at relatively low cost and over a short timescale. The fact that they can allow anonymity means that it is possible to gain information from individuals on sensitive issues that they would be otherwise unwilling to discuss in a research setting. Surveys are frequently the only way to obtain details of past history from large populations.

- Interview surveys

The interviewer can clarify the meaning of questions which may encourage the interviewee to respond appropriately rather than not responding to a question. Telephone surveys can raise other issues such as difficulties in obtaining representative samples because of ex-directory numbers, uncertainty about whom exactly you are talking to and the possibility of not knowing the name of the interviewee if 'random digit dialling' (RDD) is used. (RDD is a way of selecting telephone numbers where some of the last digits are generated randomly.)

As with any method of data collection, questionnaires have strengths and weaknesses and these are set out in Table 22.4.

EPIDEMIOLOGICAL RESEARCH

Epidemiology is the study of the distribution and determinants of health-related states or events (including disease), and the application of this study to the control of diseases and other health problems. (World Health Organization at: www.who.int/topics/epidemiology/en/)

This makes epidemiology important in maintaining healthy populations. Epidemiology can provide valuable information to support healthcare planning, through enabling

Table 22.4 Strengths and weaknesses of questionnaires

	Strengths	Weaknesses
Practical issues	• Time-saving for respondent • Cost-saving for researcher • Geographical • Size of sample • Analysis can be pre-planned	• Requires a lot of development time to be well designed • Unconditional responses/response forced • Reporting accuracy – recall for past; present • Social desirability – selecting response options that respondent thinks are socially acceptable • Context of completion may influence response • Implications of mode of delivery • Interaction between interviewer/interviewee? • Assumes respondent can read and write • Non-representative when non-response is high
Relative anonymity/easier for:	• Embarrassing issues • Issues of a personal nature	• Face-to-face completion or interviewing might elicit more information, especially on personal/sensitive issues • Who is actually completing the questionnaire?
Self-completion/potential for:	• Reducing potential bias from interaction with an interviewer	• Misunderstanding questions • Misinterpreting response choices

the development of strategies that prevent disease occurrence and by supporting the implementation of management strategies for those with disease. For example, **epidemiological research** can support the implementation of immunisation programmes and changes in healthcare treatments.

Epidemiological research is often concerned with the collection of large data sets. Large quantities of data are essential if they are to be used to support recommendations for healthcare practice and management. Data collection can be done in a number of ways, including: surveys, case studies, case control studies, documentary analysis, cohort studies, RCTs and experiments (Bowling, 2009). Chapter 25 discusses other methods of data collection.

CHAPTER SUMMARY

• Surveys provide a descriptive account of the phenomenon or enable an existing body of information to be further developed.

Table 22.5   Example of the main features of experiments and surveys

Experiments	Surveys
Address explanatory or predictive research questions, in the form of hypotheses	Address descriptive research questions; may involve hypotheses but not always
Design and methods are planned in advance of conducting the study	Design and methods are planned in advance of conducting the study
'Objectivity' is claimed	'Objectivity' is addressed
Investigate 'cause' and 'effect' relationships	Consider 'association' between variables but unable to infer 'cause' and 'effect' relationships
Involve the 'planned manipulation' of variable(s)	Executed in a 'natural' setting with no deliberate manipulation of variables
Involve deliberate 'control' to eliminate explanations of the 'effect' other than the 'cause'	Minimal 'control' is present through the selection of an accessible population, the study sample and the measurement tool
Participants constitute a convenience sample who are randomly allocated to 'groups'	Participants constitute a random sample from an accessible population
Involve predominantly the collection of quantitative data; some qualitative data may be collected	Involve predominantly the collection of quantitative data; some qualitative data may be collected
Concerned with the generalisation of findings; data analysis involves statistical hypothesis testing	Usually concerned with generalisation of findings; data analysis may or may not involve statistical hypothesis testing
Use reliable and valid measurement tools	Usually use reliable and valid measurement tools
May involve major ethical issues	Usually involve minor ethical issues
Formal consenting procedures are followed	When data are collected through postal questionnaires, consent may be implied through a returned/completed questionnaire

- Surveys yield quantitative data which can be generalised to a population of interest.
- Key features of a survey include sampling to enable cases to be randomly selected, some control and a pilot study.
- The most commonly used data collection methods for surveys are questionnaires and structured interviews.
- Closed questions provide information that produces quantitative data, whereas open questions lead to qualitative data.
- A questionnaire provides measures of aspects such as attitudes, attributes, behaviours, beliefs, health status, knowledge, psychological traits or states – that are implicit or explicit in the research question.
- There are several stages in the development of a sound questionnaire.
- A pilot study is essential to 'test' a questionnaire before its use in the main study.
- Researchers often underestimate the time required to develop a sound questionnaire.

SUGGESTED FURTHER READING

de Vaus, D. (2014) *Surveys in Social Research*, 6th edn. Crows Nest, NSW: Routledge. This book gives guidance on how to plan, conduct and analyse surveys. The links between the theory and practice of research are clearly explained. There is no expectation of an understanding of statistics and the tools you need to develop an appropriate understanding of them are given.

Hunter, L. (2012) 'Challenging the reported disadvantages of e-questionnaires and addressing methodological issues of online data collection', *Nurse Researcher*, 20 (1): 11–20. This article takes you through the processes of developing online surveys and highlights the advantages and disadvantages of conducting a survey in this way.

Punch, K.F. (2003) *Survey Research: The Basics*. London: Sage. This does what it says on the label, by providing a succinct overview of survey research. It takes you through the processes involved and could be used as a handbook when undertaking a survey yourself.

WEBSITES

Survey Monkey: www.surveymonkey.com/ – a free online survey software and questionnaire tool

The Economic and Social Research Council: www.restore.ac.uk/orm/questionnaires/quesads. htm – provides online questionnaire advantages and disadvantages

To access further resources related to this chapter, visit the companion website at http://study. sagepub.com/mouleaveyard3e

REFERENCES

Babbie, E. (2011) *The Practice of Social Research*, 13th edn. Belmont, CA: Wadsworth.

Bowling, A. (2009) *Research Methods in Health*, 3rd edn. Maidenhead: Open University Press.

de Vaus, D. (2014) *Surveys in Social Research*, 6th edn. Crows Nest, NSW: Routledge.

Hunter, L. (2012) 'Challenging the reported disadvantages of e-questionnaires and addressing methodological issues of online data collection', *Nurse Researcher*, 20 (1): 11–20.

Knapp, T.R. (1990) 'Treating ordinal scales as interval scales: An attempt to resolve the controversy', *Nursing Research*, 39: 121–3.

McColl, E., Jacoby, A., Thomas, L., Soutter, J., Bamford, C., Steen, N., et al. (2001) 'Design and use of questionnaires: A review of best practice applicable to surveys of health service staff and patients', *Health Technology Assessment*, 5 (31). York: NHS R&D HTA Programme. Available at: www.hta.ac.uk/project/937.asp (accessed March 2016).

McDowell, I. and Newell, C. (1996) *Measuring Health: A Guide to Rating Scales and Questionnaires*, 2nd edition. New York: Oxford University Press.

Moser, C.A. and Kalton, G. (1993) *Survey Methods in Social Investigation*, 2nd edn. London: Heinemann Educational.

Oppenheim, A.N. (2000) *Questionnaire Design, Interviewing and Attitude Measurement*, 2nd edn. London: Pinter.

Parahoo, K. (2014) *Nursing Research Principles, Process and Issues*, 3rd edn. London: Macmillan.

Sim, J. and Wright, C. (2000) *Research Design in Healthcare: Concepts, Designs and Methods*. Cheltenham: Stanley Thornes.

Streiner, D.L. and Norman, G.R. (2008) *Health Measurement Scales: A Practical Guide to their Development and Use*, 4th edn. Oxford: Oxford University Press.

23
INTERVIEWS

Learning outcomes

This chapter will enable you to:

- appreciate the differences between quantitative and qualitative interviewing
- explain the use of group interviews
- explain the use of telephone interviews
- understand the advantages and disadvantages of interviews as a data collection method
- understand the power issues associated with interviewing

Many research questions aim to explore issues such as individual views and beliefs about service provision, patient experience of care delivery and staff perceptions of a new way of working. The interview is a data collection approach used by researchers to address such questions. In an interview situation, the researcher as 'interviewer' holds a conversation with a purpose, asking the 'interviewee' questions with the intent of finding out specific information (Polit and Beck, 2014).

In this chapter, we consider different approaches to interviewing, explore the power issues researchers must consider when interviewing and review the advantages and disadvantages of the technique as a data collection method. The chapter will draw on research examples to support the discussion.

HOW DO YOU CONDUCT AN INTERVIEW?

Most of us will have some experience of interviews. We have probably been involved in a range of 'informal' interviews, for example when visiting the doctor we provide information in response to a series of questions about our health. We may have experienced more formal interview situations. Examples would include being interviewed for a place on a course or for a new job. As a nurse or healthcare professional, you will have experience of participating in and leading interviews, using interview techniques to gather information about patients as part of the initial assessment or admission process.

Despite some familiarity with the process of interviewing, it is suggested that nurses will require some development to employ interview techniques with the sophistication required to support measurement within research (Burns et al., 2012). In particular, you will need to give attention to generating interview questions to ensure there is a structure to the discussion. The questions asked in a research interview are designed to enable the researcher to access particular information that will be needed to answer the overall research questions (King and Horrocks, 2010). The researcher will also need to plan to collect the data, either through a face-to-face interview or by other media such as a telephone or Skype conversation (via a computer).

Generating the interview questions

When developing interview questions, it can be useful to involve those with knowledge of the research area in the initial thinking and/or piloting of the questions (Burns et al., 2012). For example, in the research presented by Moule et al. (2011) (see Research example 23.1), members of the Early Stroke Discharge team helped develop some of the interview questions used.

Research example 23.1

Interviews

Interviews were the sole method of data collection in a project undertaken by Moule et al. (2011). The project explored the experiences of Early Stroke Discharge (ESD) team members engaged in the implementation of rehabilitation care in one community and key stakeholders associated with the change. The team had been established with funding from the closure of 10 hospital beds, and included a range of allied health professionals and a nurse.

In total, six team members were interviewed. These included: the team manager, a physiotherapist, an occupational therapist, a nurse, a speech and language therapist and a dietician. Four external key stakeholder interviews were conducted with staff in NHS commissioning in the Primary Care Trust, the intermediate care service and the social care department of the local council.

The interviews lasted approximately one hour each and though guided by the semi-structured interview framework, the conversations allowed the participants to fully share their experiences and reflections.

The ESD team interviews either took place at the team members' place of work, at the university or, in one case, in the respondent's home. Key stakeholders were interviewed in the workplace, at the university or, when a face-to-face meeting was not possible, by telephone. The interviews were digitally recorded and transcribed.

The research questions were generated with input from the ESD team. Before each interview, participants received an interview guide consisting of sample questions. This was used to help them reflect on experiences of working as part of, or with, the ESD team.

Topics addressed with the ESD team respondents included:

- the formation and development of the team and how this linked with local, regional and national policies and frameworks
- the functioning of the team: roles, hierarchy, organisation, strategy

(Continued)

(Continued)

- relations with others, including patients, carers, staff outside the team, wider organisations
- the difficulties and challenges faced
- successes and areas for improvement.

Topics raised with external stakeholders included:

- the role of the respondent's own organisation in supporting stroke patients and carers
- the respondent's involvement in the working of the ESD team and the functioning of the team in relation to existing services and care delivery processes
- feedback received from patients and their carers
- the effectiveness of the team in achieving their objectives
- lessons to be learned and areas for further development/improvement.

Researchers can also involve service users and carers in the development of interview questions, or in their review. This can be particularly important where researchers are interviewing patients or members of the public. When developing questions for interview, it is important to consider a number of factors (see Research example 23.2).

Research example 23.2

Factors to consider when developing interview questions

- The language used should be easily understood.
- The language should avoid being prejudicial.
- The questions should be appropriate for the audience.
- Ambiguity in the question should be avoided.
- A question should ask about one thing at a time.
- Leading questions should be avoided.

In developing the interview guide or schedule, it is useful to include opening questions, which help relax the participant. These might include explaining the study and verifying the participant's understanding of the process. Early questions should also be easy to answer – factual data for example. We see this later on in the interview guide used by Pollard et al. (2010) (see Research example 23.4), where the opening questions ask for organisation and interviewee data. The main questions that require more thought can then be asked. The interview would normally end with a series of more simple questions and checking whether the participant has anything further to add before ending the discussion.

Conducting the interview

Preparation of the interviewer and interviewee is vital (King and Horrocks, 2010). Researchers should be organised for the event, checking recording equipment is available and working. Interview times, the method of collecting interview data and location must be communicated to interviewees in advance. It can be helpful to provide refreshments and ensure a comfortable and accessible environment is made available.

Rehearsing the interview can be a useful exercise and aid the development of technique, skills and refinement of the interview questions. A pilot interview also allows a test of the location or mode of data collection if using telephone or online methods, and ensures that the mode of data collection/location used is conducive to recording conversation (Polit and Beck, 2014). Researchers should also prepare interviewees by providing clear instructions for attendance or engagement in a telephone conversation. In some cases, researchers provide the interviewee with the interview questions prior to the interview date to allow for preparation. At this time, they can also provide consent forms or project information. Additional considerations are required for group interviews, where researchers need to be able to identify the contribution of individual participants, perhaps through allocating numbers or providing instructions asking participants to identify themselves before speaking.

QUALITATIVE INTERVIEWS

Interviews are used in a number of research designs; this said, the approach is seen most frequently in qualitative studies such as phenomenology, evaluation and case study research (for further information on these research designs, see Chapters 16 and 19). The technique is used when the researcher is trying to address questions which relate to exploring personal experience, personal accounts, perceptions, beliefs and opinions. It can also be used to access attitudes. The research example provided illustrates the use of qualitative interviewing to capture the experiences of a group of healthcare professionals and key stakeholders involved in a new service development.

When reading research papers, you will see that a range of terms may be used to describe qualitative interviews, including open, unstructured, in-depth and ethnographic. In this project, we see the use of broad interview prompts and open questions. This allowed the researchers to seek out the participant's perceptions, experiences and opinions, and to undertake a conversation, guided by the opening questions.

In some research approaches, such as ethnography, one open question may act as a prompt for the entire conversation; this allows the participant to drive the interview direction. In this approach, the structure will come from the researcher following up particular issues or areas of interest raised by the participant. It is suggested that in taking this approach the researcher will gain an understanding of social life through interpreting the meaning individuals attach to their experiences (Seidman, 2012).

The project also used both face-to-face and telephone interviewing. This reflects common practice where interviewing often occurs in a face-to-face context, yet the use of telephone interviewing has long seen an increase in popularity (Smith, 2005). Interviewing using other modes of interactive technology via the Internet, through, for example, Skype is also increasing as it offers resource savings whilst still accessing interview data (James and Busher, 2012; Janghorban et al., 2014).

Recording

A digital audio recording was taken in this research (Moule et al., 2011). Interviews need not always be recorded; however, a recording can be used to develop a verbatim or word-for-word transcript. This is needed if researchers want to include quotes from participants to support analysis.

As part of ethical approval processes, it is normally the case that participants should consent to being recorded (King and Horrocks, 2010). They should receive a research information sheet explaining what the research is about and their involvement in it prior to taking part. As part of the consenting process, participants are given the opportunity to refuse to take part in the interview or can agree to take part but refuse to be recorded. In these cases, the conversation should not be recorded. If consenting to recording, then as part of the process the researcher should record the participant confirming consent prior to asking any questions.

When qualitative interviewers want participants to talk about particular experiences, they need to ensure the discussions remain focused on particular topics, and they may need to use questions that re-focus the direction of the conversation. This digital recording (Mould et al., 2011) was also transcribed 'verbatim' or word for word and allowed team analysis, looking for key emergent themes. Either the researcher or a transcription service can produce a verbatim account of the recording and complete transcription.

Rigour

Even though Moule et al. (2011) used some prompt topic areas, we can see that the interviews did not aim to achieve standardisation in the way the data was collected. Allowing the expression of individual thoughts, feelings and experiences enhanced the quality of the data. To maintain rigour in qualitative interviewing, the participant's accounts are presented within any research report or paper, often as anonymous verbatim quotes. This reassures the reader that the data presented reflects the participant's 'voice', allowing the reader to 'hear' the participant's spoken word, a position which is seen to empower the participant by presenting their words in the research (Griffiths, 1998). The researcher often reports seeking verification of the interpretations of data with participants. This might involve asking participants to comment on draft transcripts of the interview and the analysis of this. Such presentation may also be supported by the researcher's reflexive account of the research journey (see Chapter 13).

Ethical issues

Moule et al. (2011) secured ethical approval from the Faculty Research Ethics Committee and the project was registered with the Trust Research and Development Unit (see Chapter 7 for further explanations). Informed consent was obtained from all participants. They were given an information sheet about the evaluation and all signed a consent form prior to the interview.

As the team was small and members were potentially identifiable, the research team discussed issues of anonymity at the outset. The team suggested it might not be possible to anonymise data in such a way as to fully protect the identity of individual members. Whilst the research team presented the findings in a way that would not be attributable to individuals, anonymity could not be fully guaranteed. Key themes generated were therefore returned to the participants for comment and all participants were offered the opportunity to check and change drafts of the final report.

Moule et al.'s project also raises issues of safety for the researchers, particularly as one interview was conducted in a stranger's home. Most organisations have a 'safe researcher policy'. In this case, the organisation's policy recommends notifying the research office of the intended visit and providing contact details. To maintain safety, the researcher informed the rest of the team of the intended interview, including location, and carried a mobile phone and panic alarm.

Reflexivity

Qualitative researchers will often engage in reflexivity during the interview process. This means the researcher will reflect on how individual assumptions, beliefs and emotions impact on their research (Corbin and Strauss, 2015). It is seen as an integral part of the qualitative research process. Being reflexive encourages the researcher to think about their role as an active participant in the research and as a producer of knowledge, rather than as a detached bystander. It requires the researcher to examine themselves as a researcher inside the research relationship. The use of reciprocity in the research interview is one way of supporting reflexivity. This is when the researcher shares their feelings and experiences with the participant, an approach that can be used in feminist research (McNair et al., 2008) and in grounded theory (Corbin and Strauss, 2015).

Continual reflection can impact on the processes of data collection and analysis. It challenges the researcher to reflect on assumptions made about knowledge, what we know to be right. Through reflection new insights can be developed that influence the researcher and the findings. The researcher may document reflections in a research diary or web log and present data from these alongside new knowledge.

Reflective exercise

You have probably been interviewed yourself, either for a place on a course, a job or possibly by a researcher. You also are likely to conduct interviews yourself, asking patients for information or interviewing relatives. Think about your most

(Continued)

(Continued)

recent interview: Did the interviewer help you relax at the start by opening with a conversation and easy questions? What types of questions were you asked: open or closed? Did the interviewer use a pre-determined set of questions throughout or explore particular answers you gave? What were the questions about? What did you think about the place/situation of the interview, e.g. was the interview carried out face-to-face or by telephone or Skype? Is there any way in which you feel the interview could have been improved? What could you learn from that interview to use in your own practice?

QUANTITATIVE INTERVIEWS

Quantitative research designs can be supported through structured and semi-structured interviews. Such interview approaches will involve the use of a pre-determined data collection tool, as seen with structured observations (see Chapter 24), often referred to as an interview schedule (Lodico et al., 2010). The interview may be conducted by telephone, online or in face-to-face contexts, and this includes interviews as part of survey research that might occur in settings such as the supermarket. The interviewer controls the speed of the interview and presents the same set of questions to participants in the same order. Frequently, the questions used offer limited response options, though there can be occasional open response questions. (see Research example 23.3).

Research example 23.3

Structured interview questions

- How frequently do you visit your GP?

  Daily   weekly   monthly   yearly

- How do you travel to see your GP?

  By car   motorbike   bus   train   bicycle   walking

Research example 23.4

Semi-structured interview

Pollard et al. (2010) completed a pilot study that included two phases of data collection. The first phase involved nine agencies delivering services for children and young people, in which one manager from each of two local authority and seven voluntary sector organisations was interviewed using a semi-structured tool developed by the research team with input from service users. The study provided an insight into how agencies delivering services for children and young people used research and evaluation about workforce issues to develop and enhance professional practice. The interviews were conducted by five members of the research team using the same semi-structured data collection tool, and an extract is shown below.

Organisation detail	Size (no. of workers)	Location and type (inner-city/urban/rural/sector/national/local)	Scope of practice	Research strategy? Links/partnerships (HEIs/research centre, etc.)
Interviewee detail	Title	Role	Decision-maker	If interviewee not decision-maker, who?
Training and development	CPD Stakeholders	Team development Stakeholders	In-house training Type + stakeholders	Other Type + stakeholders
Encouragement for use of research evidence	Support		Barriers	
Research-informed practice/project	Description Research base	Rationale	Process (who involved, how implemented)	Benefits Challenges
Impact on practice	Description	How identified	Effect (maintain/change existing practice)	Effective methods for using research
Example of good practice				

Data collected in this semi-structured interview was used to inform sampling for a second stage of data collection – case studies.

We can see that the data collection tool asked specific questions about the organisation and role of the individual being interviewed. It also asks some questions about the training and development being offered, what supports and hinders the inclusion of research evidence use in practice, and then seeks to extract examples of how research has been used and impacted on practice. These questions allow more scope for the respondents to highlight particular areas of good practice, and access more qualitative data.

Using the pre-determined semi-structured interview tool above allowed for a standardised approach to data collection across the research team, minimising error and difference. To aid the process of collecting standardised data, it was useful to pilot the data collection tool. Inviting completion by a sample of participants prior to the main study aided development of the reliability and validity of the measure (Burns et al., 2012). It should be remembered, however, that the researchers also aided the validity of the instrument by helping the participants interpret the questions, so that they were able to provide more relevant answers.

In this project, the researchers were not trained to ask questions in the same way, though providing interviewer training can help increase reliability. It may also be desirable to ensure inter-rater reliability is achieved (see Chapter 24). Using the semi-structured interview schedule enabled Pollard et al. (2010) to yield consistency in responses, measuring what they intended to measure across a number of participants.

FOCUS GROUP INTERVIEWS

Focus group interviews are usually held when the researcher wants to access the opinions and experiences of 5–10 participants simultaneously (Stewart and Shamdasani, 2015). The approach can be a time-efficient way of obtaining the views of a number of participants at once and has the potential to enable rich dialogue. There are, however, some potential challenges for the researcher. Organising access to a number of participants at one time can prove difficult; Barbour and Schostak (2005) also report that problems with group dynamics can affect contributions, with some individuals being more verbose than others. Additionally, maintaining confidentiality can be more problematic. Focus group interviews tend to form part of qualitative research designs and can be part of evaluative research, participatory action research and feminist approaches (Morgan, 2012) (see Chapters 16, 18 and 19).

Research example 23.5

Focus group

Moule et al. (2010) completed research in higher education institutions which explored student experiences and use of learning opportunities mediated through technology. Ethics approval was secured through the host university and copies of this were sent to the participating institutions. The study employed mixed methods of data collection and included focus group interviews involving a total of 41 students across six sites.

The groups were facilitated by two researchers and recorded. The focus group participants had been invited to take part prior to site visits, with students receiving research information sheets and consent forms ahead of the data collection day. The students were asked to introduce themselves prior to recording and submit completed consent forms. The students were asked a series of open questions such as:

- Can you tell us what sort of e-learning you use in your course?
- How were you prepared to use e-learning in your course?
- Can you tell us about your experiences of using e-learning?
- Do you have any ideas about how e-learning use might be developed?
- How do you think you might use e-learning in the future?

The focus groups yielded data that, when analysed, thematically led to the identification of three main themes: 'pedagogic use', 'factors inhibiting use' and 'facilitating factors to engagement'. It transpired that student engagement with e-learning was mainly to access data, with minimal use of interactive technologies.

Focus groups were selected as a method of data collection for a number of reasons. First, they allowed the researchers to access the views of a number of students at one time and were therefore resource-effective. Second, the discussions led to rich data capture as student input was often prompted by the comments of fellow students. Third, the use of focus groups meant there was time available to collect data from staff and undertake documentary analysis during the case study visit. As the groups were facilitated by two researchers and recorded, this enabled effective management of the discussion and ensured all the students were able to participate.

TELEPHONE INTERVIEWS

Research example 23.2 explored the experiences of Early Stroke Discharge (ESD) team members engaged in the implementation of rehabilitation care in one community and key stakeholders associated with the change (Moule et al., 2011). It included the use of telephone interviews with some of the external stakeholders, which reduced travel time and research costs, and afforded access to participants who were widely dispersed. Telephone interviewing can also encourage participation, as the approach is less intrusive and time-consuming for participants, which makes the approach attractive to busy individuals. Despite the potential benefits, the use of the telephone interview needs some consideration. It is suggested that training in interview technique will be required, and there is some concern that the method may not produce the quality of data accessible in face-to-face interview settings (Babbie, 2015). If a standardised data collection tool is used, this will need to be subjected to the same reliability and validity tests as those described in the design of quantitative interview methods, i.e. being piloted and subjected to inter-rater reliability testing.

WHAT ARE THE POWER ISSUES IN INTERVIEWS?

Interviews are often conducted between those of unequal status, power or position. For example, medical and nursing staff working as researchers in a mental health setting may interview vulnerable clients. In the research example above (Moule et al., 2010), members of university staff were interviewing students, therefore introducing an unequal power relationship to the focus groups. There may also be issues arising from differences in race, culture, accent and other personal characteristics that have the potential to affect the power relationships in an interview.

Potential power issues should be reviewed as part of the process of securing ethical approval, to ensure participants are not open to coercion or manipulation. However, the effect of potential differences in power relations on the interview can be hidden or unknown. For example, feminist researchers have criticised unequal power relations within interviews that can relate to differences in status but also in gender (Maynard and Purvis, 1994). Researchers suggest women can remain subordinate in focus groups and interviews and suggest they, the researchers, should aim to achieve symmetry in an interview (Doucet and Mauthner, 2008 ; Hollway and Jefferson, 2013).

One way of balancing the relationship within an interview is to ensure participants understand the study and their role within it so that they are protected from harm.

Table 23.1   Potential strengths and weaknesses of interviews

Strengths	Weaknesses
● Can be a flexible technique allowing the researcher to explore issues in depth	● Individual qualitative interviews can be time-consuming and costly
● Potential to ensure questions are understood, enhancing validity	● Power issues can affect data collection
● Potential for the researcher to seek clarification of meaning from the participant	● Researchers can introduce bias into the interview, especially with less structured interviews
● Structured interviews can collect a large amount of data from a large sample	● Researchers need interview skills to collect quality data
● Focus groups can be time-saving and generate increased dialogue	● Research safety can be an issue
● Telephone interviewing can be resource-saving and attract increased participation rates	● Researchers may collect powerful data which affects them personally
● Response rates can be high	
● Can be a more inclusive data collection method	

It is good practice to provide written research information, which explains the scope of the project, the expectations of the participants and how the data will be collected, stored and disseminated, prior to the event. In a structured or semi-structured interview, informing the participants may include providing the interview questions prior to the event, as reported in the research above (Moule et al., 2011).

WHAT ARE THE ADVANTAGES AND DISADVANTAGES OF INTERVIEWING?

There are a number of strengths of using interviews as a method of data collection, and many have been mentioned in discussing the research examples above (see Table 23.1).

CHAPTER SUMMARY

- A research interview requires skill and training to elicit the quality information needed to answer the research question(s).
- The research interview is a powerful method of collecting data that can enable the researcher to access in-depth, personal information and explore important questions relating to experience and perceptions.
- Interviews can also be guided through an interview guide or more structured interview schedule, enabling the researcher to access a large volume of data from a large sample. Interviews can also be conducted with groups, where, with a well-managed process, researchers can obtain a variety of views and quality data.
- Interviewing can also be undertaken by telephone or Skype, reducing costs and time taken.
- There are a range of ethical and power issues to consider, especially in relation to unequal power status and ensuring neither respondents nor researchers are harmed.

- Interviewing is a popular method of data collection and will be used by a range of researchers, either as the sole method of data collection, or as one within a mixed methods approach.

SUGGESTED FURTHER READING

Brinkmann, S. and Kvale, S. (2015) *Interviews: Learning the Craft of Qualitative Research Interviewing*, 3rd edn. Los Angeles: Sage. This book covers the theory and practice of interviewing. It supports anyone undertaking qualitative interviewing, ethical issues, transcribing data and data analysis.

McKinney, K., Holstein, J., Marvasti, A. and Gubrium, J. (eds) (2012) *The SAGE Handbook of Interview Research*, 2nd edn. Thousand Oaks, CA: Sage. pp. 177–904. This is a detailed text, which covers the history of interviewing through to current techniques. It includes data analysis and ethical issues.

Stewart, D. and Shamdasani, P. (2015) *Focus Groups: Theory and Practice*, 3rd edn. London: Sage. This text includes information on the design, preparation and conduct of focus group interviews. It covers the role of the facilitator and the ways of managing focus groups.

WEBSITES

Social Research Update, University of Surrey: http://sru.soc.surrey.ac.uk/

To access further resources related to this chapter, visit the companion website at http://study.sagepub.com/mouleaveyard3e

REFERENCES

Babbie, E. (2015) *The Practice of Social Research*, 14th edn. Belmont, CA: Wadsworth Cengage Learning.

Barbour, R. and Schostak, J. (2005) 'Interviewing and focus groups', in B. Somekh and C. Lewin (eds), *Research Methods in the Social Sciences*. London: Sage. pp. 41–8.

Burns, N., Grove, S. and Gray, J. (2012) *The Practice of Nursing Research: Appraisal, Synthesis and Generation of Evidence*, 7th edn. St Louis, MO: Elsevier Saunders.

Corbin, J. and Strauss, A. (2015) *Basics of Qualitative Research. Techniques and Procedures for Developing Grounded Theory*. Thousand Oaks, CA: Sage.

Doucet, A. and Mauthner, N. (2008) 'Qualitative interviewing and feminist research' in P. Alasuutari, L. Bickman and J. Brannen (eds), *The SAGE Handbook of Social Research Methods*. London: Sage. pp. 328–43.

Griffiths, M. (1998) *Educational Research for Social Justice: Getting Off the Fence*. Buckingham: Open University Press.

Hollway, W. and Jefferson, T. (2013) *Doing Qualitative Research Differently: A Psychosocial Approach*, 2nd edn. London: Sage.

James, N. and Busher, J. (2012) 'Internet interviewing', in K. McKinney, J. Holstein, A. Marvasti and J. Gubrium (eds), *The SAGE Handbook of Interview Research*, 2nd edn. Thousand Oaks, CA: Sage. pp. 177–192.

Janghorban, R., Roudsari, R-L. and Taghipour, A. (2014) 'Skype interviewing: The new generation of online synchronous interview in qualitative research', *Qualitative Studies on Health and Well-being*, 9. Available at: www.ncbi.nim.nih.gov/pmc/articles/PMC3991833/ (accessed 3 November 2015).

King, N. and Horrocks, S. (2010) *Interviews in Qualitative Research*. London: Sage.

Lodico, M., Spaulding, D. and Voegtle, K. (2010) *Methods in Educational Research: From Theory to Practice*, 2nd edn. San Francisco, CA: Wiley.

Maynard, M. and Purvis, J. (eds) (1994) *Researching Women's Lives from a Feminist Perspective*. London: Taylor & Francis.

McNair, R., Taft, A. and Hegarty, K. (2008) 'Using reflexivity to enhance in-depth interviewing skills for clinical researchers', *BMC Medical Research Methodology*, 8: 1–8.

Morgan, D. (2012) 'Focus groups and social interaction', in K. McKinney, J. Holstein, A. Marvasti and J. Gubrium (eds), *The SAGE Handbook of Interview Research*, 2nd edn. Thousand Oaks, CA: Sage. pp. 161–76.

Moule, P., Ward, R. and Lockyer, L. (2010) 'Nursing and healthcare students' experiences and use of e-learning in higher education', *Journal of Advanced Nursing*, 66 (12): 2785–95.

Moule, P., Young, P., Glowgoska, M. and Weare, J. (2011) 'Early Stroke Discharge team: A participatory evaluation', *International Journal of Rehabilitation and Therapy*, 18 (6): 319–28.

Polit, D. and Beck, C. (2014) *Essentials of Nursing Research: Appraising Evidence for Nursing Practice*, 8th edn. Philadelphia, PA: Lippincott Williams & Wilkins.

Pollard, K., Moule, P., Evans, D., Donald, C., Donskoy, A. and Rice, C. (2010) *User Engagement in the Co-production of Knowledge for Knowledge Exchange in Health and Social Care*, Project Report. Bristol: University of the West of England. Available at: https://eprints.uwe.ac.uk/15246/ (accessed 3 November 2015).

Seidman, I. (2012) *Interviewing as Qualitative Research: A Guide for Researchers in Education and the Social Sciences*. New York: Teachers College Press.

Smith, E. (2005) 'Telephone interviewing in healthcare research: A summary of the evidence', *Nurse Researcher*, 12 (3): 32–41.

Stewart, D. and Shamdasani, P. (2015) *Focus Groups: Theory and Practice*, 3rd edn. London: Sage.

24

OBSERVATIONS

Learning outcomes

This chapter will enable you to:

- appreciate the differences between structured and unstructured observation
- understand the participant observer role
- understand the ethical issues that arise from the use of observation as a data collection tool in healthcare research
- understand the strengths and limitations of using observation as a data collection tool

Observation is one of the key ways in which nurse and healthcare practitioners collect data to inform their practice and care delivery. This may often involve observing how patients look, how they are moving and how they are behaving. Observation can also be a useful data collection tool in research. Researchers interested in studying a range of human behaviours and actions may use observation as a sole method of data collection or may use a mixed methods approach, perhaps combining observation with interviewing or a questionnaire survey.

In this chapter, we review the two main types of observation methods researchers are likely to use, referred to as structured and unstructured observations. Research papers are used to illustrate these approaches. We consider issues of observation sampling and explore how observation data are recorded. Finally, we review the main strengths and limitations of observation as a method of data collection in nursing and healthcare research.

WHAT IS OBSERVATIONAL RESEARCH?

Nursing practice includes the use of observation skills, drawing to different degrees on the four senses – touch, sight, smell and sound – to formulate patient assessment. Though nurses will often base judgements on what they see and hear, data collection tools such as temperature recording devices and blood pressure recording machines can provide detailed physiological measurement data to support assessment. Nurses become competent in their use of observation and use these skills, and tools, to collect patient data and support care delivery.

Used in research, observation is viewed as one of the most important methods of data collection (Jones and Somekh, 2011), which aims to provide a direct record of human behaviour and action. In contrast to some of the less formal observations undertaken in practice situations, researchers approach observation methods in a systematic and purposeful way, as they are charged with collecting particular data in order to address research questions.

Observations can be used in different research designs, such as qualitative and quantitative research, and may be used in conjunction with other data collection methods such as interviews and questionnaires. The selection and use of observation methods in any research design should be appropriate to the research question(s) being asked. Research questions requiring the exploration of phenomena such as communication, non-verbal interactions and activity, which might include the delivery of psychomotor skills, can usefully employ observations. Observation can be focused on recording the behaviours of individuals and groups, but in some cases the intention may be to observe other factors that affect care delivery, such as resource availability or the use of guidelines and tools to support practice. Research questions seeking to explore issues of experience, beliefs and knowledge, are best addressed through other forms of data collection, such as interviews (see Chapter 23) and questionnaires (see Chapter 22).

Observations can be used as either the sole method of data collection or within a mixed methods approach. Mixed methods or research that includes the triangulation of data sources has become increasingly popular within nursing and healthcare research. This reflects the complex nature of the research, which often demands the use of multiple data sources in order to allow the exploration of research questions. Mixed methods approaches can improve the validity of a study, as they draw on multiple reference points to address research questions and avoid the potential biases of using a single data collection method or source. Mixed methods will also allow the researcher to verify 'what they see'. Basing interpretations on and drawing conclusions from observation alone can be limiting to the researcher. Often, the researcher needs to understand what they see, as well as describe it. For example, Manias et al. (2005) created an observation schedule to support research that looked at how graduate nurses used protocols to manage patients' medication. The data recorded gave detail on the action taken by nurses, but the additional use of interviews allowed the researchers to understand and interpret the nurses' behaviour, something observations alone could not have revealed.

In general, there are two different observation methods available for use, described as structured and unstructured approaches.

STRUCTURED OBSERVATIONS

The research team, often including service users, will have agreed the phenomenon or subject of the observation and either obtained a suitable data collection tool that has been used previously or developed one for the purposes of the research. The observation tool is likely to be highly structured and can include a checklist of tick-boxes or rating scales (for further explanation, see Chapter 24). The research example below includes the use of a pre-designed and structured tool to support the observation and recording of basic life support skills.

Research example 24.1

Example of structured observation

Moule et al. (2008) completed a pilot study to investigate whether a computer-based learning package, followed by practical instruction and traditional classroom methods, was comparable in developing knowledge and skills in basic life support with automated external defibrillator use.

Structured observation formed part of the study which aimed to:

- measure the number of ventilations and compressions without errors and compare between the groups
- measure the time taken to deliver the first shock and compare these recordings between the groups
- observe performance in the 30 procedural steps involved in resuscitating a collapsed casualty and compare between the groups.

Methods

Eighty-three mental healthcare professionals were allocated to one of two groups for the research: 28 completed an e-learning package and the remaining 55 received delivery of the same content in a classroom setting. Both groups were able to practise basic life support skills using a Laerdal© Recording Anne Manikin (Laerdal (UK) Limited, Kent, UK) for one hour before testing. Staff from the groups were tested individually and were given the same scenario, and asked to attend to a collapsed person without signs of life. A telephone and automated external defibrillator were some distance away from the manikin, but available for use.

Collecting the data

The Laerdal© Recording Anne Manikin software (VAM version 1.12.11), calibrated before use, collected the measurement of performance on chest compressions, ventilations and airway management. The Cardiff test (Whitfield et al., 2003) was used to collect the observation data. The test was pre-validated and included 30 sequenced steps to assess performance of basic life support and automated external defibrillator use. One observer completed the Cardiff test checklist.

The types of questions included on the test were:

Switch on automated external defibrillator	2. Performed	1. Not performed
Compressions: Average number of compressions of the chest delivered (obtained from the manikin data)	Insert number	

Results

Analysis of the 30 observed procedural steps revealed a small variation in performance between the groups, though these were not statistically significant differences. The e-learning group was slightly better than the classroom group in 21 of the 30 steps and performed particularly well in initial safety checks before using the automated external defibrillator.

In the study above, we can see that the use of a structured observation tool can aid reliability in data recording, as the researcher is making judgements about particular behaviours or events within defined parameters. However, there can still be issues of inter-rater reliability, where two or more researchers may interpret the same situation differently and thus select different question responses. Research papers will often report pilot work that measured the degree of inter-rater reliability seen. Two or more observers would be asked to record their interpretations of the same event or behaviour. The findings would be subject to statistical analysis using, for example, a Cohen's kappa test (see McHugh, 2012). Achieving a score of 1.00 indicates total agreement between observers and a score of 0.60 or less would be less reliable than desired, as it suggests that only 6 out of every 10 events observed will be scored the same. For example, Whitfield et al. (2003), when developing the Cardiff test used above, recruited six observers to evaluate performance using the test. A Cohen's kappa score showed inter-observer reliability was 0.7 or 70 per cent (satisfactory), for 85 per cent of the variables in the tool. This level of reliability meant it, the tool, could be 'reliably' used within the pilot study to record participants' performance in the steps in the skill of basic life support.

The research example above also shows us that observation tools can be used to provide a numerical score, giving the ability to measure. Consequently, if a highly structured tool is used, where the results can be readily qualified, the approach can support quantitative research designs (see Chapter 11).

Whilst structured observation enabled the research team to achieve the initial research aims, it is clear that if the team had been interested in explaining why the participants performed the skill in the way they did, or indeed if there had been research questions about the experience of learning through electronic or classroom needs, then the researchers would have needed to collect data through other means as well, such as interviews.

The presentation above included key information to help with a critical review of the study. The researchers provided detail on what was observed and how these observations were recorded. The validity of the tool is discussed, including how inter-rater reliability was established, and there is reference to the consistency of test application. Detail on the context of the observational test is also provided. This level of detail enables you, as the reader, to complete a critical review of a paper. It will be difficult to draw conclusions about the quality of a piece of observational research if you are unclear how the data was collected, how the tool used was validated and what was observed. It is also important to know what the context or setting of the research was and the role of the researcher within that environment. All of these factors can have an impact on the quality of the data collected.

Research example 24.2

Structured observation as part of a qualitative mixed-methods study

Vaismoradi et al. (2014) explored how nurse leaders support safe care delivery from the perspectives of nurses and nurse leaders in Iran. Using a purposive sample of

20 nurses (16 nurses and four head nurses) in total, semi-structured interviews and 10 hours of structured observation were conducted. The observer occupied a non-participant role on both medical and surgical wards, recording the activities of the head nurses. The researcher recorded the performance of daily tasks and facilitation of care delivery. Observation notes were also recorded. The notes were read and divided into meaningful units. The observational data was used with the interview data to support theme development.

Observation sampling

Structured observations are applied in relation to either time sampling (choosing a particular timeframe to record observations) or event sampling (selecting events to observe, which requires some knowledge of patterns of events) (Polit and Beck, 2014). In our Research example 24.1 above, the structured observation was applied to events, recording responses to a collapsed and unresponsive casualty. The entire event was captured on the structured observation sheet and was the sampling unit. In this case, all events were captured, whereas in our Research example 24.2 the researcher selected the events or sampling units for observation, which included 10 hours of observations.

If observing how drugs are administered, the researcher may want to sample particular 'drug rounds' as the events. Manias et al. (2005), mentioned earlier, created an observation schedule to support research that looked at how graduate nurses used protocols to manage patients' medication. They centred the observations on a two-hour period when medications were administered. They could have structured the observations around particular days of the week or specific times of drug administration, such as looking at all of the lunchtime rounds across a week or taking all drug administration events within a day.

Vaismoradi et al. (2014) above were interested in observing staff interactions; they could have used a time sampling frame to structure the observation period, perhaps making observations at five-minute intervals across a certain time period. The periods of observation become the sampling units. There may be other factors which affect the selected time period of observation. For example, the researchers may want to structure the observation periods to include a specific time of the day when staff are felt to engage in interactions with the multi-disciplinary team. This may include undertaking observations of the morning ward round or afternoon patient handover. In a community setting, the researcher may want to observe team meetings occurring at the start of the day.

Intermittent observation sampling periods may not always yield the data required. In some circumstances, the researcher may need to undertake continuous observations throughout a 24-hour period. This approach would be necessary if the researcher was interested in recording unpredictable behaviour, such as observing changes in behaviour. Longer observation periods would form the sampling units, when it is hoped that any changes in behaviour might be observed.

Research example 24.3

An observation schedule of interactions with a multi-disciplinary team

Time/Patient	Betty	Jenny	Julia	Elaine
0900	A, D	K	C	J
0905	/	K	M	J
0910	/	K	M	L
0915	G, E, F, D	K	B	L

etc.

Key:

A = healthcare assistant	B = student nurse
	D = ward manager
C = qualified nurse	F = registrar
E = junior doctor	H = cleaner
G = consultant	J = dietician
I = social worker	L = occupational
K = physiotherapist	therapist
M = other	

UNSTRUCTURED OBSERVATIONS

In contrast to structured observations, **unstructured observations** are not guided by a pre-determined checklist schedule; rather, the researchers are trying to remain open to record events or behaviour which occurs naturally. However, though described as unstructured, this approach to observation is not completely unguided. The researchers are guided by the research questions and will have a focus to their data collection, but are not tied to completing specific data collection tools. This approach is often referred to as **naturalistic observation**, with the researcher adopting the role of participant observer, taking part in the daily functioning of the setting under observation (Polit and Beck, 2014).

Research example 24.4

Unstructured observation

Research undertaken by Eriksson et al. (2010) employed an open observation approach. The observations took place in an intensive care environment, with the observer taking a non-participant observation role (see below). The research aimed to collect observational data, which would allow the research team to interpret the interplay between a critically ill patient and their next of kin. The participants met a number of selection criteria including: they were ≤ 18 years old; the reason for admission was a serious or acute illness; they were within an intensive care environment for ≥ 48 hours; they were ventilated for ≥ 24 hours; and relatives visited at least once. The next of kin visits were unrestricted. The patients were cared for in a two-bedded room, by two nurses.

Family members provided informed consent prior to the study, and consent was subsequently sought from the patients following initial treatment.

Data was collected by the lead researcher, who was not involved in the hands-on care delivery, but had an administrative and education role on the unit. The data collected focused on the interplay between patients and family members, recorded over periods of time, with the maximum being two hours. The recordings were unstructured reflective notes, with a transcript of the interaction being recorded and analysed by considering the text as a script for a play with a discussion of the context (scene), people (actors) and actions (plot).

The findings suggested that the intensive care environment inhibited interplay. The environment was felt to be designed to enable the delivery of medical care and the use of technical machinery, rather than being conducive to interactions which are also important to recovery.

The above example demonstrates the strengths of the non-participatory observation role. In this role, the researcher was able to concentrate on recording interactions between patients and relatives and ensure observational data were captured. The researcher also avoided the potential difficulties of undertaking participatory research, where the researcher has to occupy a dual role of professional care-giver and researcher. Those in participatory roles may find tension occurs as they aim to collect research data whilst delivering care. This can create ethical issues and affect the quality of either care delivery or data recording. However, non-participant observations also bring some potential disadvantages. The presence of a non-participant observer can create the 'Hawthorne effect' in research (described in more detail below), where a participant changes their behaviour in response to being 'observed'. The impact of the 'Hawthorne effect' is lessened through the use of extended two-hour observation slots over a period of 48 hours.

The research above provides insight into the type of observation, level of participation and involvement with participants. These are important factors to consider when you complete a critical review of a research paper of an observational study. Information on the research aims, selection of participants and criteria for inclusion are also provided by Eriksson et al. (2010) to allow readers to judge the appropriateness of the design. The researchers also provide information on the ethical principles being followed to protect vulnerable participants. When reading other research papers, you will need this level of explanation to help with the critical review.

Observer roles

Ethnographic research designs (see Chapter 15) have relied in part on participant observation, with its inclusion also seen in other qualitative designs such as grounded theory (see Chapter 15) and case study research (see Chapter 19). Early anthropological studies (Malinowski, 1922) describe the participant observer role used to study people in their natural environments, and Leininger (1998) suggests there are four phases of observation–participation. These include:

- Phase one: primarily observation.
- Phase two: primarily observation with some participation.

- Phase three: primarily participation with some observation.
- Phase four: reflective observation of impact.

This model would see the researcher having a period of initiation into the research setting, getting to know the research environment and participants, with observation being the focus here. Gradually, participation increases, as the researcher learns from the group and environment and then from their own experiences as participants in the group. Final reflections allow consideration of the entire observational period. Obviously, the role of the participant observer may differ according to the context of the research; in some settings, it may not be possible to adopt a role that involves participation in patient care delivery.

Classifications of the observer role were offered by Gold as long ago as 1958, when it was suggested that an observer could operate as a complete participant, participant-as-observer, observer-as-participant or complete observer. This definition is problematic in today's research environment as the complete participant was described as acting without revealing a research interest, as a covert (hidden) observer. It is inconceivable that ethical approval would be granted today for any research design that included 'hidden'/covert data collection, such as that described by Clarke (1996), who used eavesdropping as part of secret participant observation to look at the concept of the therapeutic community in a mental health forensic unit. It is more probable that researchers would operate in an overt (open) role and be known to the research participants, using observations as one of a range of data collection methods within one study, and undertake the study for a limited time period, given the costs of using prolonged observation methods.

DATA RECORDING

The presence of researchers in a healthcare, or any other, environment will always have an impact on those being observed, affecting behaviour and possibly performance. Held up as the 'Hawthorne effect', the impact of the observer on the performance of the observed has been reported over many years. The phenomenon originates from management research conducted in the USA in the 1930s that considered the effect of increased lighting provision on productivity in the Hawthorne factory of Western Electric. The researchers concluded that increases in worker productivity were linked to the effect of observation rather than environmental changes (Roethlisberger and Dickson, 1939). Obviously, the length of observation period and the degree of intrusion brought about by the researcher role assumed would affect the extent to which the 'Hawthorne effect' impacts on the research environment. The longer the period of observation, the more likely the researcher is to 'blend in' with the environment.

The advent of technology often replaces the need to take field notes and may enable researchers to capture data without having to physically locate themselves in the research environment. Visual recordings are available (see Jones and Somekh, 2011) and may help in achieving inter-observer reliability, though are not necessarily as responsive and spontaneous as field-based researchers.

ETHICAL ISSUES

The use of observation as a method of data collection brings with it a number of ethical issues. Observation is an intrusive form of data collection, where researchers can spend long periods of time observing, recording and drawing interpretations from periods of activity, behaviour and communication. Ethical approvals for observation studies would require the researcher to gain informed consent from the participants, as seen in the research by Eriksson et al. (2010). In this case, consent from family members was secured initially, followed by consent from the patients when they had recovered from the initial intensive care period. When informed consent is in place, the researcher is required to maintain confidentiality; however, the reporting of observations can compromise both the maintenance of confidence and anonymity. In these cases, participants should be warned in advance before they agree to participate (see Chapter 8). Researchers may also find themselves in situations where information needs to be disclosed in the public interest, when the health and safety of anyone has or could be compromised. For example, had Eriksson et al. (2010) observed unsafe practice, the maintenance of confidentiality would have been reviewed.

Observation studies can also create situations where the researcher is faced with ethical dilemmas. When we watch nature programmes, the recording often portrays animals in danger, but the cameraman continues to film and the producers don't intervene. The observer in a patient's home or hospital environment may experience situations when patients are in danger. In these cases, the researcher will act to prevent harm to the patient rather than maintaining a non-participant role. In many cases, the need to take action to prevent, for example, a fall or accident, will be clear; in other situations, the need for intervention will be less clear and left to researcher judgement.

WHAT ARE THE ADVANTAGES AND DISADVANTAGES OF OBSERVATIONAL RESEARCH?

There are a number of strengths of using observation as a method of data collection, and many have been mentioned in discussing the research examples above (see Table 24.1).

CHAPTER SUMMARY

- Researchers interested in studying a range of human behaviours and actions may use observation as the sole form of data collection or combine it with other methods as part of a mixed-methods approach.
- Observation methods can be employed in both quantitative and qualitative research studies.
- Structured observation tools, such as that used by Moule et al. (2008), provide standardised data used to address specific research questions in a quantitative study.

Table 24.1 Potential strengths and weaknesses of **observational methods**

Strengths	Weaknesses
• Observation methods can be used to collect data from real-life situations and events • Real-time events/natural environments can be recorded • Can be focused on recording the behaviour of individuals and groups • Used as one of a range of data collection methods, observation methods have the potential to verify individual perceptions of practice with actual conduct	• Research using observation methods can be time-consuming and costly • Potential difficulties can arise when trying to access research environments • Inter-rater reliability scores need consideration • Observers can bias data collection by focusing on preferred issues • The 'Hawthorne effect' can impact on the research outcomes • Observation methods are intrusive and require careful ethical consideration • Observer attention to detail can relax over time • The observer may 'miss' crucial data, particularly in busy environments or if consideration is not given to positioning relative to activity

In this study, a pre-designed and validated tool was employed to measure the development of competency in a specific skill.

• In contrast, observations in a qualitative design are more likely to be unstructured, allowing the researcher scope to respond to what is observed in the local environment. Eriksson et al. (2010) recorded reflective notes of the interactions between critically ill patients and their family members in an intensive care unit, with a transcript of the interaction being recorded and analysed by considering the text as a script for a play, with a discussion of the context (scene), people (actors) and actions (plot). This allowed the researchers to draw themes and theories to inform future practice.

• Researchers using observations must be mindful of particular ethical issues that can arise, particularly around the invasion of privacy, intrusion and the potential difficulties of maintaining confidentiality and anonymity. These can be particularly pertinent when using unstructured observation over a prolonged period of time.

SUGGESTED FURTHER READING

Robinson, S. (2013) 'The relevancy of ethnography to nursing', *Nursing Science Quarterly*, 26 (1): 14-16. This article offers useful insight into the relevance of ethnography as an approach in nursing practice.

Pillsbury Pavlish, C. and Dexheimer Pharris, M. (2012) *Community-based Collaborative Action Research: A Nursing Approach*. London: Jones & Bartlett. This text provides information that can be accessed at introductory level. It looks at community-based action research, providing a framework for action research, which can be used to support health outcomes and systems improvement.

Bradbury, H. (ed.) (2015) *The SAGE Handbook of Action Research: Participative Inquiry and Practice*, 3rd edn. London: Sage. This is a book which includes the theory and practice of action research, and a helpful range of exemplars.

WEBSITES

Social Research Update, University of Surrey: http://sru.soc.surrey.ac.uk/

To access further resources related to this chapter, visit the companion website at http://study.sagepub.com/mouleaveyard3e

REFERENCES

Clarke, L. (1996) 'Participant observation in a secure unit: Care, conflict and control', *NT Research*, 1 (6): 431–40.

Eriksson, T., Lindahl, B. and Bergbom, I. (2010) 'Visits in an intensive care unit: An observational hermeneutic study', *Intensive and Critical Care Nursing*, 29 (1): 51–6.

Gold, R. (1958) 'Roles in sociological field observations', *Social Forces*, 36: 213–17.

Jones, L. and Somekh, B. (2011) 'Observations', in B. Somekh and C. Lewin (eds), *Theory and Methods in Social Research*, 2nd edn. London: Sage. pp. 131–9.

Leininger, M. (1998) *Qualitative Research Methods in Nursing*. Philadelphia, PA: W.B. Saunders Co.

Malinowski, B. (1922) *Argonauts of the Western Pacific*. London: Routledge & Kegan Paul.

Manias, E., Aitken, R. and Dunning, T. (2005) 'How graduate nurses use protocols to manage patients' medication', *Journal of Clinical Nursing*, 14 (8): 935–44.

McHugh, M. (2012) 'Interrater reliability: The kappa statistic', *Biochem Med*, 22 (3): 276–82.

Moule, P., Albarran, J., Bessant, E., Pollock, J. and Brownfield, C. (2008) 'A comparison of e-learning and classroom delivery of basic life support with automated external defibrillator use: A pilot study', *International Journal of Nursing Practice*, 14 (6): 427–34.

Polit, D. and Beck, C. (2014) *Essentials of Nursing Research: Appraising Evidence for Nursing Practice*, 8th edn. Philadelphia, PA: Lippincott Williams & Wilkins.

Roethlisberger, F. and Dickson, W. (1939) *Management and the Worker*. Cambridge, MA: Harvard University Press.

Vaismoradi, M., Bondas, T., Salali, M., Jasper, M. and Turunen, H. (2014) 'Facilitating safe care: A qualitative study of Iranian nurse leaders', *Journal of Nursing Management*, 22 (1): 106–16.

Whitfield, R., Newcombe, R. and Woollard, M. (2003) 'Reliability of the Cardiff Test of basic life support and automated external defibrillation', *Resuscitation*, 59 (3): 291–314.

25

OTHER METHODS OF DATA COLLECTION

Learning outcomes

This chapter will enable you to:

- appreciate how tests, scales and measurements are used to collect data
- understand the strengths and limitations of different methods of data collection
- demonstrate the use of critical appraisal questions to review data collection methods
- understand the ethical issues that arise from the use of different methods of data collection

In earlier chapters (22–24), we discussed some of the main methods of data collection, including questionnaires, interviews and observations. In this chapter, we present other data collection tools available to nurse researchers, demonstrating the application of a variety of methods to the research setting.

TRIANGULATION IN DATA COLLECTION

Triangulation of data source and method is increasingly popular in research studies within nursing and healthcare, as researchers are often investigating complex issues that benefit from the use of multiple data sources or mixed methods. Triangulation is thought to improve the validity of a study, by drawing on multiple reference points to address research questions. Studies that employ triangulation in data collection are hoping to overcome the potential biases of using a single data collection method or source. Further discussion on the use of mixed methods in research is presented in Chapter 21. It is worth highlighting here, however, that in reviewing methods of data collection it should be remembered that different combinations of approaches could be employed within one study.

USING TESTS, SCALES AND MEASUREMENTS

Often, nurse researchers need to collect data in a way that allows for mathematical measurement, using tests and **scales** as part of interview schedules or questionnaires. Scales are measurement instruments that can be used to obtain an overall score. There are many scales available for use in healthcare research (see Bowling, 2005). Physiological measures are also important in research and are used in daily practice to collect patient data. The most frequently used nursing measurements include recording temperature, pulse and blood pressure. Though full discussion is beyond the scope of this book, it is worth mentioning the use of scales in health economic evaluations, which are becoming more important in addressing issues related to the allocation and use of healthcare resources. Health economists are often part of research and evaluation projects where there is a need to evaluate the financial benefit of a particular service. Health economists draw on a range of standardised tools to undertake an evaluation of impact and benefit (see Bowling, 2005). This chapter considers those tests, scales and measurements most commonly used in healthcare research.

Vignettes

Vignettes allow the researcher to present descriptions of incidents or situations, conjuring up images of real-life scenarios, to which the participants can respond. The scenarios can elicit information as to the participant's perceptions, opinions or knowledge about a particular situation (Polit and Beck, 2014). Though usually written up, the vignette can be presented as a digital recording or acted out in real life. Participants are usually asked either to respond to an open question about the scenario, such as 'What would you do now?', or are asked to answer a closed question that relates to recording a measurement on a scale or selecting a multiple-choice response (see Research example 25.1). The approach offers a way of exploring situations that may not be readily available in practice and a more resource-effective way of capturing how individuals might behave in certain situations. It should be noted, however, that actual behaviour may vary from that recorded in response to a contrived event.

Research example 25.1

The use of a vignette

Lawton et al. (2011) used vignettes to collect data from a sample of 98 mothers who had at least one child aged between 0 and 4 years. The study sought to investigate how the outcome of care and relationship with a care provider impact on decisions about making a complaint and aspects of responsibility and blame. Four vignettes were included in a questionnaire. The vignettes were developed using previous research findings and through discussions with midwives, breastfeeding support workers and women attending new mother and baby support groups. A senior community midwife, who provided final expert

(Continued)

(Continued)

review for accuracy, also verified them. The mothers were invited to rate each vignette using a 5-point rating scale, which addressed areas such as appropriateness of behaviour, how likely they would be to complain, how much the midwife was responsible and to blame and how serious was the outcome. They found that the seriousness of the outcome is most likely to lead to a complaint, suggesting that patients are less likely to complain because of a poor relationship with a carer.

We can see in this example that the researchers drew on existing evidence and consulted a range of key stakeholders in the development of the vignettes. In addition, expert review of the final statements was conducted. The rigour seen in development is essential to ensure robust data collection. In this design, structured responses to the vignettes were required and allowed the researchers to measure attributions of responsibility and likelihood of making a complaint. This data collection approach allowed exploration of poor practice in an ethical and rigorous way.

Rating scales

These form the most basic type of scale measurement. The researcher will compose statements that are 'rated' by the participant (see Research example 25.2) and a score is then given to the assessment or judgement made. The scales can be used to support observational measurement and can record measures of satisfaction, though caution should be exercised when constructing the statements, as extreme options are unlikely to be chosen (Burns et al., 2014).

Research example 25.2

A completed rating scale

Please rate from 1 (low) to 5 (high) the following satisfaction statements in relation to the library service:

Provision of electronic resources	(5)
Quiet working environment	(4)
Provision of inter-library loans	(1)
Range of textbooks	(3)
Opening hours	(2)

Likert scales

The most commonly used scale is that known as the **Likert scale**, composed of a number of statements on a topic, with participants being asked to identify to what extent they agree or disagree with a statement. Commonly, the statements will be both positively and negatively worded, with four or five possible responses being offered. These usually include strongly agree, agree, disagree and strongly disagree, with the fifth option being a neutral, neither agree nor disagree. The researcher scores the responses from 1 to 4 or 5, with a high score being achieved both for agreement with a positive statement and for disagreement with a negative statement. This reversal is required to ensure that a high score reflects a consistently positive attitude to the subject being measured (Polit and Beck, 2014). The scores for each statement are totalled to achieve a final score, with the higher scoring individuals having a more positive attitude to the subject. Research example 25.3 gives an example of how a Likert scale can be used.

Research example 25.3

The use of a Likert scale

Igarashi et al. (2012) undertook a cross-sectional survey in Japan involving 8,000 subjects. The research aimed to develop a scale to evaluate feelings of support and security regarding cancer care and to measure factors associated with security. A Likert scale was used to measure sense of security. The participants were asked to rate against five statements on a 7-point scale. The statements included: 'If I get cancer – (1) I would feel secure in receiving cancer treatment; (2) My pain would be well relieved' (p. 218). Results for the five items were aggregated and the researchers found participants in those regions with limited availability of palliative care services had a lower sense of security. The findings enabled the research team to develop a new scale to evaluate sense of security.

The scales used here offered 7-point scoring and the responses were used to develop a new scale. The approach allowed the team to engage with a large sample set. However, the five statements rated were all positive; there were no negatively worded statements, which might have ensured that high scores reflected a consistently positive attitude to the subject.

Visual analogue scale

The **visual analogue scale (VAS)** is most often used to measure feelings and attitudes. The scale is a line, usually 100 mm in length, with end points providing two extreme values. Frequently used as a measure of pain, the end points can be labelled as 'no pain' and 'pain unbearable'. The researcher asks the participant to mark their 'pain' on the scale, and the distance from the left end of the line to the mark is measured to provide the value.

Measuring reliability of the scale can be problematic, as a single measure is obtained for what is a complex and individual feeling. Despite this, it is suggested that the scale provides a more sensitive measure than rating or numerical scales (Burns et al., 2014). Whilst there is a range of tests and scales available, the researcher may need to develop a tailored data collection tool to answer a specific research question. Any new tool will require development and piloting to establish reliability and validity (see Chapter 13).

Physiological and biological measures

Physiological and biological measurement usually involves the use of specialist equipment, which can involve a cost to the research, and require training. Healthcare staff undertake a number of measurements as part of routine care. Radiographers complete anatomical measurement through examining radiographic images, and physiological measurement is completed by nurses when assessing a patient's pulse and blood pressure. Further measurements include the chemical composition of blood and urine and microbiological measurements of cultures and specimens (see Research example 25.4). Physiological measurements can be taken **in vitro**, when testing samples of blood in a laboratory, or **in vivo**, when recording the pulse in the presence of the participant.

As the measurements are precise and sensitive, they are objective and seen as highly reliable. Provided the equipment used is functioning with accuracy and is used correctly, the data recorded with the instrument at the same time by different researchers will be consistent. This objectivity allows the researcher to use recorded measurements to determine individual reactions to events, such as response to stress, and to compare reactions between a control and an experimental group (see Chapter 14). Though the instruments may be reliable in measuring what they are expected to accurately and consistently, they also need to be valid and collect data that is needed (see Chapter 13).

When using physiological measures, the researcher will need to consider the following:

- What factors might affect the measurement (the dependent and independent variables)? This might include age, diagnosis and effect of activity such as drinking hot fluids prior to temperature recording.
- How will data be collected? Are instruments calibrated, what is the procedure for use and has training been given?
- When will the measurements be taken (frequency and timing)?
- Can factors in the environment be controlled if needed (for example, consistency may be needed in room temperature or in physical surroundings)?

Research example 25.4

Research using physiological measures

Reimer and Mehler (2011) used physiological measures in research exploring the capability of physiological indices to determine changes in driver workload and related impact on driving safety. A sample of 26 male drivers aged between 22 and 27 years needed to meet a number of inclusion and exclusion criteria. The men were asked to drive a vehicle, and whilst doing this additional secondary tasks were introduced at three different levels of complexity. Whilst undertaking the task, physiological measures were recorded including electrocardiograph monitoring, which recorded changes in heart rate pattern. Additionally, skin conductance level changes were recorded. Both of these measures are expected to increase when aroused and workload increases. The researchers had controlled for a number of variables such as age of the men and driving experience. The frequency and timing of measurements were also considered and standardised.

The potential strengths and weaknesses of using scales, tests and measures in research are set out below.

Potential strengths:

- Scales and tests are often used in interviews or as part of questionnaires.
- Scales can be used to translate responses into a numerical score.
- Vignettes allow for the collection of data about perceived behaviour.
- Vignettes can be used to explore contrived practice situations with less instruction.

Potential limitations:

- Developing the reliability of a scale or test can be problematic.
- Measurements usually involve the use of equipment, bringing a cost to the researcher and training requirements.

USING DOCUMENTS

Documents are socially produced material that can include written records, photographs, video and audio recordings. The range of documents available for use in research is therefore vast, and includes official government statistics through to private diaries, letters and photographic records.

Types of documents

The main types of documents used are public records. These can include records of births, deaths and marriages, census material and the UK Electoral Register, political and judicial records such as records from court cases and budget or fiscal records, and documents from government departments including crime statistics or educational records. These records include quantifiable data, and are perceived as being objective data. However, it should be remembered that data collected to meet government agendas might reflect the political biases of the time.

The media publish case law in the *Times Law Reports*, with the mass popular media presenting a view of social practices and values through broadsheets and tabloids, magazines, television and radio. These are often written or produced for mass audiences, appealing to the readership and viewing public. Literature and the arts can provide public material for analysis, though as documentary sources these are often under-used (Bowling, 2005).

Personal papers, diaries (see the section later in this chapter on diaries), letters and photographs or video recordings reconstruct events and tell individual stories. These are often private records, collected unofficially.

Within healthcare, researchers have access to a number of documents that fall into official and unofficial realms, including patient case notes, nursing care plans, and patient letters or diaries of treatment experiences. Researchers also draw on literature published online and in journals or textbooks. Some of the material collected in the health service over a number of years becomes archive data (see the section later in this chapter on archive material).

The analysis of documentary sources can be either quantitative, when extracting data from statistical records, or qualitative, in considering diary narratives. These documentary records can inform both quantitative and qualitative research designs (see Chapter 11).

Issues of document use

There are several advantages in the use of documents. Data are generally free from researcher bias, as documents are constructed without researcher input. Additionally, they can be convenient to access, there are fewer ethical issues involved and there can be resource savings. Databases often provide large sources of data with records reflecting information gathered over time.

Despite these benefits, researchers have criticised documentary research because those documents falling outside official statistics are seen as subjective and reflecting society's biases (Bowling, 2005). Researchers have to be convinced of the accuracy and representativeness of any documents used. The potential strengths and weaknesses of using documents in research are set out below.

Potential strengths:

- Can remove the potential for researcher bias.
- Can be cost-effective.
- Can be an efficient approach to collecting data.

Potential limitations:

- Data may be incomplete and unusable, as it was not originally collected for research purposes.
- There may be inaccuracies, bias or errors in the data.

It is possible for documents to be falsified and they can provide an inaccurate account of events. Accounts in diaries, letters or literature may be exaggerated or distorted and be affected by the biases of the writer. The researcher will also need to consider whether the available documents constitute a representative sample of the scope of documents as they originally existed or whether particular documents are missing, which can be the case when materials are archived.

LIFE HISTORY AND BIOGRAPHICAL MATERIAL

Life histories and biographical material report individual life experiences often accessed through in-depth interviewing (see the section earlier in this chapter on interviewing). Denzin (2009) discusses the life history approach as a methodology that emerged from anthropology. The approach reconstructs and interprets an individual life story. Interviews are recorded and transcribed verbatim. Diaries, historical data and observations may also inform the development of a biography. Researchers may explore a patient's life history or that of staff.

Strengths and limitations of the technique

Life histories can provide rich data about an individual's experience of particular episodes or a complete life. Used to collect biographies from patients, histories can provide an understanding of life with particular illnesses and impairments. When considering staff, work experiences help us understand identity and roles in nursing.

Though offering potentially rich data, collecting data through interview or written accounts relies on the participant having the ability to recall intimate detail from past events.

Research example 25.5

The use of the life history technique

Bheenuck (2010) used life histories to explore the lives and experiences of 10 individuals who arrived in Britain in the 1960s and 1970s as student nurses. Originating from previous British Colonies, the narratives sought to explore why the nurses had decided to leave their country of birth and capture their experiences of adapting to life in a new country as migrant workers. The participants had worked in the National Health Service for more than 30 years and used life stories to record their career history and experience of the health service. Through this, their personal experiences, reflections on life after work and concept of 'home' were presented. The study suggests the migrants had contemplated a return to their country of birth, though none had taken action on this.

The use of life histories in the study obtained through in-depth interviewing has enabled the recording of important historical data for the profession of nursing and for key migrant populations. As highlighted above, the approach taken here relied on participants' recall of feelings and experiences over a considerable period of time, and on the collection of retrospective data from the past. This can limit collection of life histories in certain populations, such as those needing care for dementia, where there are long-term memory problems or issues with recall.

CRITICAL INCIDENT TECHNIQUE

Critical incident technique involves asking participants about key events they have experienced and collects observations of human behaviour in defined situations, so, for example, collecting observations of how nurses communicate with adolescent patients. The technique originates in the work of Flanagan (1954) who described the method as having five key steps: determine the study aims; plan how incidents will be collected; collect data; analyse data; and interpret and report data. Originally, the methodology used trained observers to collect data; however, more recently, the method has relied on the use of retrospective reporting. Over a number of years, it has been used to collect descriptions of specific events, either positive or negative, through observations, interviews and self-reporting. Using the technique, the researcher can explore actual activities that might relate to care delivery, management or education experiences.

Strengths and limitations of the technique

Critical incident technique draws on descriptions of actual events, capturing the real-life situation and acknowledging the context and pressures of the actual practice or education environment. Its main strengths are its flexibility and adaptability; however, whilst used globally, it is suggested that there are inconsistencies in the use of methodology and terminology, which have a potential impact on the rigour of use. One example of this is the inconsistency in sample size, with some studies involving 10 participants and others including over 1,000 (Bradbury-Jones and Tranter, 2008). A further weakness in the design is linked to the reliance on participants' recall and memory – participants will need to remember specific examples of effective and ineffective practice. There may also be reluctance among participants to report negative experiences or ineffective practice. An example is the use of the technique given in Research example 25.6.

Research example 25.6

Critical incident technique

Eriksson et al. (2016) used critical incident technique analysis when looking at patients' experiences and actions when describing post- operative pain. This Swedish study involved 22 patients from four different hospitals. The interview guides were developed using a critical incident technique framework. They included questions such as: What did you/ the healthcare professional do during the incident? What influenced the incident? What happened next? They also explored how the incident had made the patient feel, how they were thinking and what they were doing and why.

DIARIES

Diaries have been used as part of historical research, looking at past recordings of individuals such as Samuel Pepys, who recorded diaries of seventeenth-century London. Researchers also use diaries as part of qualitative research designs to ask participants to record current events, keeping a record over time of feelings, experiences, events, actions and reflections.

Use of diaries to collect data

Diaries written or recorded at the time of an event are thought to offer greater data accuracy than interviews, as recall is more likely to be precise at the time of the experience than some time after the event. Burns et al. (2014) suggest diaries allow researchers access to data that is difficult to collect through other methods. Diaries can be used to collect data about behaviours at home (eating habits, exercise patterns) and symptom experience (pain, medication needed, mobility issues).

Diary recording can be very structured, such as recording the time taken to achieve something or ticking off a checklist. A participant might be required to complete a health diary, recording symptom experience by answering structured questions such as 'Did you experience pain? Yes/No'. The degree of structure can vary, often with questions acting as a prompt for more open responses. Conversely, it is suggested that diaries can be completely unstructured, asking individuals to record their day, providing sensitive descriptions of their daily life (Polit and Beck, 2014) (see Research example 25.7).

Research example 25.7

The use of diaries in data collection

Thomas (2015) used unstructured diaries to collect qualitative data from student nurses to explore professional socialisation. The students used both informal and unstructured approaches to completing a daily diary. The approach was taken to reduce researcher interaction and its potential impact on the data. The students were asked to record fully their experiences of being a student nurse in their first clinical placement.

Some of the students recorded their emotional reactions to events. The diary recordings were treated anonymously and were transcribed to allow coding analysis. Following an initial period of data collection and analysis, Thomas did make some suggestions to the students about which of their clinical practice experiences to record, such as asking them to note how they responded to being left alone in the clinical area.

Aspects to consider when using diaries for data collection

Burns et al. (2014) report acceptable validity and reliability in the use of health diaries when compared with interviews. To try to improve validity and reliability, the researcher must consider whether a diary gives scope to collect data of interest, determine the degree of structure required of the diary, and pilot-test the tool. A pilot test will enable the researcher to review the clarity of completion instructions and ensure that any structured questions are robust. The period of data collection should be determined. Daily diaries may be completed over the period of a few days or weeks as in the example above. Weekly diaries, however, might be collated over a longer period.

Participant fatigue can be an issue in diary collection, with incomplete diaries returned or non-completion being problematic. Researchers can employ a system of reminders to encourage completion, and it is suggested that diary completion rates can be high (80–88 per cent) (Burns et al., 2014). It is also thought that the completion of health diaries in particular can affect participants' behaviour as they become more aware of their behaviour and implement change (Burns et al., 2014). The potential strengths and limitations of diary use in research are set out below.

Potential strengths:

- Diaries can offer historical insight.
- There is the potential to provide an intimate description of everyday life.
- Diaries can access data that is not easily recorded by other tools.

Potential limitations:

- Participants' co-operation can be an issue.
- The quality of recording can be variable.
- Diary completion can lead to a change in participant behaviour.

USING ARCHIVE MATERIAL

Researchers use archive material to draw on data from the past. The use of archive material may form part of historical or retrospective studies (see Chapter 19). Historical studies will draw on data from the past, such as photographs or records, to understand events at a particular time in history. Such analysis may generate new knowledge that can inform current practice, but may not necessarily seek to do so. For example, analysis of student nurse training data archived some 35 years ago will provide a description of the student nurse population at that time which could be contrasted with the current student population, though it has a primary aim of describing previous nursing cohorts. Burns et al. (2014) suggest that, as part of the process of completing historical research, an inventory of sources will be needed, as the researcher may be drawing on a number of different materials.

Retrospective studies will take a current issue, such as the implementation of a new nursing role, and explore past events that may have impacted on its development. The aim is therefore to use archived material to try to understand and inform present practice.

Sources of archive data used may include written or audio documents, diaries, interview data or photographs (see Research example 25.8). As discussed earlier, the researcher drawing on these data sets will need to consider issues of accessing archived material and confirm the authenticity and completeness of the data.

Research example 25.8

The use of archived documents

Reeves et al. (2010) explored some of the socio-historical issues related to the leadership of interprofessional teams. Drawing on a range of historical documents from the UK and North America, they traced the evolution of medical and nursing professions from craft guilds to the current professional groups. The analysis showed how individual professions have developed on the basis of their differences and separateness rather than on their ability to work together. It is suggested that the historical development of these professions leads to ongoing tensions and difficulties in leading interprofessional teams.

Here, we can see that the use of historical documents has provided key information about the development of two healthcare professions. Whilst using historical data can pose problems, especially if archives are incomplete, it is apparent that reviewing the past can help us understand and inform present and future practice.

Strengths and limitations of use

There are a number of concerns associated with the use of archive material in research. The researcher is relying on previously collected data that was not collated for research purposes. There may therefore be inaccuracies and instances of missing data. The data can present biases and be subjective, though this will depend on the type of data used.

The use of existing materials in research also brings benefits. The researcher will not have been involved in data collection and is not expecting individuals to recall events or experiences. Provided access to materials can be negotiated, data collection can be less time-consuming and readily achieved. Ethical issues may also be reduced.

The potential strengths and weaknesses of using historical and archive materials in research are set out below.

Potential strengths:

- Draws on existing and historical material.
- Removes the potential for researcher bias in data collection.
- Can be cost-effective.
- Can be an efficient approach to collecting data.

Potential limitations:

- There may be issues with data access.
- Data may be incomplete and unusable, as it was not originally collected for research purposes.
- There may be inaccuracies, bias or errors in the data.

INTERNET AND WEB-BASED TECHNIQUES

The Internet has been one of the fastest growing phenomena in recent years. Within healthcare, it is being used to access information and to support expert discussion forums. The World Wide Web, originally developed for research use, offers scope for educational provision across international healthcare environments. There is no wonder that its use within research is increasing. The Internet can be used to access information that can aid in the development of research, sourcing background literature or information, research design and statistical procedures. It is also used to aid data collection, often through the use of email or through providing online data collection sites, accessed through a web address. These sites are secure and provide flexibility in data collection, allowing participants to upload information or complete online data collection tools when they choose. They can also be accessed through a range of mobile devices.

Whilst there remain some limitations of use, the Internet/web can support the completion of questionnaires, diaries or blogs (web-based logs), focus groups and discussion forums, and can facilitate use of the email system to collect text data. There is even scope to undertake observational research online, recording observations of interactions and conversations taking place within chat rooms, wiki (development of a paper/document online) and virtual classrooms.

Issues of use

There are many potential benefits in the use of email, the Internet and the web to collect research data. These include being able to access international participants;

having scope to access large numbers of participants at a low cost; flexibility for participants in the completion of data collection material; and the potential to generate qualitative and quantitative data. There can also be benefits in resource savings, reducing the data collection period and facilitating ease of online analysis. Additionally, there is flexibility to use data collection methods that are either asynchronous (not real-time) or synchronous (real-time).

The possible limitations of online use relate to the need for participants to have access to computer hardware with an Internet connection. Though the numbers with Internet access are increasing at home, in the workplace, Internet cafes, libraries and through mobile devices, a number of participants may be excluded from online data collection for a number of reasons. These can include a lack of information technology (IT) skills, an inability to access computer or mobile hardware and limits set by employers to Internet connections. There are additionally issues to overcome in ensuring that participants have the necessary web addresses and passwords to enable access to data collection sites or tools. A number of healthcare staff and service users may also be reluctant to engage in online data collection processes, preferring either paper-based tools or a more personal approach.

Researchers using Internet or web-based data collection techniques will need to ensure that they have the technological support to develop data collection materials and support their use, including addressing any emergent technical issues. Development costs may be incurred, though these need to be offset against likely resource savings in researcher data collection time, travel costs and photocopying. The potential strengths and weaknesses of using the Internet for data collection are set out below.

Potential strengths:

- Can offer flexibility to the participant.
- Scope to reach dispersed samples or large numbers.
- Can be used to collect qualitative and quantitative data.
- Can reach some sample groups, i.e. the elderly and disabled, who may otherwise be unable to take part in research.
- Can be cost-effective and save researcher time.

Potential limitations:

- Excludes those unable to access the web or Internet.
- Excludes those with limited IT skills.
- Will incur some set-up costs.
- Computer-based or mobile device data collection techniques will not appeal to everyone.

This chapter has presented a range of data collection tools available to the researcher, some of which can be incorporated into questionnaires or used in interviews. Many of these tools and techniques offer ways of collecting current and retrospective data. It is clear that the use of technology is increasing and is likely to do so in the coming years.

Whilst it may exclude some members of society from research, it offers a number of benefits of scale and can support effective resource use.

CHAPTER SUMMARY

- There are a number of data collection tools available to the nurse researcher.
- Each data collection technique has its own strengths and weaknesses when used in research.
- Researchers need training in the different approaches to data collection.
- The Internet is providing a new approach to data collection that can enable ease of access to worldwide research participants through computer and mobile technology.

SUGGESTED FURTHER READING

Bowling, A. (2005) *Measuring Health: A Review of Quality of Life Measurement Scales*, 3rd edn. Maidenhead: Open University Press. This text introduces a range of measurement scales that are used to record quality of life in patients. It particularly considers the application of measures across a range of patient groups.

Bowling, A. (2014) *Research Methods in Health: Investigating Health and Health Services*, 4th edn. Berkshire: Open University Press. This book covers a wide range of methods used in healthcare research and includes an evaluation of healthcare services, health economics and assessment of health needs.

Bradbury-Jones, C. and Tranter, S. (2008) 'Inconsistent use of the critical incident technique in nursing', *Journal of Advanced Nursing*, 64 (4): 399–407. This article considers the methodological and technical inconsistencies in the use of critical incident technique and makes recommendations for future development of the technique.

WEBSITES

Assessment Psychology Online: www.assessmentpsychology.com/testlist.htm – a database of many psychological tests.

To access further resources related to this chapter, visit the companion website at http://study.sagepub.com/mouleaveyard3e

REFERENCES

Bheenuck, S. (2010) 'The ethics of writing life histories and experiences of overseas nurses in post-colonial Britain', in A. Bathmaker and P. Harnett (eds), *Exploring Learning, Identity and Power through Life History and Narrative Research*. Oxford: Routledge. pp. 70–83.

Bowling, A. (2005) *Measuring Health: A Review of Quality of Life Measurement Scales*, 3rd edn. Maidenhead: Open University Press.

Bradbury-Jones, C. and Tranter, S. (2008) 'Inconsistent use of the critical incident technique in nursing', *Journal of Advanced Nursing*, 64 (4): 399–407.

Burns, N., Grove, S. and Gray, J. (2014) *The Practice of Nursing Research: Appraisal, Synthesis, and Generation of Evidence*, 7th edn. St Louis, MO: Saunders Elsevier.

Denzin, N. (2009) *The Research Act: A Theoretical Introduction to Sociological Methods*. New Brunswick, USA: Aldine Transaction.

Eriksson, K., Wikstrom, L, Findlond, B., Arestedt, K. and Broston, A. (2016) 'Patients' experiences and actions when describing pain after surgery: A critical incident technique analysis', *International Journal of Nursing Studies*, 56: 27–36.

Flanagan, J. (1954) 'The critical incident technique', *Psychological Bulletin*, 51 (4): 327–58.

Igarashi, A., Miyashita, M., Akizuki, N., Akiyama, M., Shirahige, Y. and Eguchi, K. (2012) 'A scale for measuring feelings of support and security regarding cancer care in a region of Japan: A potential new endpoint of cancer care', *Journal of Pain and Symptom Management*, 43 (2): 218–25.

Lawton, R., Gardner, P. and Plachcinski, R. (2011) 'Using vignettes to explore judgements of patients about safety and quality of care: The role of outcome and relationship with the care provider', *Health Expectations*, 14 (3): 296–306.

Polit, D. and Beck, C. (2014) *Essentials of Nursing Research: Appraising Evidence for Nursing Practice*, 8th edn. Philadelphia, PA: Lippincott Williams & Wilkins.

Reeves, S., Macmillan, K. and Van Soeren, M. (2010) 'Leadership of interprofessional health and social care teams: A socio-historical analysis', *Journal of Nursing Management*, 18 (3): 258–64.

Reimer, B. and Mehler, B. (2011) 'The impact of cognitive workload on physiological arousal in young adult drivers: A field study and simulation validation', *Ergonomics*, 54 (10): 932–42.

Thomas, J. (2015) 'Using unstructured diaries for primary data collection', *Nurse Researcher*, 22 (5): 25–9.

26

QUANTITATIVE DATA ANALYSIS TECHNIQUES

Learning outcomes

This chapter will enable you to:

- understand different meanings of the word 'statistics', and discuss the role of statistics in relation to research
- understand different types of data, and their measurement
- discuss key features of graphical and numerical summaries
- discuss basic concepts of hypothesis testing, interpretation of ensuing results and their practical importance
- appreciate the use of computers for data analysis
- consider ethical issues in regard to the analysis of quantitative data

Previous chapters (see Chapters 13–18 and 21–25) have discussed a range of methods that nurse researchers use to collect data for the primary purpose of addressing their research questions or hypotheses. Data analysis is the process through which researchers manage the collected data to identify key patterns or features that are important when answering (or attempting to answer) research questions. To the novice researcher, the literature might seem to contain a bewildering variety of methods for data analysis. It is true that you are likely to come across many statistical tests and you will not be familiar with them all. The important point is that you are able to recognise what the purpose of the statistics is and what the use of statistics has achieved in the papers you read. At a more advanced level, you might appraise the use of the statistics used.

This chapter provides an introduction to some fundamental principles and concepts for the analysis of quantitative (or numerical) data. It explores ways of summarising and presenting data, and introduces inferential statistical methods. It also

Note: this chapter was originally authored by Mollie Gilchrist and Chris Wright and has been updated for this edition by Helen Aveyard.

considers different meanings and implications of statistics and related ethical issues. Details of specific methods can be found in texts such as those listed at the end of the chapter.

STATISTICAL METHODS

The word **statistics** has several meanings in everyday language. We are all familiar, in everyday life, with official statistics such as numbers of births and deaths. Nurses routinely meet statistics in their everyday practice – for example, bed occupancy in a ward or the number of daily admissions or discharges. The term also refers to quantities that summarise various characteristics of numerical data – for example, 'mean' waiting time for a colonoscopy, 'range' of weight loss in patients with cancer. Such statistics are useful for administrative purposes, such as in scheduling routine procedures in hospital day units. A broader use of the term encompasses methods that are used to collect, analyse and interpret quantitative data to inform decision making when accounting for variation in, for example, human behaviour or response to treatment.

In the context of this chapter, the phrase 'statistical methods' is used to refer to procedures that have been developed specifically for the analysis of quantitative data. An understanding of basic principles will enable you to read and critique articles or reports in which such techniques have been employed, and to identify:

- the use of appropriate and inappropriate methods to analyse data
- well-reported results, as well as misreported or misleading results
- valid and incorrect interpretations of results
- overstated generalisations of findings.

In general, statistical methods are categorised as descriptive or inferential. Descriptive statistics are employed in all studies in which quantitative data are collected, whereas inferential statistics are applicable when seeking to generalise findings from the study sample to a wider population. These are discussed in later sections.

Choice of method depends on the type of data collected which, in turn, is dependent upon the methods employed for their collection. Appropriate selection is also influenced by the research question and research design. This interrelationship means that methods for data analysis must be planned at the outset, alongside development of the research question, design and data collection methods. Failure to pre-plan the method of analysis could result in a collection of data that cannot be analysed to address the research question. In this chapter, we are using the RCT undertaken by Heilmann et al. (2016) to illustrate how statistics can be used in a study. Heilmann et al. (2016) evaluated an intervention to reduce anxiety in patients undergoing coronary bypass surgery. They presented descriptive statistics to summarise the results of the study and inferential statistics which indicate the extent to which the results of the study can be inferred to the wider population.

TYPES OF DATA

A research study will include the collection of data on several attributes (also termed 'variables') – for example, gender, blood group, degree of pain, satisfaction with treatment, temperature, weight, size of leg ulcers and volume of urine. Data collected on these attributes might take different values for different participants and, broadly speaking, are labelled as one of two types: categorical or continuous.

Categorical data

Gender and blood group are examples of 'categorical' variables, where each participant in a study belongs to only one of the categories. Data would comprise the labels associated with each category, such as male or female in the case of gender. This type of data is said to be at a **nominal** level of measurement, which is classed as the lowest level.

Sometimes, a meaningful order is apparent in the possible responses associated with a variable. For example, when questioned about satisfaction with the outcome of treatment, a Likert scale might ask for responses from 'strongly disagree' through to 'strongly agree'; or responses to a question on the degree of pain experienced before treatment might range from 'none', 'mild', 'moderate' to 'severe' and 'intolerable'. Data measured at this level are termed **ordinal**; they belong to named and ordered categories. It could be said that someone who responded that they had 'moderate' pain before treatment reported a higher degree of pain than a person who responded using the 'mild' category and lower than a person who reported pain in the 'intolerable' category.

For ease of handling, categorical data are often coded or scored prior to data analysis, especially when using computer software. For the variable gender, for example, 'male' might be represented by 0 and 'female' by 1. Degree of pain might be coded as 0 for 'none' through to 5 for 'intolerable' pain. Care needs to be taken to distinguish these coded numbers from the measured numbers outlined below. Numbers that denote different responses at a nominal level of measurement are purely labels reflecting distinct categories or responses. At an ordinal level, however, larger numbers represent more of some attribute (or less, depending on the coding) compared with lower numbers.

Continuous data

Continuous data comprise numerical information, expressed in terms of basic dimensions such as distance, time, pressure, temperature and weight. Measurement of most physical or physiological attributes (e.g. body temperature, blood pressure, body weight) produces quantitative data. Other examples include: years since diagnosis of a disease; time (days) since discharge from hospital; and number of asthma attacks per week. Here, the numerical values are said to be measured at an **interval** or **ratio level** of measurement.

An interval level of measurement is named, ordered and measured on a scale marked in equal intervals. For example, a body temperature of 40°C is higher than one at 37°C which, in turn, is higher than one at 34°C (that is, the scale is ordered). In addition, the difference between 40°C and 37°C is equal in some sense to the difference between

37°C and 34°C (that is, equal intervals have the same meaning). However, 0°C is not an absolute zero, so we could not say that a room at 40°C was twice as hot as a room at 20°C.

A ratio level of measurement is named, ordered and measured on a scale marked in equal intervals and has an absolute zero. This absolute zero enables us to compare relative sizes of scores, as well as differences in scores and order of scores, and makes ratio the highest level of measurement (that is, portrays the most detailed information about attributes). For example, in considering a situation of three people who weigh 80 kg, 60 kg and 40 kg, we can report that the first person is heavier than the second, who is heavier than the third, and that the difference in weight between the first and second person is the same as that between the second and third person. In addition, it could be reported that the first person is twice the weight of the third person. For the purposes of the statistical analyses presented in this chapter, there is no need to make a distinction between interval and ratio levels of measurement. They are termed 'scale' in some data-handling software packages, such as Statistical Package for the Social Sciences (SPSS).

The above examples relate to the objective measurement of attributes to produce continuous data. However, the nurse researcher will be interested in many attributes that might be considered more subjective – for example, pain intensity, general health status, physical disability and handicap, psychological well-being and quality of life. Researchers have expended much effort, over many years, developing standard tools to quantify subjective estimates of attributes that cannot be measured directly. Two popular types of tool are the visual analogue scale (VAS) and rating scales. Estimates of subjective pain intensity were first explored with use of a VAS by McDowell and Newell (1996). Participants translate assessment of their pain onto a line (100 mm in length) and their pain is scored 0 to 100, with 0 indicating no pain and 100 indicating 'pain as bad as could be'. Theoretically, the resultant scores are recorded at an ordinal level of measurement, although some research has demonstrated that a ratio level may be assumed (McDowell and Newell, 1996). The Barthel Index is a rating scale comprising 15 items (revised version) that was developed to monitor performance of people with chronic conditions and to estimate how much nursing care was required (McDowell and Newell, 1996). Scores on individual items are summed to produce a total score. Many researchers treat the resultant data as being measured at an interval level.

Careful consideration should be given to the meaning of results from analyses on data collected using these types of tool since, for some, the overall score might not satisfy all the common rules of arithmetic that are used in many statistical analyses. In all instances, however, results are meaningless when data lack validity (that is, when the data do not measure what they purport to measure) and reliability (that is, when data are not reproducible or consistent), and, therefore, judicious choice of measurement tools is essential.

It is evident that the type of data is an important consideration in the choice of descriptive and inferential statistics used for the analysis of quantitative data. Figure 26.1 lists the variables collected in a study by Seers et al. (2008), and considers their type and level of measurement.

A paper by Seers et al. (2008) reports a study to determine the effectiveness of a single session of nurse-administered massage for the short-term relief of chronic non-malignant pain and anxiety. The paper contains data collected from variables at each of the levels of measurement discussed above. Some of these are listed below:

Categorical

Nominal (named categories): profession, gender

Ordinal (named and ordered categories): verbal rating pain intensity scale

Continuous

Interval/ratio (measurement with equal units/intervals between data points): for example age (years), pain intensity (Pain Rating Index)

Figure 26.1   An example of study variables and their levels of measurement

DESCRIPTIVE STATISTICS: TECHNIQUES FOR DESCRIBING QUANTITATIVE DATA

The aim of the first part of the results section in any study is to give the reader a 'picture' of the data collected. The numerical data are organised and summarised to portray or describe important features. This description usually involves numbers and percentages that are presented in words (for example, the percentage of bedridden patients who have bed sores), tables and/or **charts**. A few meaningful numbers (called 'summary statistics') are presented to summarise the overall data set. Summary statistics include: sample size; counts or frequencies (often expressed as percentages for comparison purposes); maximum and minimum values, and values such as percentiles and quartiles; **measures of central tendency** (**averages**); and **measures of dispersion** or spread of data (variability). A measure of central tendency provides a value around which data cluster, and a measure of variability provides a value indicating how closely the data cluster around this central value.

Summary statistics enable the reader to gain a rough idea of the comparability of participants in different groups. This could be of particular interest when two different groups of people are involved, for example when comparing the characteristics of the intervention group with the control group at the beginning of an RCT. Summary statistics are given in a table in their paper which allow the reader to compare the characteristics of the different groups in the trial.

Choice of summary statistics depends on the level of measurement of the data, as outlined above. Table 26.1 summarises some appropriate summary statistics dependent on the level of measurement of the data, and definitions of some summary statistics are given in Figure 26.2.

Table 26.1　Summary statistics associated with different levels of measurement

	Nominal (named categories)	Ordinal (named and ordered categories)	Interval/ratio (measurement with equal units/intervals between data points)
Averages (measure of central tendency of data)	Mode	Median* Mode	Mean* Median Mode (not so useful)
Variability (measure of dispersion or spread of data)		Range* Interquartile range (IQR)*	Standard deviation (SD)* Range IQR

* Most useful measure for a given level of data

Averages:

Mode = most frequently occurring value

Median = middle value, when all data is placed in order

Mean = sum of all values divided by the number of values

Other location measures:

Lower quartile = middle value of the ordered data from minimum to median value

Upper quartile = middle value of the ordered data from median to maximum value

Measures of variability (dispersion) of data:

Range = maximum value − minimum value

Interquartile range (IQR) = upper quartile − lower quartile

Standard deviation = an 'average' distance of all values away from the mean

Variance = (standard deviation)^2

Figure 26.2　Definitions of some summary statistics

Note: Further properties of these measures can be explored in the resources listed at the end of the chapter.

TABLES AND CHARTS

Tables can be used when it is important that the reader has the exact figures, for reference purposes, say. They often contain basic demographic information about the sample and/or summary statistics for the variables under study – for example, Heilmann et al. (2016) describe the number of people, their nationality, gender, marital status, education, religion and household arrangements for participants in each arm of the trial. Percentages can be useful for comparison purposes, but it is important to give the actual numbers

All charts should:

- Have a relevant and succinct title.
- Have clearly labelled axes, showing any measurements used.
- Use a careful choice of scale – often multiples of 2 or 5 are used, rather than multiples of 3 or 7, say.
- Use scale breaks for 'false origins' – particularly when the vertical axis does not start at zero.
- Use carefully chosen plot symbols and connecting lines – more importance appears to be given to a solid line than to a dashed line, for example. See Takase et al. (2006: 755) for a clustered bar chart using different line styles.
- Show all relevant study information, e.g. sample size (Chatfield, 1995)

In addition, they should:

- 'Stand on their own' without the need for reference back to the text – there is the possibility of figures being taken out of context and misinterpreted, for example.
- Use of 3-D charts on paper should be avoided, as they are mathematically incorrect, although many modern computer packages allow the use of interactive charting to 'move around' a 3-D plot, thus permitting exploration of 3 variables.
- 2 or 3 charts are preferable to 1 'busy' one.

Figure 26.3   Chart checklist

Note: See Watson et al. (2006: Ch. 4) for a good discussion about data presentation and an exploration of potentially misleading charts.

too. After all, 70 per cent conveys a sizeable quantity, but when it refers to a sample size of 10, this is only 7 people.

Charts give an instant visual representation of the relative size of figures – it is said that 'a picture tells a thousand words'. Suitable charts for summarising data include: pie and bar charts for categorical data (such as a bar chart for the number of nurses who work in different specialist areas); histograms, box and whisker plots (for example, a box plot of pain scores for people with different types of arthritis); and line graphs for quantitative data (especially when data are collected over time). Heilmann et al. (2016) used a flow chart to illustrate how participants were followed up throughout their study. They also display socio-economic data and end points of anxiety measurements visually.

All charts should have certain elements to aid the interpretation of information presented in them. Figure 26.3 lists some of these features.

CORRELATION

A **correlation coefficient** is a measure of the strength of association between two variables and can take values between 0 (no correlation) and ±1 (perfect correlation). Correlations can be positive (that is, both variables increase or decrease together, for example blood pressure increasing with older age) or negative (that is, as one variable increases, the other decreases, such as physical agility decreasing with longer duration of rheumatoid arthritis).

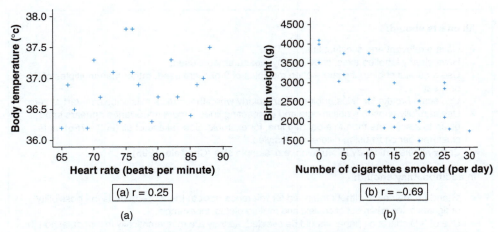

Figure 26.4   Scatter diagrams illustrating (a) weak positive and (b) moderate to strong negative linear relationships, together with their associated correlation coefficients

A Pearson's coefficient of linear correlation (usually denoted by r) is often used when data are measured at an interval/ratio level. This correlation assumes that proportionate changes occur in the two variables being considered. The researcher can check whether this assumption is reasonable by plotting one variable against the other on a graph called a 'scatter diagram'. Figure 26.4 shows two scatter diagrams and associated values of the correlation coefficient. Figure 26.4(a) plots heart rate horizontally against body temperature vertically of 25 adults. The widely scattered markers illustrate a weak positive linear relationship, confirmed by the low value (0.25) of the correlation coefficient. A moderate to strong negative linear relationship (confirmed by the correlation coefficient of −0.69) between birth weight and number of cigarettes smoked per day by the mother during pregnancy is demonstrated in Figure 26.4(b).

It is important to note that a linear relationship does not imply a causal relationship between two variables. Additional, independent, evidence would be required to support such a claim. For example, an increase in ice-cream sales in summer can be shown to be linearly related to a decrease in the size of household gas bills, but one cannot say that a change in the number of ice-cream sales causes a change in gas bills.

When data have been collected at an ordinal level of measurement, the strength of association can be measured using Spearman's coefficient of rank correlation (usually denoted by r_s). This variation of Pearson's coefficient does not assume that a linear association exists between the two variables and, therefore, can also be used to measure the association between two variables when the data have been collected at interval/ratio level and a scatter diagram indicates non-proportionate changes to the two variables.

INFERENTIAL STATISTICS

Researchers who collect quantitative data through an experimental design or a survey usually do so with the intention of making inferences about a wider population of people (or institutions, objects or events) on the basis of data collected from a sample of people; that is, they will predict the extent to which the results found in their study apply to wider populations. For example, Heilmann et al. (2016) randomly assigned 253 adult patients who were due to undergo coronary artery bypass surgery, into two groups. One group received standard care and the other group received an intervention to manage anxiety. This intervention had been developed by the researchers and the aim of the study was to determine the effectiveness of this intervention. Descriptive statistics were used to describe the anxiety level in each group – those who received the intervention and those who did not. The researchers found decreased anxiety in the group who had received the intervention. Heilmann et al. (2016) then used inferential statistics to determine whether this decrease in anxiety levels could be expected in the wider population of patients undergoing coronary artery bypass surgery, rather than just those in the study. In order to determine this, Heilmann et al. (2016) used the ANOVA test for analysis of variance and chi-square tests. These tests determine whether the difference in mean anxiety levels of the two groups could be explained by chance. Heilmann et al. (2016) found a significant difference between the anxiety reported by those in the intervention group compared to those in the control group and therefore inferred that this was unlikely to be due to chance. This allows us to assume that the reduced anxiety is due to the intervention and therefore if people receive this intervention in the future, they will experience less anxiety than if they did not receive the intervention.

In practice, generalisation is influenced by several aspects within a study protocol, including: research design, sampling method, inclusion and exclusion criteria, recruitment strategy, willingness of participants to volunteer, conditions pertaining to any intervention under study, sample size, data collection tools and their administration, completeness of the collected data, and data analysis. Inferential statistics use sample data to make generalisations about a population of which the sample is representative, through testing statistical hypotheses.

STATISTICAL HYPOTHESES

In the study by Heilmann et al. (2016), the researchers conducted the research because they believed that the intervention would decrease anxiety in those undergoing coronary artery bypass surgery. This prior belief (or assumption) is called a 'research hypothesis' and is stated at the design stage in a study (see Chapter 9).

At the data analysis stage, the research hypothesis is translated into two statistical hypotheses, called the 'null' and 'alternative' hypotheses:

- *Null* hypothesis: the intervention has no effect on anxiety for people undergoing coronary artery bypass surgery.
- *Alternative* hypothesis: the intervention has an effect on anxiety for people who are undergoing coronary artery bypass surgery.

The statistical hypotheses are part of the analysis method. They describe the two possible and complementary situations in the population from which the sample was drawn and of which it is representative. The alternative hypothesis states that the intervention has an effect in the population – implying that differences between groups in the data are due to a real effect in the population. Although unlikely, the intervention might have increased the level of anxiety rather than decreased it, hence the non-directional wording (named two-tailed or two-sided) of the alternative hypothesis. If, however, some theory or substantial prior evidence existed that precluded a situation in which the intervention might increase the level of anxiety, then a directional alternative hypothesis would be stated (one-tailed or one-sided):

- *Directional alternative* hypothesis: the intervention decreases the level of anxiety for people who are undergoing coronary artery bypass surgery.

The null hypothesis represents the prior assumption in **statistical hypothesis testing**. This is usually the situation that the researchers believe to be false. It is an assumption of no effect or no change – implying that differences between groups in the data are due to chance or random error and are not due to a real effect in the population. It may seem odd that researchers suggest a null hypothesis – one they believe to be false. However they do this because in statistical theory, it is not possible to prove a hypothesis – only falsify one. By falsifying a null hypothesis, they indirectly support the hypothesis – the one they believe in.

SAMPLING VARIATION

By definition, a sample is a subset of the population from which it was selected (Chapter 12). Hence, differences between groups in the data collected from a sample are unlikely to be identical to the differences you would see if you were able to observe every single person in the entire population. Differences between the sample statistic and the population effect are called 'sampling error'. Further, the observed difference between groups is likely to be different when calculated from a second sample randomly selected from the same population. This difference across samples is called 'sampling variation'. The theory of sampling variation is the basis on which statistical hypothesis tests are developed.

STATISTICAL HYPOTHESIS TESTING

Conventional statistical hypothesis tests are based on the prior assumption that the null hypothesis is true. This statement can be verified or refuted using data from a random sample drawn from the population of interest. Large differences between groups in the data provide evidence that the null hypothesis is false, whilst small differences cast no doubt on its truth. The dilemma lies in determining what magnitude could be considered to be sufficiently 'large' to support a decision to reject the null hypothesis in favour of the alternative hypothesis, in the existence of sampling error.

Statistical hypothesis tests (such as those in Figure 26.5) enable the researcher to make a decision about the null hypothesis and to state a probability that the decision is wrong. These wrong decisions are the Type I and Type II errors that are reported in the literature. There are two possible statistical decisions:

- Reject the null hypothesis in favour of the alternative hypothesis.
- Do not reject the null hypothesis in favour of the alternative hypothesis.

These decisions are illustrated in Figure 26.6, against the 'true' situation in the population.

The null hypothesis is rejected when the chance (or probability) of obtaining at least as extreme an outcome as the observed data are smaller than some selected value. Otherwise, the null hypothesis is not rejected. The computed value of chance is the p-value reported in research studies and the selected cut-off value for decision making is the significance level. The choice of significance level is based on tradition or the importance of a Type I error and should not be influenced by the data in a study. Hence, the significance level is specified at the design stage. Conventionally, it is set at 5 per cent, and is associated with a p-value of 0.05 for making a decision.

Types of statistical hypothesis tests

In general, statistical hypothesis tests may be termed **parametric** or non-parametric methods. Their use requires certain assumptions to be satisfied, as summarised below for frequently used hypothesis tests:

- *Parametric methods*
  For example: t-test of difference between mean values of two populations, one-way ANOVA (analysis of variance) test of differences between mean values of two or more populations.

Instruction for use: Start from the top, answer the questions and follow the appropriate lines until you reach one of the test boxes

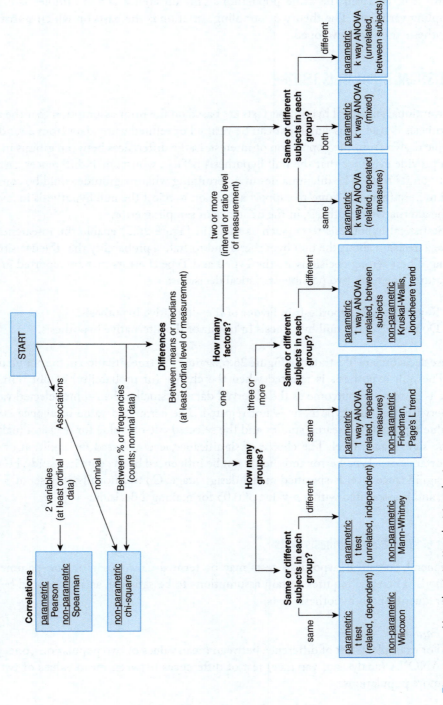

Figure 26.5   Hypothesis testing decision chart

	Situation in the population	
	No effect (null hypothesis is true)	**An effect exists** (null hypothesis is false)
Reject null hypothesis	Incorrect decision Type I error (Significance level)	Correct decision (✓) (Called the 'power')
Do not reject null hypothesis	Correct decision (✓)	Incorrect decision Type II error

Decision on the basis of data from a random sample (vertical axis label)

Figure 26.6   Statistical decision against 'true' situation

- o   data measured on at least an interval level
- o   data (in each group) constitute a random sample from a normally distributed population, i.e. data are distributed mostly around a central value with a few lower and higher values, forming a bell-shaped pattern
- o   equality of group variances (called homogeneity).

- *Non-parametric methods*
  For example: chi-squared test of independence between two attributes used to classify the data, Mann-Whitney U test of difference between median values in two populations.

- o   data measured on at least a nominal level
- o   does not require assumptions of normality and homogeneity
- o   requires independence between cases.

Interpretation of results from statistical hypothesis tests

When the null hypothesis is rejected, the data provide evidence of an effect that is larger than that expected by chance. However, the magnitude of the observed effect might or might not be of importance in clinical practice. There is a difference, then, between a result that is *statistically significant* and one that is *clinically important*. Further research needs to be conducted to estimate the order of magnitude of an effect that is clinically important. Research methods have been developed to estimate clinically important changes for some outcomes and in some populations.

Ideally, the size of a minimal clinically important effect needs to be known at the design stage. From this, a sample size can be determined (using statistical techniques) that enables an effect of clinical importance to be detected as statistically significant. An effect that is not statistically significant might have occurred by chance and, therefore, provides no evidence to inform practice.

An alternative approach to statistical hypothesis testing is to estimate the magnitude of effect in the population through a 'confidence interval' that is computed from the data in the sample. A **confidence interval** is stated as a lower value and an upper value that bound the magnitude of effect in the population with a stated confidence. In this way, the interval indicates how small or large the effect might be in the population.

Confidence intervals help practitioners to relate findings from research to their potential usefulness to practice. The width of the confidence interval is determined by the variability in the data (i.e. is associated with the standard deviations of change in scores, with smaller standard deviations leading to narrower intervals), the sample size (with larger sample sizes leading to narrower intervals) and the selected confidence level (with higher confidence levels leading to wider intervals). Heilmann et al. (2016) did not use confidence intervals – they used p-values instead. However confidence intervals are often reported alongside other statistics in the results section to provide the reader with a more informative estimate of the potential benefit or otherwise of a new intervention. Confidence intervals can be quoted for other parameters, including odds ratios and risk ratios. (See Goodman and Gilchrist (2009) for more discussion around presenting results in a more useful format for interpretation.)

CHOOSING A STATISTICAL METHOD FOR DATA ANALYSIS

Choice of an appropriate test is dependent upon:

- Research question:
    - association (for example, relationship between variables)
    - difference (for example, between groups in an experimental design)
- Type of data collected:
    - level of measurement
- How many factors (1 or more):
    - variables or attributes that are deliberately controlled in an experimental design, e.g. the amount of analgesic (1 'factor'); the type and amount of analgesic (2 factors); the frequency, intensity and duration of exercise within a particular programme (3 factors)

- o attributes or characteristics across which certain outcome variables are to be compared – usually within a survey, e.g. gender (1 characteristic or factor); type of health professional and management approach for a specific condition (2 attributes or factors)

- How many groups (2 or more):

  - o levels of a factor, e.g. 250 mg, 500 mg of analgesic (2 groups within a factor 'amount of analgesic'); low, medium, high doses of an analgesic (3 groups within a factor 'amount of analgesic')
  - o sub-classification within an attribute or characteristic, e.g. male, female (2 groups within a factor 'gender'); rheumatoid arthritis, osteoarthritis, ankylosing spondylitis (3 groups within a factor 'type of arthritis')

- Same or different participants in each group.

Figure 26.7 shows a decision chart from which to choose an appropriate hypothesis test linking the above elements. The tests are not exhaustive of all statistical techniques or research questions, but represent some of the more frequently used tests of association and differences.

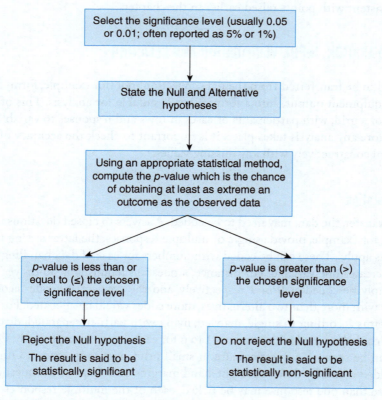

Figure 26.7   Steps in making a statistical decision

USING COMPUTER SOFTWARE FOR ANALYSIS

Most researchers use computer software to conduct analyses of quantitative data. This is due to the advent of menu-driven packages and the increased availability of data-handling software, such as SPSS. The use of computer software enables the emphasis of statistical analysis to be placed on appropriate techniques and the interpretation of results. Accuracy of calculations is assured, provided that the data have been entered correctly. However, a computer will conduct any techniques requested of it, regardless of their lack of suitability, as, currently, computers are not programmed to ask a series of questions to ensure that the analysis that has been requested is appropriate. Hence, the researcher needs to think carefully about what statistical analyses are requested and how the data need to be input.

MS Excel (or any other 'spreadsheet' package) is another program that may be used to produce basic charts and simple statistical analyses – for example, calculation of means and standard deviations. Excel is more versatile than SPSS for creating some charts, such as clustered bar charts. Some researchers prefer to enter data into Excel, from where it is possible to transfer the data into SPSS. It is important to appreciate that charts drawn using software packages can be edited, so that the default output from the computer does not have to be accepted. Most aspects of a chart can be altered to be consistent with points raised earlier in the chapter.

DATA PREPARATION, INPUT, VERIFICATION AND CLEANING

Data need to be transferred from the data collection tool (for example, form, questionnaire or equipment output) into a format that is suitable for analysis. This often takes the form of a grid, with participants or cases in rows and responses to variables in columns. Before any analysis takes place, it is important to check the accuracy of the data and to deal constructively with any missing values.

Data preparation

Prior to transfer, the data may need to be coded. Answers to closed questions in a questionnaire, for example, provide single or multiple responses, the latter arising from 'tick as many as apply'. These can be coded with numbers for ease of data handling. A single response creates one variable. For instance, a question requiring a 'no' or 'yes' response could simply be coded as 0 or 1 respectively, and the appropriate code recorded. For questions with more than two alternatives, more codes would be allocated. For example, marital status according to single, married, living with partner, separated, divorced and widowed could be coded with numbers 1 to 6 for each category respectively. Often, this coding can be seen on a questionnaire in small print next to questions. Otherwise, it can be added manually down the right-hand margins on receipt of the questionnaire.

If more than one response may be ticked, each of the multiple responses will need to be regarded as 'not ticked'/'ticked' and hence become 'no'/'yes' variables. Therefore, if a question has 10 responses, any number of which may be ticked, this translates into 10 variables, each with an answer 'yes' if ticked but 'no' if not, and coded 1 or 0, as above.

A further consideration occurs if the respondent is asked to indicate, in order, the three most important concerns in relation to an issue. This translates into three variables, indicating first, second and third choices. Responses to quantitative variables, for example, height or a mark on a VAS, are recorded with none or some decimal places, as required.

Data input

Data can be written on squared paper and totals counted by hand, but, ideally, a data set can be entered directly into a data analysis package (e.g. SPSS, SAS, Minitab), or at least a spreadsheet (e.g. MS Excel), to allow for speedy formulation of frequency tables and some summary statistics and charts. Data are input carefully, according to an agreed coding, into an already structured database (see software instructions to achieve this). Online questionnaires and some equipment provide an option to import data directly into a computer package, thus saving data input time.

Data verification

Once the data have been entered into the computer package, they need to be checked carefully for accuracy. Verification is an attempt to ensure that errors do not occur when transferring data from one source to another – for example, from questionnaire to database, or from one computer package to another. Strategies to achieve this include proofreading, checking 10 per cent of data entry and 'double entry', when data are entered twice, and comparing for agreement.

Data cleaning

Inputting errors need to be corrected. For example, if scoring on a Likert scale can range from 1 to 5, a value recorded as 6 will need investigating. A negatively worded statement on a Likert scale scoring from 1 to 5 will need its responses to be reverse-scored; that is, 1 will become 5, 2 will become 4, and so on. In addition, decisions need to be made as to how to code missing data, and data need to be checked that they are within sensible limits. Once this data set is prepared, it should be carefully stored or saved to disk as a raw data file, and another copy becomes the 'working file' that is used for subsequent analysis.

Decisions need to be made on how to deal with missing data. The most direct approach is to eliminate any missing observations, known as 'listwise deletion'. However, although simple, this does reduce the effective sample size. 'Pairwise deletion' only excludes missing values for particular calculations. Another approach is to make some sort of estimate of the missing value(s). For example, if you are asking participants to respond to several statements with a range of options, say from '1 = low' to '7 = high', it is acceptable practice to 'impute' the mean of the reported responses to obtain an overall scale score, provided that at least 50 per cent of scores have been completed. An alternative approach is to substitute the group mean of available responses to a particular variable, although this is no longer considered to be good practice. Newer, less biased methods for estimating missing values, such as 'multiple imputation', are being developed all the time. It may be possible to deduce responses to one missing question by a response to another. For example, it might be known that all the patients in one ward, where data have been collected, are female, so that a missing gender response may be completed. However, absolute honesty and openness must be adhered to at all times. It is recommended that advice about estimating missing numbers be sought from experienced researchers. The best solution is to maximise response rates, thus avoiding missing values altogether!

ETHICAL CONSIDERATIONS

Ethical issues that might arise with regard to the analysis of quantitative data include anonymity, confidentiality, deception, exploitation and risk of harm (see Chapters 7 and 8).

Data from individual participants are combined during statistical analyses and results are reported as numerical values, so anonymity and confidentiality are unlikely to be infringed. However, it is good practice to use a unique number to identify data from each participant rather than their name (especially in a computer database) and to store a list of identifiers and participants' names in a different location from the data.

Deception and exploitation might arise in several ways. In theory, deception and exploitation of participants occur when data are used for a purpose other than that stated or inferred on the participant information sheet or consent form. Whilst this would not cause harm to the participants, if the data were manipulated to fit requirements for a different purpose (or the design or data collection methods were inappropriate for the other purpose), the resultant findings might be erroneous with potential to misinform decisions based on them. The consequence could be risk of harm (physical, psychological, social or economical) to future patients, health professionals or other groups of people. A similar situation might arise when:

- results are obtained through inappropriate statistical methods (for example, incorrect level of measurement, assumptions not satisfied)
- data cases are omitted from analyses without sound justification and the researchers do not report this in a clear and honest manner
- outcome measures are not valid for the population of interest in the study
- the primary outcome is chosen after the data have been analysed to ensure that a statistically significant result can be reported
- the sample size is too small to enable differences (or changes) of clinical importance to be detected as statistically significant
- the statistical findings are incorrectly interpreted, with too much or incorrect emphasis on statistical significance and little discussion on clinical relevance.

CHAPTER SUMMARY

- Statistical methods are used to organise and summarise large quantities of numerical data.
- Statistics are used to portray or describe important features in the data, either graphically or by calculation of a few meaningful numbers called 'summary statistics' (often presented in tabular form).
- Statistical methods use data collected from a (random) sample of a population of interest to draw inferences about that population.
- Statistical methods aim to generalise findings to a population of which the sample is representative.
- Statistical methods are applicable for all experimental studies (for example, RCTs) and for many surveys and comparative studies.
- Statistical methods use probability theory.
- Statistical methods are 'deductive' in that they test a prior assumption (or hypothesis) about the population, are based on specific assumptions (a method is valid only when its assumptions are met) and are used ethically and honestly.

SUGGESTED FURTHER READING

There are a variety of textbooks to assist your understanding of statistics and we have identified a selection below. The best advice is to identify a book which you find accessible and easy to read.

Campbell, M.J., Machin, D. and Walters, S.J. (2007) *Medical Statistics: A Textbook for the Health Sciences*, 4th edn. Chichester: Wiley.

Harris, M. and Taylor, G. (2008) *Medical Statistics Made Easy*, 2nd edn. London: Taylor & Francis.

Pallant, J. (2010) *SPSS Survival Manual: A Step-by-step Guide to Data Analysis Using SPSS*, 4th edn. Buckingham: Open University Press.

Salkind, N.J. (2010) *Statistics for People Who (Think They) Hate Statistics*, 4th edn. London: Sage.

Schmuller, J. (2013) *Statistical Analysis with Excel for Dummies*, 3rd edn. Hoboken, NJ: Wiley.

Scott, I. and Mazhindu, D. (2005) *Statistics for Healthcare Professionals: An Introduction*. London: Sage.

WEBSITES

A collection of e-books for learning statistics from Massey University, NZ: http://cast.massey.ac.nz/collection_public.html

SurfStat Australia from the Australian National University: http://surfstat.anu.edu.au/surfstat-home/cont1.html

Understanding Uncertainty, produced by the Winton Programme for the Public Understanding of Risk, based in the Statistical Laboratory, University of Cambridge, UK: http://understandinguncertainty.org/

To access further resources related to this chapter, visit the companion website at http://study.sagepub.com/mouleaveyard3e

REFERENCES

Chatfield, C. (1995) *Problem Solving: Statistician's Guide*, 2nd edn. London: Chapman & Hall.

Goodman, M.L. and Gilchrist, M. (2009) 'Reading and critiquing randomized controlled trials', *British Journal of Cardiac Nursing*, 4 (10): 492–7.

Heilmann, C., Stotz, U., Burbaum, C., Feucjtinger, J., Leonhart, R., Seipe, M., Beyersdort, F. and Fritzsche, K. (2016) 'Short term intervention to reduce anxiety before coronary artery bypass surgery – a randomized controlled trial', *Journal of Clinical Nursing*, 25: 351–61

McDowell, I. and Newell, C. (1996) *Measuring Health: A Guide to Rating Scales and Questionnaires*, 2nd edn. New York: Oxford University Press.

Melzack, R. (1975) 'The McGill Pain Questionnaire: Major properties and scoring methods', *Pain*, 1: 277–99.

Seers, K., Crichton, N., Tutton, L., Smith, L. and Saunders, T. (2008) 'Effectiveness of relaxation for postoperative pain and anxiety : Randomized controlled trial', *Journal of Advanced Nursing*, 62(6): 681–688.

Takase, M., Maude, P. and Manias, E. (2006) 'Role discrepancy: Is it a common problem among nurses?', *Journal of Advanced Nursing*, 54 (6): 751–9.

Watson, R., Atkinson, I. and Egerton, P. (2006) *Successful Statistics for Nursing and Healthcare*. Basingstoke: Palgrave Macmillan.

27
QUALITATIVE DATA ANALYSIS TECHNIQUES

Learning outcomes

This chapter will enable you to:

- appreciate the processes involved in preparing qualitative data for analysis
- understand how qualitative data are interpreted
- understand how computer packages can assist the process of data preparation and analysis
- appreciate the need to establish rigour in the process of analysis

Qualitative data analysis can commence at the start of the project and the researcher will continue analysis throughout the period of data collection and beyond. In a grounded theory approach, for example, the qualitative researcher in nursing will engage in data analysis as soon as the first data are collected. Analysing data throughout the data collection period supports a constant comparative method used in grounded theory research (see Chapter 15). In this research approach, the researcher will look for evidence of themes and revise the research questions to support theory development as the project progresses (Oktay, 2012). Engaging in data analysis throughout the data collection process contrasts with the approach to quantitative data analysis we described in Chapter 26. When working with quantitative data, the researchers tend to collect all of the data before starting data analysis.

Those new to analysing qualitative data often find the process complex. Qualitative data analysis processes can raise far more issues than seen in the analysis of quantitative data. This arises as the process of preparing and analysing qualitative data relies on the individual judgements and interpretations of the researcher. Mechanisms can be built into the process to aid the 'objectivity' seen in qualitative analysis. These can include 'member checking', where research participants are involved in verifying the interpretations of the researcher, corroborating the analysis. Other validation strategies can be used, such as the provision of an 'audit trail' (see Chapter 13). This presents the research journey and approaches taken to the analysis of the data (Elo et al., 2014). Such strategies aim to support the trustworthiness of data analysis and should be an integral part of any data analysis process.

Polit and Beck (2014) discuss further challenges to the nurse researcher working with qualitative data, including the volume of effort required in the analysis of lengthy narrative materials and the presentation of data in a concise form that maintains meaning and value. Quantitative data are often presented in tabular or graphical form. This affords the presentation of copious amounts of numerical data in a concise space. In contrast, the presentation of narrative, often as verbatim quotes of the spoken word extracted from interview transcripts, can be challenging. The researcher must select specific data for presentation that will support the key issues arising from the interpretation of vast quantities of textual data.

In this chapter, we discuss the methods employed in the analysis of qualitative data. Chapter 15 presented some of the approaches used in qualitative research and identified that qualitative data was often derived from field notes generated as part of participant observation, personal diaries and the verbatim transcriptions from interviews. The discussion below reviews how researchers manage qualitative information, drawing interpretations from text-based and visually presented data.

ANALYSIS OF QUALITATIVE DATA

There is no one approach that should be used when analysing qualitative data, but an array of methods is available. These might be employed in the analysis of transcripts from interview or focus group data, field notes or documents (see Chapters 23 to 25). Qualitative data can also include digitally recorded visual images, such as photographs, video and pictures. The analysis of images would draw on further analytic frameworks. In selecting the method of analysis, the researchers should review the variety of methods available, selecting an approach that would enable the interpretation of data through a rigorous approach.

The analysis of qualitative data should be embedded in the research process, often integral to the period of data collection. This allows the process of analysis to be reflexive and iterative. The analysis of data collected initially can then inform further data collection. Within action research and participatory enquiry (see Chapter 18), data analysis is seen as an ongoing process occurring as part of reflective processes within data collection. In action research approaches, the development of practice and implementation of change are based on the initial research findings and followed by further data collection and analysis as the outcomes of new actions are evaluated (Koshy et al., 2011).

Reflexivity is part of nursing practice and needs to be a consideration within nursing research, particularly where the researcher may have the dual role of practitioner. Researching as an 'insider' being part of the culture of nursing should be acknowledged by the researcher, who will have pre-determined experiences and thoughts about practice. These can have an impact on the approach taken to the analysis of findings and requires the validation of interpretations. Researchers can attempt to 'bracket' themselves (see Chapter 15 for explanations on the use of 'bracketing' in phenomenology), trying to ensure their personal experiences are acknowledged, limiting any researcher bias in the **interpretation of qualitative data**. Researchers can also validate their interpretations externally by returning original data to participants for clarification of meaning or through the involvement of independent researchers in the process of analysis.

It is also worth noting that the analysis of qualitative data can be viewed as a series of tasks, whereas for others it is an act of interpretation, where meaning is drawn from the data. Hollway and Jefferson (2012) suggest that researchers with large amounts of unstructured data often resort to imposing structure upon it, by breaking it into manageable segments through **data coding** and retrieval methods. They criticise **computer-assisted data analysis** packages for fragmenting data in this way. A further approach to **qualitative data analysis** is offered by Miles et al. (2014), which encompasses data reduction, display and conclusion drawing and verification.

Qualitative data analysis is viewed as continuous. Data are selected and simplified from the initial field notes or transcriptions. Codes, themes or clusters are identified, transforming the data. This process involves analysis, and data are displayed or organised to allow conclusion drawing. The explanations or propositions are tentative, developing as data collection continues. When more develop, these conclusions are tested through verification processes, such as returning to the 'raw data' or gaining outside opinion. The following sections examine more closely the **preparation** of qualitative data for content and **narrative analysis**.

It should also be remembered that qualitative data, though generally in text format, could be pictorial and visual. The analysis of photographic images can be based on key observational questions such as the weather, the scenery, the interactions taking place, or can include measurements of the number of trees or number of people.

Reflective exercise

You can try and do this yourself. Look at the photograph below and analyse it using the following questions:

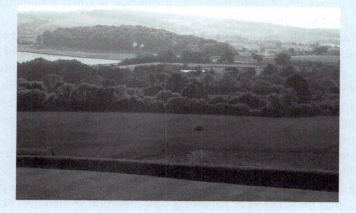

Figure 27.1

(Continued)

(Continued)

- What is the main focus of the photograph?
- What is in the foreground?
- What is in the background?
- Which season is it taken in and how do you know?
- Are there any people in the scene?
- Was the photograph taken in recent years? How do you know?

Video or digital media can be used to record skill acquisition, allowing more detailed analysis of learning by more than one researcher and by the research participants. For example, Yoo et al. (2010) videoed nursing students completing Foley catheterisation and were able to evaluate student performance. Twenty students who evaluated their own performance using a checklist developed by members of the research team reviewed the videos. The process of self-assessment enabled the students to develop self-awareness of performance.

PREPARING THE DATA

The nurse researcher will collect raw data, which could encompass text, digital recordings or visual data such as photographs and video. The types of textual data available will reflect the data collection processes involved. They could include notes taken in the field (field notes), participant diaries or documents. The researcher may have collected verbal data through recording individual interviews or focus group discussions. Data are initially prepared through verbatim transcription, providing a written record of the conversation to include all verbal interactions noted between the participants and interviewer. Visual data can be in the form of still photographs, pictures or moving images. Initially, whatever the form of data, it will exist in copious amounts and require preparation prior to analysis.

The researcher will need to have a system of storing data that enables easy retrieval. This may be a computer-based system, depending on the type of data being held; for example, digital photographs can be held in online files, whereas printed photographs, accessed from historical records, will need indexing into a document-based filing system, perhaps by month and year the image was recorded, or by location. If using a computer program for analysis, the data may need specific preparation to enable its use.

Field notes and transcripts of interviews or focus group discussions are more likely to be available electronically as word-processed documents. Field notes may need reading through before organising into more coherent notes. Detailed notes can be stored in electronic files for easy access. Following data collection at interview or focus group, the researcher will have digitally recorded conversations that require transcription. Transcription can be a lengthy process, taking a number of hours to transcribe one hour of

Project title: Experience of hospital admission

Date of interview/focus group: 17.09.2012

Site: A

Facilitator: Pam Moule

Number of participants and code: HA 23

Line No.	Speaker	Comment	Analysis
1. 2.	Interviewer	Can you tell me about your experience of hospital admission?	
3. 4. 5.	HA23	It was the first time I have been in hospital. I didn't really have any expectations.	First admission. No prior expectations.

Figure 27.2 Example of a transcription template

recorded interaction. There are different schools of thought regarding the approach that should be taken. One view suggests transcription can be undertaken by support staff and need not occupy the researcher's time. Another view would suggest that there are enormous benefits gained through the researcher taking time to transcribe the recordings. These relate to the opportunity afforded for immersion in the data, from listening to the recording and word-processing its content. However the process is facilitated, the researcher must ensure that data are prepared to allow analysis. Once data are stored in easily accessible and identifiable files, be they electronically or physically based, the researcher can retrieve them for further analysis.

Often, if a team of researchers is undertaking the analysis it is helpful to work with an agreed template to support analysis. Working with a structured template enables the researchers to identify key information about a conversation. The template below is one example that can be used. The transcription can be presented using the layout in Figure 27.2. This presentation of data enables the research team members to identify key information from recorded conversations from either one-to-one interviews or focus groups. It provides space for the researcher to record interpretations alongside the text. In numbering the lines of data transcript, the researcher is able to identify specific quotes for use in later stages of analysis and presentation of data. These electronic documents can be shared with other team members and the participants to support verification.

USING COMPUTER SOFTWARE FOR ANALYSIS

Given the vast amounts of data generated in qualitative research, computer-assisted qualitative data analysis software (CAQDAS) can support the nurse researcher in analysis. A number of packages are available for use, offering differing levels of support. Some packages merely code and retrieve, others are able to start to make connections between categories, and there are packages that have theory-building capacity. This said, none completely analyses the data without researcher input. The researcher needs to identify the codes required and suggest the links that should be identified across the data.

The most commonly used packages include ETHNOGRAPH, ATLAS Ti, NVivo and HyperRESEARCH. ATLAS Ti, NVivo and HyperRESEARCH are examples of packages that are described as having theory-building capability. All these packages have 'coding' ability, retrieving data that relates to specific codes, which can then be arranged to show relationships as determined by the researcher.

The benefits of using computer-assisted data analysis aren't necessarily linked to time-saving, but there are advantages to the researcher in the way packages organise and store information. The electronic storage and retrieval of information within the programmes is superior to that offered through paper-based working or basic word-processing packages. They facilitate access by members of the research team working in different locations, supporting ongoing interpretation across national and international boundaries if required. There is scope to copy material and store a number of versions as analysis develops.

There are, however, some concerns that the use of packages may reduce researcher immersion with the data as the process becomes more mechanical, less cognitive and more detached (Polit and Beck, 2014).

These concerns arise because the researcher is one step away from handling the data, as the processes of analysis are managed within the programme. This said, the use of computer-based packages to support qualitative data analysis within nursing research is increasing. Changing practices may reflect the development of packages, with new versions offering greater scope and enhanced usability. It should be remembered that new versions are regularly produced and each one is more sophisticated in its functions than its predecessor. NVivo version 11, for example, supports the analysis of data on the web and social media. It allows researchers to collect, organise and analyse content from interviews, focus groups, surveys and audio recordings. Additionally, nurse researchers are developing their computer-based skills. This reflects an increased use of computer packages in other aspects of research, including computer employment in data collection and dissemination. Nurse researchers also have access to a range of training materials and courses to enable their use of computer-based packages. For example, there is supportive information on the use of CAQDAS provided by the Economic and Social Research Council through their Networking Project, www.surrey.ac.uk/sociology/research/researchcentres/caqdas/.

CONTENT ANALYSIS

As part of analysis data is organised and managed, the researcher is able to retrieve key areas of information. The process of analysis is therefore one of making sense of the data. **Content analysis** is the simplest form of data processing. It is a process that involves labelling the data for retrieval.

The nurse researcher starts with the textual or visual data. Taking interview transcripts as one example of textual data, the researcher will have a number of pages of data to analyse. The content of the data is explored, reducing the data by the process of 'coding'. This can be approached using one of a range of computer packages, or through manual processes. The process of coding is one where the researcher is retrieving the data, which can then be organised into categories and themes or constructs. Thus, the process relates to Miles et al.'s (2014) interpreting and conclusion drawing. Different researchers may approach the process of coding in different ways.

Moule et al. (2008) analysed interview data by initially reading through the transcripts and identifying keywords to reflect their individual interpretations of the data. These initial thoughts were then shared with other members of the research team. This was achieved by each member noting key issues on Post-it® notes. These were then arranged on a wall and reviewed by the team. The researchers then attempted to develop the codes into categories and themes, linking codes in ways that were meaningful. This research explored mental health nurses' experiences of using computer-based learning in the clinical setting. A team of three researchers analysed two focus group transcripts. Initially, the researchers were provided with electronic copies of the transcripts for coding. Each researcher read through the transcripts, identifying keywords to describe the content, producing a list of about 30 codes. The team then met to share their initial coding, which was presented on flip-chart sheets. It was clear from this stage of analysis that there was some consistency across the team, with a number of the key areas being identified by several members, though often different terminology was used to present the same issues. The team then agreed a common terminology and reviewed areas where there were differences in interpretation. Links across the data were then explored, building the coded data into categories and then these into themes. Research example 27.1 provides an example of the coded data from this research that relates to one theme, 'Meeting individual learning needs', with examples of data relating to two categories shown – flexibility of use (B1) and revision aid (B2).

Research example 27.1

Transcript data (Moule et al., 2008)

Interviewer: Okay then? So really what we wanted you to talk about was em, because you've already used the learning approach in relation to the basic life support with automated external defibrillators, we wanted to get a feel of your experience of using that, so …

Laura: I suppose from my point of view I'm quite experienced in using computers and IT so I found using the actual e-learning fairly simple. I don't know if everybody would though, and that's one thing I noted. I found it quite easy to use; it ran quite freely to some extent. There was some difficulty. In some

(Continued)

(Continued)

> of the e-learning when I was doing it, some of the video work was sticking, or not coming through quite properly and I suppose it's not downloading properly and it made it quite difficult to follow. **B2** But luckily I knew what I was doing anyway so I wasn't a new learner, I'm quite experienced in basic life support and AEDs so, I knew what I should be seeing so I can kind of guess what should be happening, so that was a bit awkward ...

Sophie: **B1** I went and did it at home because I felt that it would just be easier for me and quieter ...

[Additional text removed]

Sophie: **B1** I actually took a whole afternoon off to do mine and very much the same I felt that when my ... because when you are staring at that computer screen it can be a bit tedious, so I felt I could go off and have a cup of tea or walk around the garden whenever I felt like it, or re-go over bits I don't quite understand. So I think that was quite good, and you know you can read it at your own pace, I found it quite good for that reason.

[Additional text removed]

Liz: **B1** I did it all in one hit so I was a bit sick really. [*laugh*] With the ... on the background the fact that I had my day off to do it in one hit and I found that the easiest way to do it. I'm a bit more different, (a) I know the subject, but (b) once I start something I kind of like to complete it really. I found it quite easy.

At the initial stage of analysis, the researchers had coded the sentences in Research example 27.1 as data that showed the computer-based learning was flexible to use (B1) and that the package had been used as a revision tool (B2). Looking across the transcript, there were several examples of data that could be coded in this way, as shown in the three areas of text highlighted as (B1) above. Further analysis enabled the researchers to look at the coded areas for links. In the example above, the coded areas of 'revision of learning' and 'flexible way of learning' were seen to link, as supporting the way individual staff were learning. Thus, they were presented as categories of a theme, 'Meeting individual learning needs'. The research included two focus groups as part of its design and therefore the team chose to use manual analysis rather than a computer-assisted data analysis package. Had a computerised package been used, the researchers would have specified the links that should be made between the categories and themes, getting the programme to retrieve the data within this hierarchical structure rather than approaching this manually.

Reflective exercise

You could try to analyse the abstract of data below. What do you think are the key themes? Can you see a link between the themes?

Transcript	Code
We are using a programme that includes goal setting so women can learn from each other and from us so women set their own goals.	
Our belief is that they do better when they set their own goals and decide what to do, rather than being told what to do and this is more sustainable in the long run.	
The women told us the times that were best and how they wanted us to run it.	

If you try and code these sentences, you will see that the overall theme is related to being women-centred, developing a programme that allows women to set the agenda.

NARRATIVE ANALYSIS

Narratives and stories are collected through open interviews as part of research approaches that seek to understand the lived experience of participants. Narrative may also be generated in the field naturally as part of participant observation (see Chapter 24).

Those undertaking narrative analysis are concerned with the structure of the story, and the content. They will review how the story was organised. They will be interested in how the story was started and progressed, reviewing why it was told in a particular way, how the story was developed and brought to a conclusion. Transcriptions of the story will be read several times to identify the structure and facilitate analysis. Narrative analysis can form part of the analysis of textual data within research.

Discourse and conversation analysis aim to make sense of conversations. Conversation analysis can be employed to interpret digital recordings. Recordings are transcribed and analysed in detail to show overlaps in conversation, pauses and intonation. Conversation analysis describes and analyses the language of social interaction that takes place in conversation between people. Discourse analysis also seeks to make sense of conversation, but is interested in broader issues of the rules of conversations, mechanisms guiding discussion, power issues and gender positions. This form of analysis might be used to explore discourse between nurses and patients or members of the interprofessional healthcare team within the workplace. There are a range of approaches that researchers can use to analyse discourse which may involve some coding to facilitate management of the data. Ethnomethodologists who are concerned with questions about how people function in their everyday lives use conversation and discourse analysis. Communication is viewed as the basis of maintaining social order and is therefore analysed in order that roles, relationships and social norms might be understood.

INTERPRETING THE FINDINGS

This chapter has given some examples of how qualitative data can be stored and retrieved to enable its interpretation. As mentioned, there are a number of frameworks available to support the nurse researcher in the interpretation of qualitative data. Colaizzi (1978) devised such a framework, now frequently used, that provides a set of steps that can be applied in the analysis of phenomenological data that recounts the lived experience of the participant (see Research example 27.2 and Chapter 15). Colaizzi (1978) advised a process of analysis that involved six main steps. This was extended to include a seventh step as set out below (see Edward and Welch, 2011):

1. Transcribing and reading the interviews that are validated by the participants.
2. Extracting initial key data as statements.
3. Formulating meaning from the statements.
4. Looking for links in the data that are clustered into themes.
5. Ensuring that the themes represent the entire data set.
6. Researcher interpretative analysis of any symbolic representations in the form of a metaphor collected during the interview such as painting, poetry, music.
7. Validating the themes by returning the interpretations to the participants.

Step 6 is newly introduced and may not necessarily appear in research using the framework as seen in the example below.

Research example 27.2

Use of the Colaizzi framework

Bowen et al. (2015) used Colaizzi's framework to analyse data from 18 interviews with African–American women who were overweight and obese. The study used a phenomenological approach (see Chapter 15) to explore the lived experiences of being overweight and obese. The interviews were transcribed. The transcripts were read by the researchers who extracted significant statements and then formulated meaning from them. The statements were organised into clustered themes. The major themes included: impact of health conditions, incongruent perceptions and a desire for independence. The researchers did not implement the seventh stage and the results were not verified by the participants.

We can see that those analysing the data followed the steps of Colaizzi's framework. The main themes offer a description of the lived experiences of obese and overweight American–African women. Further analytical frameworks used within phenomenology include those of Giorgi (1985) and Smith et al. (2009).

Strauss and Corbin (1998) offer a comprehensive analytical framework to support the interpretation of data within a grounded theory approach (see Chapter 15). The method includes three types of coding:

● Open coding: data are broken into parts and compared for similarities. This generates the categories that are similar actions, events and objects that are grouped together.

Table 27.1   Framework for qualitative data analysis (Miles et al., 2014)

Activity	Description
Data reduction	Working with field notes or transcriptions, the data is subjected to selection and simplification. There is focus, as part of analysis, with transformation of the data. This process is continuous, occurring throughout the project.
Data display	The organisation of the data, displayed to allow conclusion drawing. This can be as text, verbatim quotes, graphs, charts or diagrams that show links and interrelationships.
Conclusion drawing/ verification	Starting at the data collection stage, the researcher begins to draw meaning from the data. Initial patterns in the data are noted, regularities and irregularities, possible explanations are outlined, causation patterns outlined. Final conclusions are made when data collection is complete and the research verifies these through confirming the conclusions.

- Axial coding: categories and sub-categories are linked around the axis of a category.
- Selective coding: this involves the integration and refining of the theory.

These frameworks are amongst many, including that previously mentioned, developed by Miles et al. (2014). This framework includes three interrelated activities that can occur concurrently (see Table 27.1).

Operationalising this process involves the researcher coding the data to identify data that enter the display. Further data reduction may be required as more categories emerge and the initial conclusions are drawn. This may lead to further data collection to verify the conclusions.

Lockyer et al. (2008), when analysing focus group data, employed this approach to data analysis. Nursing staff in surgical settings completed online-based learning in cancer care and were then asked to discuss their experiences. The excerpt in Table 27.2 shows how the data were displayed as a verbatim transcription. The complete transcript was read and re-read to gain initial understanding of the data. The data was then coded, reducing the data to support initial conclusion drawing. A further focus group was conducted and the data displayed and coded in the same way. Once both were coded,

Table 27.2   Example of a focus group transcript

Interviewer:	Tell me about the experience you have had of the online cancer nursing course. If you could just ... just tell me, maybe, what the experience has been – whenever you want to start.	
Jane:	I was just going to say, I think it was quite daunting at first because I looked at it and thought, Oh my God but when I actually worked through it and	Daunting

(Continued)

Table 27.2   (Continued)

	kind of studied the questions,	
	I thought Oh, well I do know some of the things, and	
	then kind of – you know –	Reinforced
	go through all the Internet questions and – you	learning
	know – reinforcement –	
	also learned new as well, but just sort of – pre-empted	New
	what I did know, and I didn't really realise I did this.	learning
Sue:	I was just going to say exactly the same thing. The	
	thought of it was actually ...	
	the thought of it was actually more work than it	
	actually was ...	
Interviewer:	Thank you very much. [nervous laughter]	
Sue:	I kept thinking I would have to put hours to one side	Daunting
	to do it, so I put it off and put it off, thinking this is	Flexible
	going to take ages, but then actually you could just	learning
	dip in and dip out, you didn't have to spend hours and	
	hours doing it each time. So then, kind of ... it was just	
	the thought ... the thought of ...	
Jane:	When you first put the first bit through, it was about	Daunting
	five pages wasn't it? – of the questions,	
	and you think – crikey! And I don't know this many ...	
	vignettes and bits you'd be able to do and then bits	
	you wouldn't. It's going to take ages. Probably be able	
	to do another lot – you know – do a second lot, but	
	actually, it was quite ... the actual site itself was quite	
	user friendly and it didn't take as long as I thought. You	User
	know when you went to it and it said 'username' and	friendly
	'password' and I thought my God, I can't do any of this,	
	and then I realised it was just the number, and again it	
	wasn't as daunting as I thought it was going to be – I	
	thought it would be a lot more complicated.	
Interviewer:	Right. And that is ... sort of ... the beginning part. Were	
	you talking about the programme ...	

Theme/sub-theme structure:

Learning experience   – student centred (flexibility, new learning, reinforced learning)

– need for preparation (daunting)

links were established across the data from both transcripts. This process again involved reducing the data and producing new displays to support ongoing conclusion drawing. Further data reduction took place with three key themes emerging, with sub-themes.

CHAPTER SUMMARY

- Qualitative data analysis often occurs throughout the project.
- Researchers are often working with vast amounts of data.
- A number of methods/frameworks exist that can support the researcher in data analysis.
- Audio data are prepared for analysis through transcription.
- A number of computer packages exist that can code and retrieve data and facilitate theory-building following researcher instruction.
- Textual data can be subjected to 'coding' or narrative analysis.
- The interpretation of findings can be verified through expert review or member checking.
- Verification processes support the maintenance of **rigour** and **trustworthiness**.

SUGGESTED FURTHER READING

Boeije, H. (2010) *Analysis of Qualitative Research*. London: Sage. This book covers three main areas: What is analysis? How to analyse? What to expect? Usefully, the text includes a section in each chapter on 'Doing your own qualitative research', which is useful for the more novice qualitative researcher.

Gibson, W. and Brown, A. (2009) *Working with Qualitative Data*. London: Sage. This text covers the transcription and presentation of data, working with image, text, video and audio data. It also provides insight into the use of technology in data analysis and how to write and present data.

WEBSITES

Information on the use of CAQDAS provided by the Economic and Social Research Council through their Networking Project: www.surrey.ac.uk/sociology/research/researchcentres/caqdas/.

Ethnograph : www.qualisresearch.com – qualitative data analysis software

Atlas.ti : www.atlasti.com – qualitative data analysis software

NVivo : www.qsrinternational.com – qualitative data analysis software

To access further resources related to this chapter, visit the companion website at http://study.sagepub.com/mouleaveyard3e

REFERENCES

Bowen, P., Eaves, Y., Vance, D. and Moneyham, L. (2015) 'A phenomenological study of obesity and physical activity in southern African American older women', *Journal of Aging and Physical Activity*, 23 (2): 221–9.

Colaizzi, P. (1978) 'Psychological research as a phenomenologist views it', in R. Valle and M. Kings (eds), *Existential Phenomenological Alternative for Psychology*. New York: Oxford University. pp. 48–71.

Edward, K-L. and Welch, T. (2011) 'The extension of Colaizzi's method of phenomenological enquiry', *Contemporary Nurse*, 39 (2): 163–71.

Elo, S., Kaariainen, M., Kanste, O., Polkki, T., Utriainen, H. and Kyngas, H. (2014) 'Qualitative content analysis: A focus on trustworthiness', *SAGE Open*, 1–10. Available at: www.sgo.sagepub.com/content/4/1/2158244014522633.full-text.pdf (accessed December 2015).

Giorgi, A. (1985) *Phenomenology and Psychology Research*. Pittsburgh, PA: Duquesne University Press.

Hollway, J. and Jefferson, T. (2012) *Doing Qualitative Research Differently: A Psychosocial Approach*, 2nd edn. London: Sage.

Koshy, E., Koshy, V. and Waterman, H. (2011) *Action Research in Healthcare*. London: Sage.

Lockyer, L., McGuigan, D. and Moule, P. (2008) 'Web-based learning in practice settings: Nurses' experiences and perceptions of impact on patient care', *Electronic Journal of E-learning*, Special Issue: e-Learning in Healthcare, 5 (4): 279–86.

Miles, M., Huberman, A. and Saldana, J. (2014) *Qualitative Data Analysis: A Methods Sourcebook*, 3rd edn. Thousand Oaks, CA: Sage.

Moule, P., Albarran, J., Bessant, E., Pollock, J. and Brownfield, C. (2008) 'A comparison of e-learning and classroom delivery of basic life support with automated external defibrillator use: A pilot study', *International Journal of Nursing Practice*, 14: 427–34.

Oktay, J. (2012) *Grounded Theory*. Oxford: Oxford University Press.

Polit, D. and Beck, C. (2014) *Essentials of Nursing Research: Appraising Evidence for Nursing Practice*, 8th edn. Philadelphia, PA: Lippincott Williams & Wilkins.

Smith, J., Flowers, P. and Larkin, M. (2009) *Interpretative Phenomenological Analysis*. London: Sage.

Strauss, A. and Corbin, J. (1998) *Basics of Qualitative Research: Techniques and Procedures for Developing Grounded Theory*, 2nd edn. Thousand Oaks, CA: Sage.

Yoo, M.S., Yoo, I.Y. and Lee, H. (2010) 'Nursing students' self evaluation using a video recording of Foley catheterization: Effects on students' competence, communication skills and learning motivation', *Journal of Nursing Education*, 49 (7): 402–5.

PART 4
SHARING RESEARCH

28
PRESENTING AND DISSEMINATING RESEARCH

Learning outcomes

This chapter will enable you to:

- identify the key components of a research report
- appreciate how to develop a paper for publication
- understand the publication process
- discuss how to develop and deliver a conference presentation and poster
- understand the range of methods available to use in disseminating research

The dissemination of research findings to the nursing and healthcare professions is a key component of the research process and one that should not be neglected. Nurses completing research need to plan their dissemination strategy as part of the research process, considering how to present the research to a range of interested audiences. Presentation may include a final written report, often required by those funding the research. Researchers often produce papers written for academic and professional audiences and can undertake international, national and local dissemination through presentation at conferences and research meetings. Additionally, dissemination may include podcasts, information leaflets or the production of specialised materials for audiences such as service users. A number of presentation options are available to the researcher and different approaches may be taken to dissemination that reflect the scope of the research. Developing a dissemination strategy will ensure that the research findings are presented in the public domain and are accessible to practitioners and a range of audiences.

In this chapter, we discuss the most common methods of dissemination, including the research report, academic papers and conference presentations.

DISSEMINATION OF RESEARCH

The research report

The **research report** is the presentation of the research journey. A report is usually required by the research funding body and may need to be written to a specified outline brief. It would usually include detail of the research process, outcomes and recommendations for future practice and research. A report may also be required for local, unfunded or small-scale research, though the scope of this may vary and alternative forms of output may be acceptable, such as a published paper in a peer-reviewed journal.

When there is a requirement for a formal report, the research team should understand what content is expected, when it should be produced and to whom it should be sent. Though report structures may vary, commonly the headings suggested in Table 28.1 are used. When completed, an International Standard Book Number (ISBN) can be obtained, often accessed through library or administration staff, which gives a unique identifying number to the report. The ISBN is usually 13 digit numbers presented as a barcode that enables ease of identification and tracking.

Table 28.1   Suggested research report structure

Heading	Content
Executive summary	Provides an overview of the report content, including main findings and recommendations for practice.
	This could be developed at the start to aid thinking about the report content and then revised once the report is completed.
Introduction	Should include the rationale for the study; research aims, questions/hypotheses should be stated here (see Chapter 9).
Literature review or background	The key literature including background policy should be included here. This may encompass current and previous knowledge. The depth of presentation will depend on the audience, with some funders requiring minimal information (see Chapter 6 and 20).
Research design	The overall research design is presented (see Chapters 11, 14-19).
Ethical approval	Any ethical approval processes involved should be presented, including reference to ethics committee approval, information provision, informed consent (see Chapters 7 and 8).
Sampling	The sampling approach used, sample size and any power calculations guiding this should be included. Any sampling issues should be discussed here and raised as part of the study limitations. The composition of the final study sample should be presented (see Chapter 12).
Data collection	The approach to data collection is presented, including presentation of data collection tools used, location and processes.
Data analysis	The handling of data is discussed, how it was stored and processed, including the use of any statistical tests, processes of qualitative analysis and rationale for these (see Chapters 26 and 27).

Heading	Content
Results	The presentation of quantitative results in the form of charts, tables and graphs is included in the report, either in total or as a selection. Qualitative findings are presented within the discussion.
Findings/discussion	In reports presenting qualitative data, this section will present the findings as part of a discussion. In reports presenting quantitative research, this section will discuss an interpretation of the results, providing evidence for support where available in the current literature.
Limitations	Here, the authors should refer to any limitations of the research design and process, identifying how these might affect the interpretation of the results.
Conclusions	The author discusses what the findings mean for further research and practice.
References	All literature referred to in the report is included here.
Appendices	These are included as appropriate, such as sample raw data or data collection tools.

Alternative modes of presentation

As mentioned above, the final research report remains a requirement for many funded research projects. It provides key information about the research activity and findings for the funder and other audiences. There are, however, some areas of research where different modes of presentation are becoming more acceptable or being offered as alternatives to the final report. It may well be the case that small-scale projects are looking for other outputs as part of the dissemination process.

Alternative outputs might include the **publication** of a **research paper** in a peer-reviewed journal, electronic publication of web pages or a You Tube clip, a podcast (a verbal presentation that can be downloaded onto mobile devices such as a mobile phone) or the dissemination of any products of the research such as teaching materials or guidelines. Some funders of educational research, where the dissemination and sharing of newly produced teaching materials or other research outputs are prioritised above a traditional report, are requesting such outputs. Nurse researchers must be clear at the outset of the research what the desired outputs are, and plan to deliver these on completion of the project. Calls for project proposals will often outline specific deliverables that may encompass more than a final report (see Chapter 10).

Dissertations and theses

Nurses studying at undergraduate (BSc), Master's (MSc) and doctoral level will often be required to present their research as a dissertation or thesis. The dissertation can be the final written assessment of a BSc and MSc programme, written to meet specific learning outcomes and to certain criteria. For example, a dissertation can address research questions through a literature review or primary research, presented with an abstract and chapters that include the background, methodology, discussion of findings to answer the research question and a concluding chapter that presents implications for nursing practice and further research.

The thesis is a more in-depth piece of written work presented as part of the written examination of a professional doctoral programme, such as an EdD (Doctorate in Education) or doctoral studies (PhD, Doctor of Philosophy). A number of texts are written specifically to guide those producing a thesis (see Oliver, 2014; Greetham, 2014; Murray, 2011). The length of a doctoral thesis varies between 40,000 and 100,000 words and can be written over a period of two to five years. The structure of the thesis will be determined by the research approach taken, but is likely to include chapters on background literature, research design, data collection, data analysis, discussion of results, theoretical development, conclusions and recommendations for practice and research.

WRITING UP RESEARCH PAPERS

Dissemination strategy

The authors of research reports and papers should conceive the dissemination strategy at an early stage and this should include publications, conference and other presentations. In writing any paper for publication, the authors must be confident of the integrity of the publication content, avoid plagiarism and present the results in such a way as to protect anonymity and confidentiality. Any possible conflicts of interest that exist for the author must also be considered, and the authors must avoid simultaneous submission of a paper to a number of journals for publication.

A dissemination plan can be developed prior to commencing the research, as part of an application for funding or support. If this is not the case, then the team should discuss and develop a dissemination strategy early on in the research and identify the authorship of papers. This should include mapping the potential publications and authors' contributions, which may allow for novice writers to work alongside more experienced writers and will enable time for negotiations and agreement of authorship that reflect the contributions made, avoiding later conflict. It is customary practice to disclose each author's contribution to a paper prior to acceptance. This enables publishers to determine whether those credited with authorship have made a significant contribution to the paper and the development and implementation of the research. Authors are also asked to return a completed copyright assignment form, often at the stage of submission. This ensures the reviewing journal has the right to publish the paper should it be accepted, and prevents simultaneous submission to a number of journals. The submission process can involve authors making statements regarding the research ethics of a project, which might include confirming whether the study was presented to an ethics committee, the outcomes of this and any processes involved such as provision of written information and securing of informed consent (see Chapters 7 and 8).

Editors are expecting to receive a paper that assigns credit to other authors and funders where needed and presents accurate findings. Authors should ensure that any presentation conforms to acceptable ethical practices, being honest in its content and presentation. This will require careful construction and proofreading, involving the statistician if required and team members. Team members should also, as a matter of good practice, declare any conflict of interest and identify any funding received in the paper.

What, who for, where?

One of the main ways of disseminating research findings is through publication. Research papers may also present other aspects of the research such as the literature review, methodology and ethical discussions. The process of publishing multiple journal papers from one piece of research is known as 'salami slicing'. The decision as to what should be written may come early on in the research process, or develop as the research continues and is completed. Authors must, however, ensure they do not self-plagiarise if writing more than one paper for publication from the same piece of research.

The nurse researcher will need to consider the target audience for the research, as this will help determine suitable journals for publication. A number of audiences may be interested in various elements of the research. For example, research in the field of cancer care education could have three potential key audiences: practitioners in cancer care, educationalists in universities and healthcare settings, and researchers. Each paper should be presented differently, with the emphasis tailored to the target audience, and can be submitted to journals that reflect this (see Table 28.2). There may also be a requirement among some professionals to write for those journals that have high academic ranking, or Impact Factor ratings. The Impact Factor gives an indication of the standing of the journal in the field and is a measure of the number of citations it receives. Writing for journals with a higher impact rating can be a strategy for nurses attached to academic institutions likely to be submitted by the institution as part of an exercise that measures research quality, the Research Excellence Framework (REF). In the REF, national and international experts will grade the quality of published research and further research funding will be awarded according to the institutional grading achieved. However, it should be noted that those reviewing REF submissions are most concerned with the quality of the individual papers, and it is the originality, rigour and significance of the work which is most important.

Table 28.2   Possible journals to consider

Focus	Journals
Cancer care practitioner	*European Journal of Cancer Care* (http://onlinelibrary.wiley.com/journal/10.1111/(ISSN)1365-2354)
Education	*Nurse Education Today* (www.nurseeducationtoday.com)
	Nurse Education in Practice (www.nurseeducationinpractice.com)
Research	*Journal of Advanced Nursing* (http://onlinelibrary.wiley.com/journal/10.1111/(ISSN)1365-2648
	Nurse Researcher (http://journals.rcni.com/journal/nr)

It should also be remembered that the range of publications available is vast, and unless the researcher is familiar with the journals in the field an initial search is required to include a review of the aims, objectives, philosophy and journal contents.

Following contributors' guidelines

Having identified the target journal for a particular paper, the researcher needs to obtain a copy of the guidelines for authors and use these to inform the writing. Guidelines can be available in published journals and are usually held online. In relation to the journals in Table 28.2, key information is available on the websites identified. Prior to writing, all authors should have access to these guidelines, have agreed different writing responsibilities and the timeframe for the work, and have dealt with any ethical issues of writing as discussed below. Novice writers will benefit from the support of more experienced authors drawn from within the team or of supervisors and research advisers. It is vital to check through the paper for errors prior to submission, and all referencing should be checked for accuracy.

Paper submission

Contributors' guidelines should also state how to submit a paper. Papers are usually submitted electronically via the journal website. As part of the submission process, authors may need to provide information such as authorship details and evidence of ethical approval. A statement is often needed to authenticate author contributions; this may need electronic signatures or some form of verification from all those involved. Receipt of the submission will be confirmed by the journal and then the process of review is commenced. This usually starts with initial consideration by the editor. Editors can decide to reject a paper at this stage, but hopefully will forward the paper for full review by two or three independent reviewers selected from a panel who have appropriate subject and/or methodological expertise. The review process can take a number of weeks. Reviewers are often academics or practitioners, who are provided with a set of key questions to guide the review process. The types of questions reviewers are asked to address include:

- Does the paper meet the aims and scope of the journal?
- Are the presentation criteria met?
- Is the content accurate and up to date?
- Is there scientific rigour in the research?
- What contribution does the paper make to the field?
- Should the paper be published in the journal?

Revise or rethink

There are generally four possible outcomes from the review of an academic paper:

- Acceptance without change (this is rare).
- Acceptance with minor revisions (requires changes and resubmission to the editor and /or reviewers).

- Acceptance with major revisions (requires changes and resubmission to reviewers as well as to the editor).
- Rejection (the reviewers feel the paper is not appropriate for publication in the journal).

Depending on the outcome, there will be various actions required. Acceptance without change will result in you receiving 'galley proofs' of the paper at some stage to check and return. This is important, should be done carefully and quick replies are often needed to meet a tight publication deadline. These proofs are a copy of those that will appear in print, so they need to be accurate. It may be several weeks before the paper appears in the journal, though in the interim electronic versions may be made available online. Acceptance with minor or major revisions requires some thought. Feedback from the reviewers will be helpful in identifying what amendments are needed, and the authors need to agree who will make these changes prior to resubmission. These should be done as quickly as possible and checked carefully before resubmission.

Rejection rates can be high and the feedback provided should help the researcher make decisions about what to do next. It might be that the paper needs further development or restructuring prior to submission to a new journal. The research team may also need to review the emphasis of a paper or reconsider the target audience. Difficulties with presentation and content will need addressing prior to forwarding to other journals. It should be remembered that not all research can be published and occasionally researchers may not secure publication despite submitting revised papers to a second or third journal.

PREPARING CONFERENCE PRESENTATIONS

Conference abstracts

Conference calls appear throughout the year, often advertised online and through mailings. Conferences are held internationally, nationally and locally. More conferences are including virtual access to enable global attendance. A novice researcher may want to select a conference where new presenters are encouraged to attend and present to small audiences in a less formal way. This can be facilitated in conferences that run along a themed approach, where a smaller number of delegates attend one themed group to hear presentations about one particular area such as technology-enhanced learning. The presenters and delegates are able to get to know each other throughout the conference as they deliver their papers within the small group setting. Often, this kind of environment is supportive and less threatening than conferences where presenters speak to a large auditorium of delegates. Most conferences offer opportunities for poster display and sometimes there is a scheduled five-minute presentation of each poster. These events can also be a good way of developing presentation skills.

It is important to ensure synergy between the intended presentation and conference themes outlined in the call, before selecting which conference to submit an abstract to. Many conferences are focused on particular specialisms, such as critical care, cancer care,

Title: Evaluating a leadership programme: impact and future directions

Authors: Pam Moule, Jane Hadfield and Michele Lima

Purpose: Academics, health service representatives and service users were involved in all stages of evaluating a leadership programme delivered to nursing and other staff at one large hospital.

Methods: First stage data collection involved three Knowledge café (KC) events with 36 staff who had completed the programme. A KC is a data collection approach, which offers a way of engaging staff in conversations (Brown and Isaacs, 2005), often providing voice to those who would not normally be heard (Thunberg, 2011). The content of KC conversations was captured and thematically analysed. Second stage data collection included 15 telephone interviews with individuals who had participated in the KC. Data from this stage were also thematically analysed.

Results: Four main themes were identified from the KC and interview data. 1. *Impacts and benefits of the programme for self and organization*: The programme provided an opportunity for frontline, supervisory and senior managers to learn together. This approach meant staff had been exposed to a wide range of new ideas and perspectives. 2. *New learning applied to practice:* Participants talked about applying their learning to leadership roles. A number reported taking a different approach in their management of more challenging situations and being more confident. 3. *Ongoing support*: Participants felt the hospital learning culture could improve the transfer of learning to practice. They suggested peer support and ongoing mentorship could help. 4. *Course delivery: The* use of techniques, such as role play, provided staff with opportunities to practise skills, which were seen as challenging.

Discussion/Conclusions: The leadership programme was successful on many levels. Organising the delivery of content across groups of nursing, other clinical and non-clinical staff meant they all learned from each other and developed new insights, which they felt benefitted both themselves and the hospital. The course provided new tools and employed teaching and learning approaches that facilitated self-reflection and the development of new skills and ways of working. The evaluation also suggested there was a need to develop a wider 'learning culture' in the hospital, which would offer ongoing support for staff and help them overcome the challenges of applying their learning in practice. The findings have been used to inform the organisation and delivery of new leadership programmes in the hospital, which have included the planning of ongoing internal support to help staff applying new learning to practice.

References

Brown, J. and Isaacs, D. (2005) *The World Café: Shaping our future through conversations that matter.* San Francisco: Berrett-Koehler.
Thunberg, O. (2011) World cafes and dialog seminars as processes for reflective learning in organizations. *Reflective Practice,* 12 (3): 319–333.

Figure 28.1   Example of a conference abstract

nursing education, nursing research or methods, and will invite abstract submissions related to specified themes. For example, the British Association of Critical Care Nurses hosts an annual conference and invites calls for specific themes such as evidence-based practice, clinical practice and education.

When submitting an abstract, thought needs to be given to the probable content of the presentation. If presenting at a research-focused conference, the methodology or ethical issues are likely to be emphasised, whereas practitioners attending a clinical conference may prefer to hear more about the research results. The abstract needs to clearly link to the conference focus and any themes. For example, the abstract shown in Figure 28.1 was submitted and accepted at an international nursing conference. It was written in the required format and provides a title, presents the research under key headings that reflect the research process and includes two references.

Conference calls should include the following information that will help presenters:

- Key practical information:
    - dates of the conference
    - location of the conference
    - accommodation
    - travel
    - payment.
- Specific information:
    - aims of the conference
    - themes for presentation
    - abstract content and presentation, suggested headings, reference use, word limit
    - instructions for submission
    - review process
    - dates of notification of reviewer's decision
    - criteria for selection that should be adhered to closely.

Any submission not addressing the specified criteria is unlikely to be successful. A presenter profile may be requested, as well as information on employing organisations, funding and evidence of ethical approval for any study presented.

Oral presentations

If the abstract is selected for an oral presentation, the conference organisers will contact the presenter, providing details of the date, time and location of the presentation. Details of the facilities available should also be provided. Commonly, presenters use PowerPoint presentations to present key information; alternatively, presenters can read a paper or other text, such as poems. A presenter needing Internet access should ensure this is available prior to the conference.

The content of the presentation needs to be developed to reflect the detail of the accepted abstract, and consideration should be given to the amount of time available for the presentation and questions. A 20-minute time slot will allow for a presentation that includes approximately ten PowerPoint slides. A PowerPoint presentation would include an opening slide, featuring the logos of any funding bodies and the presenter's employer, and should follow a corporate design if one exists. PowerPoint presentations allow for the use of images, video and, if Internet connection is available, the ability to demonstrate and link to the web. Given the limited scope of the presentation, it is unlikely that the entire research project will be presented, but emphasis will be placed on certain aspects of the research dependent on the audience. The content may emphasise the research methodology, ethical issues or findings.

Some conference organisers request access to the PowerPoint slides ahead of the conference. In these cases, the slides will be loaded and available in the appropriate conference room for presenter access. Alternatively, the conference organisers may request the presentation on arrival or expect the presenters to load the PowerPoint onto the conference room computer. Whatever the process, it is recommended that presenters visit the allocated room ahead of the presentation to familiarise themselves with the surroundings, ensure they can access any PowerPoint presentation and check the availability of any other equipment needed.

More novice presenters may wish to enrol colleagues to listen to the presentation prior to the conference. Alternatively, there may be an opportunity to present the work informally to a local audience ahead of the conference. This will give an opportunity to check the timing and slide content, and refine the presentation if needed. It can be useful to have feedback on your style of presentation and mannerisms. Presenters can also take printed versions of the PowerPoint presentation, gauging the number of copies needed on the expected audience size. Presenters should have the presentation on at least one USB stick or similar device, even if it has been emailed ahead.

Poster presentations

Posters form a significant part of nursing and healthcare conferences, with a number awarded prizes for innovative presentations. Many organisers allocate specific time slots in a conference programme for a formal presentation of posters. Other conferences include more informal viewing slots, as well as setting coffee and lunch breaks around the displays. Presenters should be available to discuss the poster content at these times.

Presenters often leave contact information with posters for delegates to take, such as business cards, PDF versions of the poster and/or an abstract with contact details. Taking such steps ensures contact information is available for delegates when the posters are left unattended.

Applications to present a conference poster follow the same process as that outlined above, with an abstract being submitted in a particular format. Successful presenters will receive specific information from the conference organisers. This will include: the required poster size; whether the design should be presented as landscape or portrait; when the poster is expected to be displayed; where it will be displayed; and if a verbal presentation is required, this will be indicated. The times of scheduled poster viewings should also be identified.

Poster presentations have been a popular method of displaying research findings at conferences for some time (see the example in Figure 28.2). Given the longevity of their use, there has been a development in the style and quality of presentation, aided by the advent of computerised desktop publishing software. Many nurse researchers will have access to design and production services within their organisations, or can access these services from high street printers. There is often a charge for these services that can be considerable. This may be justifiable if the poster is likely to be used more than once, and can be displayed in workplace or education settings following use at conference. The poster may need to present a corporate image if one exists for the presenting

Conceptualising nursing through simulation
Liz Berragan

Department of Nursing and Midwifery, University of the West of England, Alexandra Warehouse, Gloucester Docks, GL1 2LG
Elizabeth.Berragan@uwe.ac.uk

Background

Simulation has become an established pedagogy for teaching the fundamental skills of nursing, providing the learner with opportunity to acquire essential skills in an environment closely representing reality.

Whilst the concept of simulation is not new, there has been an increase in its use in nurse education both nationally and internationally (Jeffries, 2007; Kaakinen and Arwood, 2009; Warland, 2011; Lasater, 2012).

The Nursing and Midwifery Council have identified standards for the safe use of simulation and its inclusion as a contributory part to practice learning (NMC, 2007).

There is still a need for robust evidence in relation to the role of simulation as a teaching and learning approach.

Aims

This aim of this study was to explore the impact of simulation on learning for first year undergraduate nursing students and focus upon:

- The evolution of simulation in nurse education.
- The student experience of participating in simulation.
- Mentor and educator views of simulation.
- Theoretical underpinning of simulation learning.

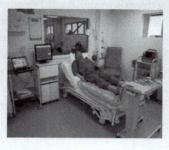

Methods and Conceptual Approach

Conducted as a small-scale narrative case study, this study explores experiences of learning through simulation of a small number of undergraduate nursing students (n=9), nurse mentors (n=4) and nurse educators (n=4).

Data was collected through semi-structured interviews supported by student reflections and observation of student OSCEs. Data analysis was achieved through thematic analysis and progressive focusing (Parlett and Hamilton, 1972).

The conceptual frameworks used for this study draw upon the work of Benner and Sutphen (2007) and Engeström (1994). Benner and Sutphen's work highlights the complex nature of situated knowledge in practice disciplines such as nursing. They suggest that knowledge is integrated within the curriculum through pedagogies of formation, interpretation, contextualisation and performance.

Engeström's work on activity theory and expansive learning, recognises the links between learning and the environment of work and highlights the possibilities for learning to inspire change, innovation and the creation of new ideas. His notion of expansive learning offers nurse education a way of reconceptualising the learning that occurs during simulation.

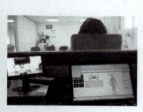

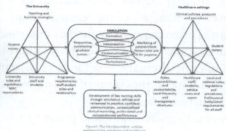

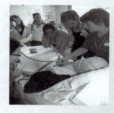

Results

Participants suggested that simulation had the potential to offer an environment in which the students could begin to practise the performance of nursing and bear witness to human events (performance) and acquire the skills of 'practical reasoning'.

They suggested that it offered the opportunity to consider the context of care (contextualisation), interpret nursing information (interpretation) and learn to develop their identities as nurses (formation). Students who demonstrated development in each of these pedagogies were successfully learning to become nurses.

Mentors and educators suggested that simulation may also offer an opportunity to support 'reflective transfer' and enable students to explore the contradictions between the activity systems of the university and healthcare settings as they learned and developed their nursing practice.

Discussion

Results from the study support the contribution of this pedagogical model towards elucidation of an effective and expansive approach to learning in nurse education. They also help to illustrate the different activity systems to which student nurses are exposed, and the expansive learning process that can occur between these systems, and is experienced by students as they learn to be nurses.(See Figure 1).

An expansive approach to learning through simulation may offer an environment where students can be supported to explore and examine the role of the student nurse and the responsibilities incumbent upon them in that role to deliver safe, evidence-based nursing care.

Clearly, if the aim of simulation is to enable students to learn and begin to develop their identities as nurses in an environment that authentically mimics the clinical nursing environment, then learning must be adequately theorised, supported and evaluated.

Conclusion

Simulation offers potential for learning nursing. In order to be effective, however, such activity needs to have a solid theoretical foundation. Taking a root and branch approach, the pedagogies of formation, interpretation, contextualisation and performance, could helpfully revise and refresh present approaches to simulation learning .

The opportunity to use simulation to explore patient care supported by these pedagogies offers an expansive approach to learning and a contrast to the linear task orientated approaches of the past. This might offer a more liberating experience for nurse educators and an integrative experience for nurse mentors and students.

Having a greater understanding of the learning that occurs through simulation experiences may enable educators and practitioners to harness the potential of simulation for the development of a competent, confident and caring nursing workforce.

References: Benner, P. and Sutphen, M. (2007) Learning across the professions: the clergy a case in point. *Journal of Nursing Education.* 46, 3, 103-108. Engeström, Y. (1994) Training for change: new approach to instruction and learning in working life Geneva: International Labour Office. Jeffries, P.R. (2007) Simulation in nursing education. New York: National League for Nursing. Kaakinen, J. and Arwood, E. (2009) Systematic review of nursing simulation literature for use of learning theory. International Journal of Nursing Education Scholarship. 6, 1, Article 16, 1-20. Lasater, K. (2012) Controversies in simulation. Personal communication. Fringe Event NETNEP 2012 Nurse Educators Conference, Baltimore, Maryland. Nursing and Midwifery Council, (2007) Simulation and Practice Learning Project: Outcome of a pilot study to test the principles for auditing simulated practice learning environments in the pre-registration nursing programme (Final report). London: NMC. Parlett, M. and Hamilton, D. (1972) Evaluation as illumination: A new approach to the study of innovatory programmes. Occasional Paper No. 9, Centre for Research in the Educational Sciences University of Edinburgh. Reprinted in G. V. Glass, (Editor) (1976) Evaluation Studies Review Annual, Beverly Hills. SAGE Publications. 140-157. Warland, J. (2011) Using simulation to promote nursing students' learning of work organization and people management skills: a case study. Nurse Education in Practice. 11, 3, 186-191.

Figure 28.2   Example poster

university, hospital or employing organisation. Usually, a poster will feature the logo of any funding body and employing organisation(s), as well as including details about the content authors and place of work.

The design of the poster needs consideration. Often, less is more. Presenting key images and text can be the most effective. Designers should remember that the content of the poster needs to be digested in five minutes, and consideration should be given to the colours used, eye-catching use of pictures or design, the use of headings and essential text (Sherman, 2010).

In designing the poster, transportability also needs thought. The most popular presentation is a poster of A3 size and above, laminated for protection, and rolling to enable transport in a lightweight and waterproof carrying tube. Preferably, the tube should travel as hand luggage if flying, though it may have to be placed in the aircraft hold.

Conference organisers may provide materials to enable display of the poster; however, it is recommended that presenters take a supply of adhesive Velcro, drawing pins or other adhesive materials and a mechanism for displaying PDFs, abstracts and business cards, such as an A4 plastic wallet.

CHAPTER SUMMARY

- A dissemination strategy should be decided as early as possible in the research process and agreed by members of the research team.
- A research report is often required by funders and would usually include details of the research process, outcomes and recommendations for future practice.
- There are a number of alternative methods of dissemination that include presentations, research papers, provision of online materials, podcasts and making available the products of research.
- Research students are usually required to present their research as a dissertation or thesis.
- Researchers need to follow contributors' guidance when producing papers and abstracts for conference presentation.
- Novice researchers may benefit from gaining feedback on submissions and presentations and can benefit by working with more experienced writers and presenters initially.

SUGGESTED FURTHER READING

Happell, B. (2012) 'Writing and publishing clinical articles: A practical guide', *Emergency Nurse*, 20 (1): 33–8. This article offers a practical approach to writing for clinical and professional journals. It also explains the editorial process.

Holland, K. and Watson, R. (eds) (2012) *Writing for Publication in Nursing and Healthcare: Getting it Right*. Chichester: Wiley-Blackwell. This is a resource for nurses and healthcare professionals thinking of publishing. The text covers a variety of media such as journal articles and book reviews. It helps the reader develop writing skills.

WEBSITES

To access further resources related to this chapter, visit the companion website at http://study.sagepub.com/mouleaveyard3e

REFERENCES

Greetham, B. (2014) *How to Write Your Undergraduate Dissertation*, 2nd edn. Basingstoke: Palgrave Macmillan.

Murray, R. (2011) *How to Write a Thesis*, 3rd edn. Maidenhead: Open University Press.

Oliver, P. (2014) *Writing Your Thesis*, 3rd edn. London: Sage.

Sherman, R. (2010) 'How to create an effective poster presentation', *American Nurse Today*, 5 (9): 13–15.

29

USING RESEARCH IN PRACTICE

Learning outcomes

This chapter will enable you to:

- appreciate the need for research to be implemented in practice
- have an understanding of some of the barriers for getting research into practice
- understand the difference between evidence-based practice and research utilisation
- have an appreciation of the different roles for nurse researchers

Traditionally, nursing practice has been learned from a combination of books, journals, individual experiences, observation of the practice of other practitioners and word of mouth. When little thought is given to the rationale behind them, such learned practices can become routine and ritualistic. In other words, a nurse does something because it has always been done that way, it says so in the procedure book or simply: 'This is the way that Sister likes it done'. Learning in this way is not necessarily a bad thing and much of the traditional knowledge being passed on is based on sound reasoning. However, there is a danger that these routine practices are never questioned and the rationale underpinning the practice has been forgotten. It is also thought that what we learn through experience is more enduring than what we are taught (Parahoo, 2014). However, experience can be narrow: consider how many patients you have cared for with one disease and the number of treatment approaches you have used for this disease. This may be good experience, but it may mean that you are unfamiliar with other treatment options and possibly reluctant to try other care approaches.

Research is different because it is a systematic enquiry that uses disciplined methods to answer questions or solve problems. Research is important for every nurse, and nursing research is needed to inform nursing practice. The evidence provided by research helps to ensure that care is safe and effective and, to some extent, enables nurses to describe and explain nursing practice.

The emphasis on practice being evidence-based has altered the way nursing research is regarded and it has become every nurse's responsibility to engage in research in some way. The expectation is that, at the very minimum, nurses will have an awareness of research. Awareness in this context requires nurses to access, read, appraise and apply research that is relevant to their practice. In other words, it is expected that nurses utilise research as part of their professional practice.

There is, however, also a need to recognise that it is not always easy to implement research findings and that the existence of a gap between research and practice in healthcare has long been recognised. Back in 1601, the benefits of limes and sauerkraut to prevent scurvy were discovered, but the British Navy did not introduce rations containing vitamin C until 1795. It then took a further 70 years for the British Board of Trade to order citrus fruits to be provided on merchant ships – a total of 264 years between evidence and practice (Berwick, 2003). Then in the twentieth century, in a speech to the World Health Organization in 1968, Lord Rothschild stated: 'If for the next 20 years, no further research were to be carried out, if there were a moratorium on research, the application of what is already known, of what has already been discovered, would result in widespread improvements in world health' (cited in Peters, 1992: 68).

Since then, the volume of research has increased and there is even more of a drive to implement research findings in practice with the advent of National Service Frameworks, the Commission for Health Improvement (CHI) and the National Institute for Health and Care Excellence (NICE), which have sought to promote the notion of evidence-based practice amongst healthcare practitioners as well as the recipients of healthcare. Associated with this has been an increasing public awareness of healthcare research in terms of the way it can lead to increased health benefits and the areas where there is still a need for more research. However, actually implementing change, getting research into practice and improving the quality of patient care are complex things which can be very demanding and is an issue that has been recognised for some time (Rycroft-Malone et al., 2002). This chapter discusses issues concerned with getting research into practice, how nurses and **healthcare consumers** influence the research agenda and research roles for nurses.

WHY SHOULD WE USE RESEARCH IN PRACTICE?

The impetus to use research in practice can be arrived at from a number of sources but essentially it is driven by the need to deliver care that is efficacious, patient-orientated and cost-effective. Some of this is because healthcare resources are limited, both in terms of financial and staff resources but also in respect of the level of knowledge of how to restore or maintain health. The imperative is for healthcare professionals to meet the challenges of delivering healthcare in the best way possible and to ensure that we actually think about the care that we provide and appreciate the expectations of our patients. Furthermore, it is illogical to spend time, effort and resources on research, only to have the findings ignored, and continue to practise on the basis of tradition and experience rather than rely on information that should improve the outcome and quality of care. Indeed the requirement to integrate research evidence in practice is now firmly stated in most professional nursing documentation across the world (Aveyard et al., 2015).

Getting research into practice, or **research utilisation**, is about applying research findings from one or more studies in practice and is unrelated to the original research (Polit and Beck, 2012). This recognises that completing a research study is not sufficient; that both nurse researchers and practitioners have responsibilities. For nurse researchers, these responsibilities focus on ensuring that their research has relevance for practice. This is not saying that all nursing research has to have a clinical orientation, but simply that the main focus ought to be on problems that practitioners identify as being relevant to them professionally and to the practice of nursing. Researchers also need to ensure that their research is based on rigorous methods and, where appropriate, is multi-centred. Associated with this is the need to consider whether studies need to be repeated to confirm findings, either with different patient groups or within different settings, to ensure that findings are robust. The role of the nurse researcher is not, however, simply about doing research. Nurse researchers also have a responsibility to ensure that their findings are published and taken to a wider audience so that they can be implemented in practice once a study has been completed.

The responsibilities of nurses in practice in relation to research focus on the utilisation of findings in their own practice and the practice of others, including healthcare assistants, learners and other healthcare professionals. This means keeping up to date by reading research reports and attending conferences where research findings are reported. In addition, you then need to apply, appropriately, your research-based knowledge in practice. These responsibilities are related, primarily, to the development of an evidence-based practice culture in healthcare, as well as being connected with the need for nurses to accept personal responsibility for professional development and a sharing of knowledge with other healthcare practitioners.

This need for research utilisation is not specific to nursing or healthcare and, as has already been indicated, is not even a contemporary issue. However, the need to put research findings into practice has taken on more significance because of the pressures on healthcare resources, alongside societal demands for 'best practice' in terms of healthcare delivery. It is, however, important to recognise that research utilisation is not synonymous with evidence-based practice (see Chapter 1).

Evidence-based practice has been described as the integration of best research evidence with clinical expertise and patient values (Sackett et al., 2005). Evidence-based practice involves making clinical decisions on the best evidence available. The best evidence is primarily gleaned from rigorous research, but also uses other sources of credible information such as clinical expertise, patient input and resources available for practice.

HOW DO YOU 'DO' EVIDENCE-BASED PRACTICE?

Evidence-based practice involves applying the best evidence to a particular case and also using professional judgement and seeking patient preference (Aveyard et al., 2013).

This involves balancing the risks and benefits of alternative treatments for each patient, alongside accounting for the patient's unique clinical condition and personal preferences.

Evidence-based practice can be said to comprise five explicit steps:

1. Identify a problem from practice and turn it into a specific question. This might be about the most effective intervention for a particular patient, about the most appropriate test or about the best method for delivering nursing care.
2. Find the best available evidence that relates to the specific question, usually through a thorough and systematic search of the literature.
3. Critically appraise the evidence for its validity (closeness to the truth), usefulness (practical application) and methodological rigour.
4. Identify and use the current best evidence, and, together with the patient or client's preferences and the practitioner's expertise and experience, apply it to the situation.
5. Evaluate the effect on the patient or client, and reflect on the nurse's own performance.

Current pre-qualifying nurse education helps students address all these stages, but specifically you need to learn how to search effectively for appropriate evidence and research through a range of literature sources (see Chapters 4 and 6) and how to critically appraise research (see Chapter 5).

You should note that evidence-based practice and research utilisation are not the same thing. The main distinction is that evidence-based practice is broader than research utilisation because factors other than research findings are incorporated. Evidence-based practice uses a variety of evidence to identify what is best at solving a clinical problem; whilst this is usually research, it can incorporate a wider range of evidence, whilst research utilisation is the use of findings from a study, or studies, into a practical application. Thus, the focus for research utilisation is to translate empirically derived knowledge into clinical practice.

Practising evidence-based nursing is not always straightforward. It involves a conscious use of current best evidence in making clinical decisions rather than relying on traditional/ritualistic practice, opinion or authority. Evidence-based practice integrates professional judgement with research findings, patient preferences and circumstances, together with any resource constraints. Evidence-based practice requires you to have the skills to identify, appraise and implement research findings appropriately for the different clinical situations encountered. This can present nurses with a challenge, but it can also act as a framework for self-directed learning that is so necessary in this age of rapid clinical advances (Polit and Beck, 2012). There are, though, resources available that can support evidence-based practice in nursing such as systematic reviews and clinical practice guidelines.

Systematic reviews are considered to give the best evidence available because all (or as much as possible) evidence relating to a clinical problem has been gathered, evaluated and synthesised (see Chapter 20) to enable conclusions to be drawn about effective practices. These are published in peer-reviewed journals that can be readily searched for (see Chapter 4 and 6) and accessed. They are also available on databases such as the Cochrane Database of Systematic Reviews (CDSR); the Centre for Reviews and Dissemination at the University of York; the Database of Abstracts of Reviews of Effects (DARE); and the Joanna Briggs Institute at the University of Adelaide.

Clinical practice guidelines should all be evidence-based and are similar to systematic reviews in that they attempt to distil a large amount of evidence into a manageable format. The main difference between systematic reviews and clinical practice guidelines is that the latter give specific recommendations for evidence-based decision making, although it is important to check that the guidelines are based on a strong evidence base. Clinical practice guidelines are developed to provide guidance in clinical practice even when there may not be reliable evidence available. Usually, a clinical practice guideline will be developed by a group, which may include researchers, practitioners and experts on the problem and will often result in a consensus decision outcome for the guideline (especially if there is limited research evidence). Hence, it is possible for different guidelines to result from the same evidence base and also because they will have to conform to different local circumstances and resources. Helping to develop clinical practice guidelines is one of the areas where you as a practitioner can combine your clinical experience with your research knowledge. Similarly, your critical appraisal skills will be useful in assessing the appropriateness of clinical practice guidelines developed by others for use in your own clinical practice. There are now also clinical practice guidelines available online, such as two in the UK: the Translating Research into Practice (TRIP) database (www.tripdatabase.com) and the National Institute for Health and Care Excellence (www.nice.org.uk); the National Guideline Clearinghouse in the USA (www.guideline.gov); and in Canada the Registered Nurse Association of Ontario (www.rnao.org/bestpractices).

ORIGINS AND DEVELOPMENT OF EVIDENCE-BASED PRACTICE

The concept of evidence-based practice emerged in the early 1990s from the increasing acknowledgement that research evidence should be seen within the context of professional judgement and patient preference; and that evidence alone is not sufficient to guide care (Aveyard et al., 2013). There are various terms currently used, for example evidence-based medicine or evidence-based nursing. There have also been various evidence-based initiatives and new terminology within the health services. These include initiatives such as Evidence-based Child Health and Evidence-based Mental Health, specialist 'evidence-based' journals, websites and web-based discussion lists.

All these initiatives rely on the assumption that a combination of evidence, professional judgement and patient choice underpin our decision making. However most people would agree that the strongest emphasis is on the use of evidence; it would be hard for a professional to justify reliance on his or her professional judgement if this was in direct conflict with a substantial body of evidence.

CRITICS OF AN EVIDENCE-BASED PRACTICE APPROACH

Some people argue that evidence-based practice constrains professional decision making and that it is too simple; promoting a 'cookbook' approach to practice. This argument is generally countered by a reconsideration of the components of evidence-based practice, of which professional judgement is central. An overreliance on evidence and negation of professional judgement might indeed promote a 'cookbook' approach; however this is not the intention of an evidence-based approach.

Other people have expressed concern that an evidence-based practice approach focuses too much on randomised controlled trials as the highest form of evidence and neglects to recognise the value of reflection in developing best practice (Mantzoukas, 2008). Again, this argument can be countered by a reconsideration of the evidence that is used to underpin practice and the role of professional judgement. Randomised controlled trials are indeed the gold standard when looking to determine the effectiveness of practice; however they are not for other research questions. Hence an understanding of the evidence that underpins practice is needed in order to promote the appropriate application of evidence-based practice.

Others argue that not all research trials are of good quality or directly transferable to practice. It is also important to appraise the evidence used in an evidence-based practice approach. If the research underpinning practice is of poor quality or was not undertaken on the patient group concerned, this should be flagged up and less reliance placed on this evidence.

USING RESEARCH AND EVIDENCE-BASED PRACTICE IN PRACTICE

In this chapter we have discussed the importance of using a research and evidence-based approach within your professional practice. This is not always easy and we have outlined some of the barriers to this and suggest some strategies to help.

Promoting user-friendly research findings

One challenge is the accessibility of research findings. There is evidence from many studies that nurses are not confident in reading research (Chien, 2010; Profetto-McGrath and Raymond-Seniuk, 2012; Uysal et al., 2015). Brooke et al. (2015) identified that many student nurses are apprehensive about understanding research and do not find research accessible. The researchers concluded that a carefully guided educational programme was paramount in reducing this. There is a general move towards increasing nurses' knowledge of research methods and making research findings more accessible. This places a responsibility on nurse researchers to ensure that their results are presented in a way that clinical nurses can readily understand them (Gunter and Osterrieder, 2012). It may lead to nurse researchers publishing or presenting findings in a range of settings and publications that they would not ordinarily consider appropriate, for example presenting results of a study on the uptake of breast or cervical screening at Women's Institute meetings.

Accessibility also refers to the fact that not all research is published. It is not uncommon for research findings to be reported at a conference rather than being published in a journal, and so they will only reach a limited audience. For some nurses, access to research findings may be associated with difficulties in actually getting the opportunity to read reports. This could be for a variety of reasons, including lack of, or limited, library/IT facilities. Simple strategies like establishing a journal club or lunchtime discussion group, where the content of a recently published research report can be discussed, may go some way to addressing these issues. In some NHS healthcare institutions, the implementation of evidence-based practice has resulted in the establishment of working groups where specific areas of nursing care, such as patient privacy, have facilitated nurses being given the time and opportunity to consider the research evidence available and hence initiate research-based changes for practice. An increasing trend is also for academic nurses/researchers to have formal links or joint appointments with healthcare institutions. In this way, practitioners can have direct contact with researchers who can provide support, advice or guidance at the level needed by practice.

Knowing when to change practice

Another challenge for nursing research is that it tends to be wide ranging and often gives rise to a plethora of individual studies, often undertaken in order to fulfil the requirements of a degree programme rather than in the context of funded research. This is changing, but it will take time to build the large body of evidence that nurses will be able to apply to all clinical problems.

Associated with this is knowing when to change practice. In most situations it would be inappropriate to implement a change in practice on the basis of a single study unless it was of a high quality and involved large numbers. Rather, recommendations for practice from a single study that appear to be applicable to your own practice should encourage you to critically appraise the study to ascertain its quality and validity. There should then be a consideration of the need for replication of the study to confirm the outcomes. Again, this highlights the need for all nurses to have some understanding of research and an ability, and willingness, to critically appraise research.

Promoting a positive organisational culture

Another challenge is the organisation itself. Every organisation has its own culture, but there will inevitably be different perspectives that influence attitudes towards the implementation of research in the clinical setting. Many researchers have identified that organisational culture is key in developing research (Chien, 2010; Profetto-McGrath and Raymond-Seniuk, 2012; Uysal et al., 2015). There may be resistance to change or a perception that research utilisation will disrupt the status quo. However, unexpected prompts may act as facilitators of research into practice, such as a directive from organisations like the National Patient Safety Agency that can provide impetus for the implementation of research-based innovations which would not necessarily have been given the required organisational support.

Research utilisation needs the support and commitment of management and recognition that it takes time to implement changes to practice. The support needed may be something as simple as facilitating time in the library or IT access in order to search the literature and identify whether there has been any other research undertaken on the topic. More tangible support may be necessary for some nurses in the form of experienced nurse researchers readily available to guide and encourage, or the option of being able to get small grants locally that could, for example, 'buy out' practitioner time to facilitate data collection/analysis or purchase time from a statistician.

Specialist nurses are also uniquely placed to facilitate a 'research aware' environment, both as active researchers and to facilitate linkages between research, policy and practice. Additionally, because specialist nurses have expertise within their own specialities and credibility with clinical nurses, it means that they have a firm base to facilitate, support, encourage, provide role models, consistency and application of research to practice for other clinical nurses, and hence help to develop research interest and expertise.

Research with impact

Further efforts to facilitate the implementation of research into practice are supported through the Research Excellence Framework (REF) (see www.ref.ac.uk/). The REF is a six yearly assessment of the quality and impact of research conducted by higher education institutions that is used to allocate public monies annually to support further research activity and excellence. The definition of impact for the REF includes changes beyond academia and in health should ideally have led to a change in practice and behaviour amongst professionals and the public. For example, research developing and testing new guidelines for care delivery would be published and implemented in practice. The new guidelines would be used by professionals and lead to a change in care with service user benefit.

The last exercise, submitted in 2014, was the first to include impact measures. Impact was assessed through a statement of achievement and activities and evidence-based case studies outlining the translation of research findings into practice and policy. The researchers wrote a case study of the research and its impact, including evidence of this. The types of evidence submitted included for example, statements about the wide use of the guidelines by practitioners, numerical evidence of use and evaluation data from service users reporting the benefits of the new guidelines. Nursing impact case studies were submitted as part of the REF by a number of higher education institutions. Examples included impact in areas such as the reduction of falls and incidence of pressure ulcer development following surgery.

Impact assessment is expected to form an even greater component of the next REF assessment, predicted to be in 2020. In addition, a number of research funders are requiring impact statements from researchers as part of a project proposal. Thus, both the REF and research funders are working to secure impact. This means that all institutions intending to bid to certain funders and make a REF submission are implementing strategies to support and record impact from their research. This in turn should help to support the impact of research in practice. Ideally it will help to ensure that research makes a difference to professionals and in particular to the public, who should benefit from the implementation of evidence-based research findings.

CHAPTER SUMMARY

- Getting research into practice is about applying research findings from one or more studies into practice and is unrelated to the original research, that is, closing the gap between the knowledge generated by research and using it in clinical practice to improve patient care.
- Evidence-based practice involves making clinical decisions on the best evidence available; it is not the same as research.
- Not all practice can be research based; where there is research evidence it should be incorporated into practice.
- Care needs to be taken to ensure that research utilisation is appropriate.
- Nurses need to recognise that research has an important role in improving patient care and be aware of when they need to seek assistance.
- Experienced nurse researchers and specialist nurses should expect, and endeavour, to encourage and facilitate colleagues to become research active.
- Healthcare organisations should promote a research culture that is inclusive for nurses.
- There is a variety of roles for nurses in research, but all nurses should endeavour to utilise available research in their practice.

WEBSITES

Council of Deans: http://www.councilofdeans.org.uk/wp-content/uploads/2014/12/Care-Transformed-web-version-1.pdf – presents a selection of impact case studies presented in REF 2014.
Hefce: www.ref.ac.uk. – includes further information of the REF 2014 submissions and outcomes.
Evidence-based nursing: http://ebn.bmj.com/content/14/3/63.extract
Nurses' Use of Research Information in Clinical Decision Making: A Descriptive and Analytical Study: www.york.ac.uk/res/dec/resources/papers/decision_report.pdf

To access further resources related to this chapter, visit the companion website at http://study.sagepub.com/mouleaveyard3e

REFERENCES

Aveyard, H., Sharp, P. and Woolliams, M. (2013) *A Beginner's Guide to Critical Thinking and Writing in Health and Social Care*, 2nd edn. Maidenhead: Open University Press.

Berwick, D. (2003) 'Disseminating innovations in healthcare', *Journal of the American Medical Association*, 289: 1969–75.

Brooke, J., Hvalic-Touzery, S. and Skela-Savic, B. (2015) 'Student nurse perceptions on evidence based practice and research: An exploratory research study involving students from the University of Greenwich, England and the Faculty of Health Care Jesenice, Slovenia', *Nurse Education Today*, 35: e6–e11.

Chien, W.T. (2010) 'A survey of nurses' perceived barriers to research utilization in Hong Kong', *Journal of Clinical Nursing*, 19: 3584–6.

Gunter, C. and Osterrieder, A (2012) 'A modest proposal for an outreach section in scientific publications', *Genome Biology*, 13(8): 168.

Mantzoukas, S. (2008) 'A review of evidence-based practice, nursing research and reflection: Levelling the hierarchy', *Journal of Clinical Nursing*, 17: 214–23.

Parahoo, K. (2014) *Nursing Research: Principles, Process and Issues.* Basingstoke: Palgrave Macmillan.

Peters, D. (1992) 'Implementation of research findings', *Health Bulletin*, 50 (1): 68–77.

Polit, D. and Beck, C. (2012) *Essentials of Nursing Research: Methods, Appraisal and Utilization.* Philadelphia, PA: Lippincott Williams & Wilkins.

Profetto-McGrath, J. and Raymond-Seniuk, C. (2012) 'Research utilization and critical thinking among newly graduated nurses: Predictors for research use: a quantitative cross sectional study', *Evidence-based Nursing*, 15 (3):73.

Rycroft-Malone, J., Harvey, G., Kitson, A., McCormack, B., Seers, K. and Titchen, A. (2002) 'Getting evidence into practice: Ingredients for change', *Nursing Standard*, 16 (37): 38–42.

Sackett, D.L., Straus, S.E., Richardson, W.S., Rosenberg, W. and Haynes, R.B. (2005) *Evidence-based Medicine: How to Practice and Teach EBM*, 3rd edn. Edinburgh: Churchill Livingstone.

Uysal, A., Terrel, A., Ardahan, M. and Ozhahrama, S (2015) 'Barriers to research utilization among nurses in Turkey', *Journal of Clinical Nursing*, 19: 3443–52.

GLOSSARY OF TERMS

Accidental sampling: see Convenience sampling.

Action research: a research approach that involves planning, implementing and evaluating change in practice.

Action research cycle: describes the continuous process of planning, acting, observing, reflecting and revising the plan characteristic of action research.

Anonymity: refers to the way we attribute information from a specific person, i.e. being unable to attribute specific data and/or what any particular participant said or did in a research study. Participants are likely to give researchers large amounts of very personal information if they are assured that they cannot be identified if quoted in any report or article.

Audit: a methodological review of existing documentation.

Average: a numerical value around which collected data values cluster; a measure of central tendency, such as mean, median, mode.

Beneficence: literally means 'doing good'. The moral principle is the obligation to do good, to remove and prevent harms and weigh possible goods against the costs and possible harms of an action.

Capacity/capability building: developing an ability to appreciate and use research for practice.

Case study: a research design that focuses on specific groups or populations, often one, and collects data using a variety of methods. The 'case' is clearly defined and limited.

Chart: a pictorial summary of numerical data that displays patterns in the collected data; a graph of data values, such as a bar chart, box and whisker plot or histogram.

Cluster/multi-stage random sampling: includes the random sampling of 'clusters' or identifiable groups, followed by further random sampling within each cluster or group.

Computer-assisted data analysis: analysis of research data using specialised computer packages.

Conference presentation: presentation of a poster or academic paper at a conference gathering.

Confidence interval: a range of values, based on sample data, that is likely to contain the estimate of an unknown population parameter with an associated confidence, e.g. 95 per cent.

Confidentiality: relates to the way information gained from participants is treated and the assurances given that it will not be revealed to anyone outside the research team.

Confirmability: a measure of objectivity of the data, the extent to which data and interpretations reflect the phenomenon under study.

Consensus technique: the consensus method involves a panel of multi-disciplinary experts who meet face-to-face to discuss and develop practice. Gaps in knowledge and resultant research priorities can also be identified as part of consensus knowledge-building.

Construct validity: the degree to which a questionnaire or scale reflects the construct that is being measured.

Content analysis: analysis of the content of textual data, often produced as part of qualitative research, to identify key themes.

Content validity: the degree to which a tool, such as a multi-item scale in a questionnaire, covers all relevant concepts about the phenomenon under study.

Convenience/accidental sampling: a convenience or accidental sample is usually taken from the local population convenient to the researcher and team.

Correlation coefficient: a measure of the strength of a relationship (association) between two variables, lying between 0 and 1 for positive correlation or between 0 and −1 for negative correlation. Positive correlation implies that values of both variables increase (or decrease) together, whereas negative correlation implies that as values of one variable increase, values of the other decrease (or vice versa).

Credibility: a study has credible findings if they reflect the experience and perceptions of the participants. Those who read the report and any published journal articles must also view the findings as credible.

Criterion-related validity: the results obtained by a measure can be validated by comparing them with the results obtained through another validated questionnaire.

Critical analysis: a structured process of identifying and evaluating the merits and/or value of research.

Critical appraisal: a structured process of identifying and evaluating the merits and/or value of research.

Critical incident technique: the technique involves asking participants about key events that they have experienced, and collects observations of human behaviour in defined situations.

Critique: exercising careful judgement or evaluation.

Data coding: the researcher applies codes to the data as part of the process of interpretation and conclusion drawing.

Data Protection Act 1998: sets out how to handle and process personal information and data collected through research.

Deductive reasoning: principles or theories are applied to a particular situation.

Delphi technique: a form of survey that collects the views of experts on a particular issue. The experts are invited to respond individually to issues and rank statements or concepts according to priority. A series of rounds of review and revision continue until a consensus is achieved.

Dependability: establishing dependability can be seen as a parallel process to that of confirming reliability in quantitative data. An audit trail of the research can assist in establishing dependability.

Diaries: researchers can use diaries as part of a qualitative research design to ask participants to record current events, keeping a record over time of feelings, experiences, events, actions and reflections.

Discourse/conversation analysis: the analysis of discourse, which includes verbal, non-verbal and written communication. This approach attempts to understand interactions between people.

Dual role of practitioner and researcher: there are potential conflicts of interest associated with the dual role of practitioner and researcher. Nurses must ensure that participants understand the role of the nurse in a research study.

Emic perspective: gaining the insider view.

Epidemiological research: research that measures the prevalence and incidence of disease in populations.

Epidemiological survey: the collection of information that will enable a description of the distribution and determination of health to be described.

Ethical principles: refer to moral norms that are basic for biomedical ethics. Ethics is a generic term for various ways of understanding and examining moral life.

Ethnography: a qualitative research approach developed by anthropologists to guide the study of culture and cultural groups. Ethnographers observe behaviour, customs, rituals, interaction and practices.

Etic perspective: entering a culture from the outside.

Evaluation outcomes: have to be appropriate to the question being asked and can be qualitative or quantitative or a mixture of both. Outcome indicators can be classified as patient-, carer-, staff- and service-based.

Evaluation research: a form of applied research that is designed to address current issues or questions about the way a service functions or the impact of services, care programmes or policies.

Evidence-based practice: the use of current best evidence in making decisions about nursing care delivery and practice.

Experimental design: a quantitative research design that tests a hypothesis through applying a treatment or condition to an experimental group. The outcomes are usually compared with a control group.

Feminist research: research conducted for the benefit of women.

Focus group: discussions with one or more researchers and between two and nine participants.

Full economic costing: the costing and charging of research undertaken within universities.

Good Clinical Practice: in research is an international ethical and scientific quality standard, and compliance with the standard should provide public assurance that the rights, safety and well-being of research participants are protected and that the clinical research data are credible.

Grounded theory: a qualitative research methodology that aims to support the generation of theory through a process of simultaneous data collection and analysis.

Hawthorne effect: occurs as a result of research participants knowing they are involved in a study.

Healthcare consumer: a controversial but now accepted term for 'patient'.

Hermeneutics: understanding the human experience.

Hierarchy of evidence: placing evidence in a hierarchy based on the rigours of the approach taken to collect information, with evidence from a systematic review of multiple well-designed randomised controlled trials at the top and personal, professional and peer expertise and experience at the bottom.

Historical data: research data used by historical researchers that can be text-based, visual or numerical.

Historical research: a research approach that examines past events to increase understanding and gain new knowledge to inform current and future practice.

Human Tissue Act 2004: for anyone involved in research with organs or tissue, the full legislation of the Human Tissue Act must be consulted and particular reference made to the consenting process.

Hypothesis: usually takes the form of a statement of the relationship between variables, and attempts to answer a question that has emerged from a research problem.

Inductive reasoning: principles or theories are developed from a situation or observation.

Informed consent: refers to the process of gaining agreement from an individual to participate in a research study, based on having been given all relevant information, in a manner that is appropriate for that individual, about what participation means, with particular reference to possible harms and benefits.

Instrument: the means by which data are collected, e.g. a questionnaire.

Interpretation of qualitative data: processes undertaken by the researcher to draw meaning and interpretation from qualitative data such as text.

Interval level: data are named, ordered and measured on a scale marked in equal intervals, for example body temperature in °C.

Interviews: a data collection technique that includes gathering information through verbal communication. Interviews can be managed in one-to-one situations, groups, over the telephone and face-to-face.

Intuition: developed insight gained through experience.

In vitro: physiological measures conducted without the presence of the participant, e.g. in a laboratory.

In vivo: physiological measures made in the presence of the participant, e.g. recording a pulse.

Justice: refers to the moral obligation to be 'fair', and requires that preference is not given to some participants over others in respect of morally relevant equalities and inequalities.

Life history: life histories and biographical material report individual life experiences, often accessed through in-depth interviewing.

Likert scale: a measurement scale that requires the participant to give an opinion on the extent of their agreement or disagreement with a series of statements.

Literature review: the selection of available documents (both published and unpublished) on a topic and the effective evaluation of these documents in relation to the research being proposed.

Literature search: aims to identify the most appropriate sources to answer a question within a field of study.

Longitudinal study: a design used to measure the effect of changes over time. It involves the collection of data at various points, sometimes from the same participants.

Measure of central tendency: see Average.

Measure of dispersion: a numerical value that indicates how closely collected data values cluster around the average; a measure of scatter or dispersion around the average, with smaller values indicating data values clustered closer to the average, e.g. standard deviation, range and interquartile range (IQR).

Mental Capacity Act 2005: researchers can undertake research with vulnerable participants or those who lack capacity to give consent provided that the requirements of the Act are fulfilled. The Act sets out duties to ensure that individuals who lack capacity are treated with due respect and their rights protected.

Meta-analysis: a statistical amalgam of the findings of a number of research studies that have been carried out on a specific topic, and usually regarded as secondary analysis of original data.

Mixed methods: using different data collection methods within one study. Usually qualitative and quantitative methods are combined.

Multi-stage random sampling: see Cluster sampling.

Narrative analysis: can form part of the analysis of textual data within research. Those undertaking narrative analysis are concerned with the structure of the story rather than focusing on the content.

Naturalistic observation: observation of phenomena in naturally occurring contexts.

Network/snowball sampling: network or snowball sampling is the approach used when nurse researchers are aiming to select hidden samples. The researcher will need to draw on networks to identify the sample, often involving a third party.

Nominal data: can be classified into named categories, which have no inherent order attached, such as male or female.

Nominal group technique: a technique of data collection where the participants meet face-to-face to try to achieve a consensus through a process of ranking and refining responses to key issues.

Non-maleficence: the principle of 'doing no harm'. For research participants, there is a duty to prevent harm (physical, psychological, emotional, social and economic) and do good; to protect the weak and vulnerable; and the weak, vulnerable or incompetent should be defended.

Non-probability sampling: non-random methods are used to select elements for inclusion in non-probability sampling. This means the researcher is unable to state the chances of elements of the population appearing in the final sample.

Nursing research: the systematic gathering of information to answer questions and solve problems in the pursuit of creating new knowledge about nursing.

Observational methods: can be used to examine phenomena such as communication, non-verbal interaction and activity in practice settings. Researchers observe practice and might record this activity in a structured or unstructured way.

Ordinal data: can be classified into named categories, which do have an inherent order attached, such as 'strongly agree' down to 'strongly disagree'.

Outcome: refers to the effectiveness or impact of any intervention in relation to individuals and communities.

Parametric methods: make certain assumptions about the distribution of data (for example, data measured at least on an interval level and following a normal distribution), whilst non-parametric (distribution-free) methods do not.

Participant information: should be presented in a manner that is comprehensible to potential participants, and should explain what question the research is trying to answer and what a participant will have to do.

Patient and public involvement in research: refers to involving patients and members of the public in research projects.

Personal knowledge: individual knowledge shaped through being personally involved in situations and events in practice.

Phenomenology: a qualitative research approach that aims to understand human experience. Researchers focus on individuals' interpretations of their lived experiences.

Pilot study: a small-scale replica or trial run of the proposed study using a small sample of participants who are representative of the study population.

Population: a group of people, documents, events or specimens about whom or which the researcher is interested in collecting information or data.

Preparation of data: preparing the 'raw data' which could encompass text, tape/digital recordings, numerical data or visual data such as photographs and video for analysis.

Probability sampling: all units in the sampling frame have more than a zero chance of being included in the final sample.

Process: refers to the activities themselves and how services are organised and delivered.

Publication: a process of preparing research papers for publication in academic journals.

Purposive/purposeful sampling: the researchers use their own judgement and knowledge of the potential participants to support recruitment.

Qualitative approaches/research: a term for research designs and methods that collect non-numerical data that is often textual.

Qualitative data analysis: the analysis and interpretation of data obtained through qualitative research approaches, which might include textual data from interviews.

Quantitative approaches/research: a term for research designs and methods collecting numerical data that is analysed using statistical methods.

Quasi-experiment: an experimental design where the research does not meet all three criteria of a true experiment. An intervention is always present, but randomisation and/or a control group might not be used.

Questionnaire: a data collection instrument that includes questions requiring written responses. These can be administered by post, via the Internet, in person or left for respondent collection.

Quota sampling: an approach to sampling where the researcher pre-determines the numbers required in each group and selects according to these specified characteristics. For example, the researcher can select the sample to meet gender and age requirements.

Randomised controlled trial (RCT): this design is the true experimental approach, with a control group, randomisation and an intervention. RCTs are usually conducted in clinical practice settings.

Rating scale: a tool that quantifies subjective estimates of attributes that cannot be measured directly and requires ratings along a continuum.

Ratio level: data are named, ordered, measured on a scale marked in equal intervals and have an absolute zero, such as weight of adults in kg.

Reading analytically: an active process concerned with learning to think.

Reliability: the consistency with which a tool measures what it is intended to. The nurse researcher is interested in three measures of reliability: the stability of a measure, its internal consistency and equivalence.

Research aims: describe the overall purpose of a project.

Research design: a map of the way in which the researcher will engage with the research subject(s) to achieve the outcomes needed to address the research aims and objectives.

Research ethics: refer to the principles that underpin ethical research. Nurses in research are expected to be guided by the principles of veracity, justice, non-maleficence, beneficence, fidelity and confidentiality.

Research ethics committee: considers applications from researchers wishing to undertake healthcare research; scrutinises research protocols; and determines whether the study is ethical. Research studies in healthcare cannot be started until ethical approval has been given.

Research Governance Framework: sets standards; defines mechanisms to deliver standards; describes monitoring and assessment arrangements; and aims to improve research quality and safeguard the public.

Research hierarchy: a kind of league table where some types of research are classed as being of 'better' quality than others.

Research literate: having the ability to interpret research findings, an essential skill for knowledge-led nursing practice.

Research objectives: describe the individual, specific tasks that need to be carried out to meet the research aims.

Research paper: a published paper written to disseminate the research findings.

Research problem: a broad topic area of interest that has perplexing or troubling aspects which can be 'solved' by the accumulation of relevant information or evidence.

Research process: a series of steps or stages undertaken by researchers in order to address research questions.

Research proposal: an outline of the research to be undertaken, detailing research aims, methods, costing and ethical issues.

Research question: a concise description of exactly what issues the research intends to acquire information about.

Research report: often required by funders at the end of a project, and would usually include details of the research process and outcomes and recommendations for future practice.

Research utilisation: about applying research findings from one or more studies into practice.

Respect for autonomy: autonomy is the capacity to make deliberate or reasoned decisions for oneself and to act on the basis of such decisions. Respect for autonomy is the norm of respecting the decision-making capacities of autonomous persons.

Rigour: the accuracy and consistency of a research design that gives a measure of its quality.

Safety of researchers: may include providing taxis, special training, counselling, mobile phones, working in pairs, overnight accommodation.

Sample: a subset of the population, selected through sampling techniques.

Sample size calculation: a mathematical calculation used to determine the size of the sample required in quantitative research, so that the study can be powered to enable a clinically important difference to be detected as statistically significant.

Sampling frame: developed to include all of the possible members of the population who might be eligible for inclusion in the final sample.

Scale: provides a numeric score to place respondents on a continuum with respect to an attribute being measured, e.g. for measuring temperatures.

Scientific knowledge: knowledge developed and verified through systematic and rigorous enquiry.

Search strategy: a carefully developed plan for searching the literature in a comprehensive manner.

Secondary research/analysis: includes systematic reviews because new data are not collected and makes use of previous findings.

Simple random sampling: a simple approach to sampling that draws on the sampling frame to select a random sample as a subset of the population.

Snowball sampling: see Network sampling.

Statistical hypothesis testing: a methodical process that uses the laws of chance to test an explicit assumption about characteristics in a population (or of differences in values across more than one population) on the basis of data collected from a sample of people drawn from that population (or populations), such as when researching the effectiveness of different approaches to managing pain.

Statistics: formally collected numerical data, such as the number of patients on a waiting list; numbers that summarise specific features in a sample of collected data, such as mean; methods used to collect, analyse and interpret numerical data, in particular to inform decision making, for example when researching the effectiveness of different approaches to managing pain.

Storage: data must be stored safely and with due regard to issues of confidentiality and anonymity.

Stratified random sampling: the researcher separates the sampling frame into subsections, such as gender groups, age groups, professional disciplines, before randomly selecting an agreed number from each group for inclusion in the study.

Structure: the organisational framework for an activity or care-giving environment.

Structured interview: an interview where the researcher has a set of specific questions to ask, often with limited response options.

Structured observation: a data collection method used where actions or events are observed and recorded in pre-determined categories or checklists.

Survey/survey design: a design that collects descriptive or correlation data from a sample of the population (such as the census that includes the entire population).

Synthesis: the rearranging of elements derived from analysis of the literature to identify relationships not previously noted.

Systematic random sampling: this approach sees the researcher drawing a random sample by selecting units from a list at pre-determined set intervals. Every unit has an equal chance of inclusion in the sample.

Systematic review: a review of a clearly formulated question that uses systematic and explicit methods to identify, select and critically appraise relevant research, and to collect and analyse data from studies that are included in the review.

Tacit knowledge: developed through practice and experience over time.

Thematic analysis: an approach to data analysis of primary or secondary sources in which text is analysed for emerging themes.

Theoretical sampling: involves a determination of the sample on the basis of the themes that emerge from data analysis; the researcher then explores these themes in more depth and/or develops a theory from these data. It is frequently used in grounded theory.

Thick description: an analysis of the group culture, a view of its patterns of working, member relationships, meanings and functions.

Tradition: ongoing use of past actions or customs which may or may not continue to have relevance and currency.

Transferability: the extent to which research findings can be transferred from one context to another by providing a 'thick description' of the data, as well as identifying sampling and design details.

Triangulation: the use of two or more research approaches, data collection methods or analysis techniques in one study.

Trustworthiness: a term used in the appraisal of qualitative research when describing credibility, dependability and transferability.

Unstructured observation: a data collection method used where actions or events are observed and recorded without pre-determined categories or checklists.

Validity: a measure of whether a data collection tool accurately measures what it is supposed to. A measure is not valid unless it is also reliable.

Visual analogue scale (VAS): a scale used most often to measure certain clinical symptoms, feelings and attitudes by getting participants to indicate intensity on a straight line, e.g. pain.

Vulnerable participants: individuals who may have compromised capacity to give informed consent due to physical, mental or psychological debility.

INDEX

Entries in **bold** represent glossary definitions